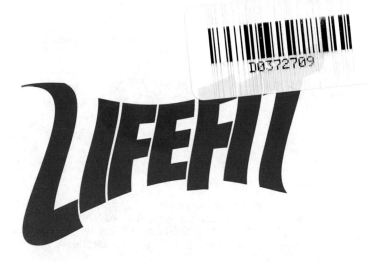

An Effective Exercise Program
for Optimal Health and a Longer Life

Ralph S. Paffenbarger, Jr., MD
and Eric Olsen

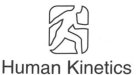

Human Kinetics

Library of Congress Cataloging-in-Publication Data

Paffenbarger, Ralph, 1922-
    LifeFit: an effective exercise program for optimal health and a longer life/Ralph Paffenbarger, Eric Olsen.
      p.   cm.
    Includes bibliographical references and index.
    ISBN 0-87322-429-9
    1. Health. 2. Physical fitness.   I. Olsen, Eric.   II. Title.
RA776.P127   1996
613.7--dc20   95-49235
                                                    CIP

ISBN: 0-87322-429-9

Developmental Editor: Holly Gilly; **Assistant Editors:** Chad Johnson and Kent Reel; **Editorial Assistant:** Amy Carnes; **Copyeditor:** Barbara Field; **Typesetter and Layout Artist:** Denise Lowry; **Text Designer:** Stuart Cartwright; **Photo Editor:** Boyd LaFoon; **Cover Designer:** Jack Davis; **Illustrators:** Studio 2-D and Keith Blomberg; **Printer:** United Graphics

LifeFit is report LX in a series on chronic disease in former college students. This report has been supported by research grants HL34174 from the National Heart, Lung, and Blood Institute and CA44854 from the National Cancer Institute, U.S. Public Health Service, Bethesda, Maryland.

Human Kinetics books are available at special discounts for bulk purchase. Special editions or book excerpts can also be created to specification. For details, contact the Special Sales Manager at Human Kinetics.

Printed in the United States of America   10 9 8 7 6 5 4 3 2

Human Kinetics
Web site: www.humankinetics.com

United States: Human Kinetics, P.O. Box 5076, Champaign, IL 61825-5076
800-747-4457
e-mail: humank@hkusa.com

Canada: Human Kinetics, 475 Devonshire Road, Unit 100, Windsor, ON N8Y 2L5
800-465-7301 (in Canada only)
e-mail: orders@hkcanada.com

Europe: Human Kinetics, Units C2/C3 Wira Business Park, West Park Ring Road
Leeds LS16 6EB, United Kingdom
+44 (0) 113 278 1708
e-mail: hk@hkeurope.com

Australia: Human Kinetics, 57A Price Avenue, Lower Mitcham, South Australia 5062
08 8277 1555
e-mail: liahka@senet.com.au

New Zealand: Human Kinetics, P.O. Box 105-231, Auckland Central
09-523-3462
e-mail: hkp@ihug.co.nz

5/3/09

For Ron + Barbara —
I'm looking forward
to dinner with you both
and having more good
conversations about
'Dangerous Women who Read'!
Warmly,
Joann Paffenbarger

For all those who wish to realize the benefits of an
active and fit way of life.

contents

preface

Throughout *LifeFit*, we have relied heavily on data from the College Alumni Health Study (CAHS) in many of our discussions about exercise, health, and longevity. The study, usually referred to herein as the "College Study," is perhaps most commonly known as the "Harvard Study." It is an ongoing, 36-year follow-up study of more than 50,000 Harvard College and University of Pennsylvania alumni* that looks at the relations among a variety of lifestyle habits—particularly exercise—and health and longevity.

Over the years, the College Study has yielded some interesting and sometimes surprising findings on the benefits of an active life. For example, the data clearly show that if you become and remain physically active, you will live longer. And most recently, the study has also provided heartening news about the benefits of change from a sedentary to an active life, clearly showing that it's never too late to benefit from becoming even a little more physically active. Data from the study, coupled with the work of others, also suggest that not only will you live longer if you are physically active, you will also live better, with more vitality, and comparatively free of those debilitating though not necessarily life-threatening ailments we associate with aging—arthritis, osteoporosis, depression, and mental decline.

LifeFit is a collaboration between Dr. Ralph Paffenbarger, "Paff" to his friends and colleagues, and Eric Olsen. Thus, throughout *LifeFit*, we refer to ourselves collectively in the first person plural, which could lead to some misconceptions, particularly as we discuss the College Study. In fact, about the time Paff was first conceiving of the College Study back in 1960, Olsen was in high school dreaming about one day becoming a rocket pilot and plying the interplanetary wastes between Earth and Mars. Whenever "we" talk about the College Study, please understand that the study is the work of a

*The study includes both men and women, but for the sake of simplicity, we'll refer to the alumni meaning both.

great many individuals at Harvard, The University of California at Berkeley, and Stanford, including Paff and his co-principal investigator, I-Min Lee, and Robert Hyde, Alvin L. Wing, James B. Kampert, Rita W. Leung, Patricia Ford, and Chung-Cheng Hsieh, plus a host of others who have contributed over the years.

Paff and Olsen didn't hit it off initially when they first met nearly 20 years ago. Paff was busy preparing himself mentally and physically for the grueling Western States 100-mile run up and over the Sierra Nevada from Lake Tahoe to Auburn, California. Olsen, who was covering the race for *The Runner* magazine, kept pestering Paff with requests for interviews about his training and research. Paff, an intensely private and modest man, thought Olsen was a nuisance.

For the next several years, though, as the College Study continued to yield important findings about the health benefits and psychological and philosophical consolations of exercise, Olsen continued to bug Paff for interviews. As a freelance writer, Olsen's beat was exercise, health, and fitness, and unfortunately for Paff—but fortunately for Olsen—they happened to live only a few blocks apart. Thus it seemed just about every time Paff would go out into his front yard to trim his roses or cut the grass, there would be Olsen asking for an interview. Eventually, Olsen's persistence began to wear Paff down. They even became good friends, and out of that friendship has grown *LifeFit*.

The underlying premise of *LifeFit* is that change from a sedentary to an active lifestyle comes most easily when it's accompanied by good information about why such a change is important, what the benefits of specific changes are, and how to implement and manage change step-by-step. Thus we've divided *LifeFit* into three parts: "Invitation to Change," "Benefits of Change," and "Program for Change."

In part I, "Invitation to Change," we discuss what's at stake at both a personal and a social level, why our changing political, social, and economic environments make appropriate changes in lifestyle more important than ever, and why each of us should make these changes for his or her own good and for the good of the community. In this section, we also take a closer look at the College Study, at our aging society and its implications, as well as at aging itself and at theories on slowing or delaying the aging process.

In part II, "Benefits of Change," we consider the specific benefits of change from a sedentary to an active lifestyle. Our purpose is to provide you with information we hope will motivate you to become more active. And if you are already active, this information should help keep you inspired to maintain your lifestyle, particularly when it's dark and cold outside and your enthusiasm for a brisk walk or bike ride or run begins to wane.

In part III, "A Program for Change," we offer a detailed exercise "prescription"—the LifeFit program—that establishes the frequency, duration, intensity, and types of exercise that provide the most benefits and the greatest gains in longevity and vitality. This section also describes, step-by-step, how to get started, how to design and customize your own program, and how to avoid injury or burnout to stick with it for a lifetime of improved health and vitality.

Of course, if you're already feeling inspired to take up or keep at an active lifestyle, you can start with part III, then refer back to the first two parts of *LifeFit* for additional inspiration or to enhance your understanding of the fundamental theories and practices underlying your active lifestyle.

If you have comments or questions about any of the information presented in *LifeFit* you can send an e-mail to us at:
103217.1426@compuserve.com.

acknowledgments

While drawing extensively on the College Study, we've also relied on the work of many others who, at different times and places, or using different approaches, have contributed much to what is known today about the physical, mental, psychological, and spiritual benefits of an active life. Among these is Jeremy N. Morris, whose study of British civil servants provided the first adequate data on the relation of higher levels of physical activity to reduced risk of heart disease. Other studies that have shed light on heart disease and other chronic "diseases of civilization" such as cancer, hypertension, and diabetes include the Multiple Risk Factor Intervention Trial (MRFIT) from Minnesota; the Framingham (Massachusetts) Heart Study; the American Railroad Study out of the University of Minnesota; the Nurses' Health Studies, the Physicians' Health Study, and the Health Professionals Follow-up Study from the Harvard University School of Public Health and the Harvard Medical School; the Seventh Day Adventist Study out of Loma Linda University; and the Alameda County (California) Human Population Laboratory.

Numerous individuals have contributed much to the field, and informed our discussion here. These include Steven N. Blair and Kenneth H. Cooper at the Cooper Institute for Aerobics Research in Dallas; H. William Kohl at Baylor; Claude Bouchard, Terence Kavanagh, and Roy J. Shephard in Canada; Per-Olof Åstrand, Kaare Rodahl, and Bengt Saltin in Sweden; Ilkka M. Vuori, Martti J. Karvonen, Pekka Oja, Rainer Rauramaa, and Jukka T. Salonen in Finland; Peter D. Wood, William L. Haskell, Marsha L. Stefanick, Abby C. King, and Anita Stewart at Stanford; James M. Hagberg, Ronald E. LaPorte, Andrea M. Krisha, and Paul Thompson at the University of Pittsburgh; Kenneth E. Powell and Carl J. Caspersen at the Centers for Disease Control and Prevention in Atlanta; Dexter L. Jung, Richard J. Brand, Marian Diamond, George A. Brooks, and Timothy P. White at the University of California-Berkeley; JoAnn E.

Manson and Walter C. Willett at Harvard; Annie J. Sasco, International Agency for Research on Cancer; Susan P. Helmrich and George A. Kaplan, California State Department of Health; Maria A. Fiatarone, Harvard and Tufts Universities; Arthur S. Leon and David R. Jacobs, Jr., at the University of Minnesota; Henry J. Montoye, University of Wisconsin; James F. Sallis, San Diego State University; Russell R. Pate and Barbara Ainsworth, University of South Carolina; Lester Breslow, University of California, Los Angeles; Barbara Drinkwater, Vashon, Washington; Lisa F. Berkman, Harvard School of Public Health; and Timothy D. Noakes at the University of Cape Town, South Africa.

In the realm of cognitive, psychological, and social benefits of activity and the biology, sociology, and demographics of aging, we've drawn on the research and writings of, among many others, Walter M. Bortz II, Cheung Fong Ha, William Morgan, Rod K. Dishman, James F. Fries, Robert Dustman, James Black, Dan Landers, Waneen Spirduso, S. Jay Olshansky, Sylvia Ann Hewlett, S. Boyd Eaton, Marjorie Shostak, Melvin Konner, George Leonard, Johann Huizinga, Mihalyi Csikszentmihalyi, James F. Fixx, George Sheehan, Kenneth Pelletier, and Timothy D. Noakes. Many thanks, and our apologies to those many scientists we have inadvertently neglected to mention.

And most important, our thanks to the college alumni and the alumni offices at the University of Pennsylvania and Harvard University. Without their continuing help and support during the past 30 years, neither the College Study nor this book would have been possible.

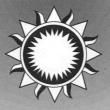

part I

AN INVITATION TO CHANGE

The goal of life is to die young, as late as possible.

—Ashley Montague

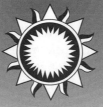

chapter 1

AN INTRODUCTION TO CHANGE

The LifeFit message is a message of hope—that it's never too late to change from a sedentary to an active lifestyle, nor to benefit from that change. Findings from the College Study show quite clearly that it's possible for even the most determined couch spud to become and remain active and vital well into old age, largely free of all those so-called diseases of civilization that leave too many of us worn out by life in our later years.

Our intent in *LifeFit*[1] is to provide a prescription for change for those who want to take up or continue an exercise program and do so efficiently, effectively, and pleasurably. We'll also provide specific strategies for starting and sticking with an exercise program for the long haul to enable you to make positive changes in your life and direct and control the changes associated with aging—that is, to slow or prevent the negative changes and emphasize the positive. We'll include specific information about the following:

- The physiology and psychology of aging and which "unavoidable" consequences of aging can be prevented or delayed through exercise and other specific lifestyle changes.

- Specific physical, psychological, and even spiritual benefits of an active lifeway to help you become motivated to take up and maintain physical activity.

- The LifeFit program, a prescription for change outlining the general frequency, duration, and intensity of exercise that provide the most benefit for effort expended.

- Advice on how to remain committed to an active lifestyle for a lifetime of benefits and how to avoid injury and burnout that can interfere with an active life.

How do we know that our information is sound and that our prescription works? We have the wisdom of the College Alumni Health Study to draw from.

WHY THE COLLEGE STUDY IS SO IMPORTANT

The College Study began 36 years ago and now represents over two million person-years of observation.[2] It is one of the larger data sets available on the subject of activity, health, and longevity and one from which meaningful conclusions can be drawn about the importance of regular physical activity in slowing the aging process.

The College Study population, of course, is mostly—but not entirely—men, and mostly white, upper middle-class men at that. An obvious question, then, is whether their experiences are relevant to women, or for that matter, to all the rest of us, men and women alike, who haven't had the social and economic advantages typical of earlier generations of elite university students.

When the study was designed, however, a variety of social and economic factors made the use of mostly male university graduates largely unavoidable. For example, Harvard didn't go coed until fairly recently, but Harvard and the University of Pennsylvania were ideal for the purposes of the study. Huge numbers of subjects were essential to produce meaningful findings, and so were records of physical exams of incoming freshmen. Harvard and Penn, in particular, were among only a handful of large universities around the country that gave entering students thorough physicals in the 1920s and earlier (Harvard started in 1916). Even fewer universities kept records of those physicals for any length of time, and fewer still had alumni offices as dedicated as Harvard's and Penn's to keeping track of graduates through current mailing addresses so we could conduct long-term follow-ups of their habits and health status. When the study was first being designed, we did review the records at several women's colleges, as well as Cal, Yale, Ohio State University, MIT, and the military academies, in the hope of finding subjects, but unlike Harvard and Penn, these schools usually didn't save records, and records were essential—standardized, comprehensive case-taking records from prior times that had been preserved and could be "exhumed," like bones from a Paleolithic dig, for current study.

As it turns out, the constraints helped; the many differences in education, income, social status, access to health care and health information that exist in a more diverse population and that might tend to confound the findings were minimized among the college alumni. Thus the alumni provide a relatively homogeneous population in which differences in health habits such as exercise, and resulting differences in outcomes such as risk of disease, can be more easily observed.

Think of the College Study not as a study for college alumni but a study of alumni, the findings from which give us clues about how the rest of us ought to be living our lives. We do think the College Study findings apply to us all—men and women alike, of all socioeconomic classes. Several other studies, particularly the Nurses' Health Studies and other large studies of women, are demonstrating that when it comes to physical activity, diet, and other health habits, what's true of men is also true of women.

WHAT THE COLLEGE STUDY TELLS US

There is no doubt, though, that the knowledge we're gaining from the College Study data has important personal as well as social implications, and the conclusions to be drawn from the data have at times been quite intriguing. But perhaps most intriguing and comforting are conclusions drawn from some of the latest College Study findings, which clearly show the benefits of change from an unhealthy way of life to a healthy one.

These most recent analyses concern specifically subjects who changed from a sedentary to an active life in adulthood, even at an advanced age. The data show compellingly that even the most resolutely sedentary of us can achieve the same health benefits by changing to an active lifestyle as are enjoyed by the habitually active. If you become and remain active, you will not only live longer, you'll live better, look better, and feel better about yourself. You will have more vitality, you'll think more clearly, and you'll sleep better. And you'll function better and be more productive, creative, and joyful.

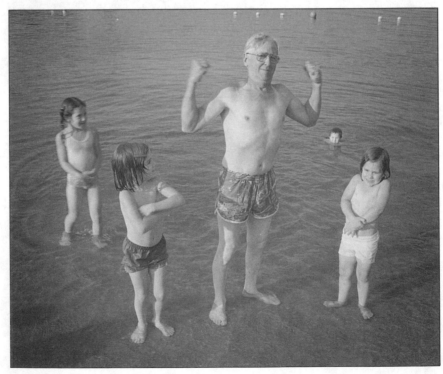

© Terry Wild Studio

OUR BASIC MESSAGE

Our message is intended primarily for men and women 40 and older, a diverse group that's beginning to confront a variety of life changes, some of them good and some not always for the better. On the downside, we 40- and 50-somethings are beginning to confront for the first time our own vulnerability; we're getting a bit gray at the temples and beginning to fret about it; we're having more and more trouble fitting into those blue jeans that may have been quite loose 15, 10, or even 5 years ago. We may find ourselves more susceptible to illness and injury and a bit stiff in the mornings. And maybe we're beginning to scale back on some of our dreams and ambitions, or rethinking them as career opportunities shift in an increasingly uncertain and rapidly changing world. Our children are growing up and beginning to leave home (or in these difficult economic times, what is sometimes worse, not leaving home). For women, menopause represents an unmistakable marker of physical and emotional change. Those of us in our sixties, seventies, and eighties are confronting even more striking life changes as we adjust our life goals still further, as we retire, and, unfortunately, as our friends and relatives begin to pass away.

Conventional wisdom would have us believe that all of these midlife or late-life changes are inevitable and that they inevitably precipitate crises of one kind or another, most notably the proverbial "midlife crisis." But it may be that the inevitability of the so-called midlife crisis is something of a myth; although many do confront striking changes with aging, even declines that may indeed lead to crisis, plenty of men and women move through their forties, fifties, or sixties untouched by any desire to recapture lost youth, drive too fast in bright red convertibles, date 22-year-olds, or move to Tahiti. Likewise, the sixth, seventh, and even later decades of life can and should be a time of new opportunity to do all those things for which we did not have time when we were busy with families, careers, and "getting ahead."

And that's the upside, and what *LifeFit* is all about. A healthy, vital middle or old age should be filled not with disease and withdrawal but with physical and mental vigor and new opportunities for self-fulfillment, freedom, social connectedness, community involvement, and personal development. Clearly, we need to break out of the rigid thinking that has always assigned development and growth to youth, career and family to middle age, and only a marginal role in society to older men and women. Already, the so-called baby-boom generation, that huge bulge in the demographers' charts, has begun to demand, by sheer force of numbers, new ways of thinking about middle age. And that generation in particular will likely redefine old age as well as create new roles for men and women in the second and third phases of life.[3] It may well be that our "new" elders—physically active, socially, intellectually, and politically involved men and women in the third phase of life, possessed of physical and mental vigor as well as the wisdom that comes only from many years of experience and learning—will play an increasing role in solving many of the seemingly insoluble environmental, economic, and social problems we now face on a worldwide scale. Wisdom, after all—the ability not to make the same dumb mistakes twice—is purely the possession of older men and women. You can't buy it. You can't fake it.

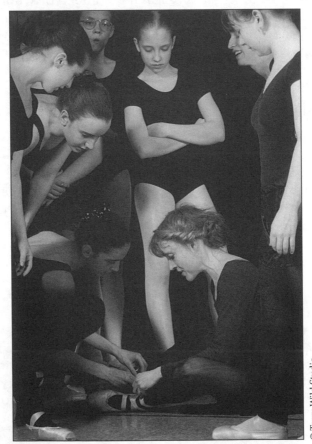

© Terry Wild Studio

NOW IS THE TIME

We think the LifeFit message is more important now than ever before. The call for a more physically active populace is hardly new, of course. In Asia, philosophers and physicians have recognized the importance of exercise in health and longevity for 4,000 years. And 2,500 years ago in the West, the Greeks proclaimed the importance of physical activity as part of a life well lived. But the call for physical activity is taking on increasing urgency: We are a "graying" nation, and we are a nation that seems determined to remain resolutely sedentary despite decades of messages to change our ways. The impending convergence of these demographic realities bodes ill.

Today, only about 22 percent of adults are active at a level recommended for any meaningful health benefits by the U.S. Department of Health and Human Services Healthy People 2000 report on health promotion and disease prevention.[4] Fewer than 10 percent of adults exercise vigorously at an intensity sufficient to promote improved cardiovascular fitness.[5] As our sedentary society grows older, our inactive lifestyles will begin to catch up with more and more of us, creating a huge population of frail older men and women, at enormous cost in suffering, lost productivity, and resources.

ESTIMATED DEATHS CAUSED BY "BIGGEST KILLERS"

Lifestyle factors are now the biggest killers. Estimated numbers of deaths caused in 1990 by lifestyle and other factors were:

Tobacco	400,000
Diet/activity patterns	300,000
Alcohol	100,000
Microbial agents	90,000
Toxic agents	60,000
Firearms	35,000
Sexually transmitted disease	30,000
Motor vehicles	25,000
Illicit drug use	20,000

Adapted, by permission, from J.M. McGinnis et al., 1993, "Actual causes of death in the United States," *Journal of the American Medical Association* 270(18): 2207-2212. Copyright 1993, American Medical Association.

Sedentary living is associated with many of the most debilitating and enormously expensive health problems afflicting us today, including heart disease, probably some types of cancer, diabetes, osteoporosis, stroke, obesity, an epidemic of back problems, and perhaps even mental decline, depression, and other mood disorders. It's not certain at this point what already-strained health care and other support resources will be available for older or sick adults 10, 20, or 30 years from now.

SOCIAL IMPLICATIONS OF SEDENTARY LIVING

Nowhere will conflict between individual aspirations and community needs, or between the young and old, be more bitter than over Social Security, as fewer and fewer workers are available to earn wages and pay taxes to support more and more retired citizens.

An even more difficult and poignant problem has begun to surface as more and more of us are living longer but need care and support from our children, who may themselves have children needing support and care. This "sandwich" generation is already being squeezed between the demands of career, children, and dependent parents, an often unbearable financial and emotional burden. Our society has developed no support systems to help these families.

Not that we could pay for them. The huge national debt siphons off billions of dollars that might be used for social programs for both young and old; the problems caused by rising needs and decreasing resources affect not only older adults needing extensive medical and support care, but future generations as well. To pay the bills, we're already shifting limited resources from such things as prenatal care, preschools, and better education to care for the frail elderly. According to Sylvia Ann Hewlett, in her book *When the Bough Breaks*, the United States is the first society in history in which the poorest population group is its children.[6]

To the degree that this spending on older adults is to provide long-term care for chronic, preventable diseases, our sedentary lifestyles are in a very real sense a "tax" on future generations. To the degree that poor health habits and resulting poor health derive from such factors as lack of education and limited access to preventive health care early in life, then as a society we've created a vicious downward cycle in which money taken from preventive health care and education for the young to support the frail elderly contributes to increasing health problems of future generations as they age, taking money from education and health promotion for the young, and so on . . . and on.

Market forces are producing profound changes in the way health care is provided and paid for, and these changes will continue with or without Washington's intervention or meddling. Already we can see that the new medical culture will be based on limiting services, as it seems clear our present economy can no longer support the old fee-for-service system and its spiraling health care costs. Managed care and capitation will reward providers for not providing specialized care, shifting the emphasis to prevention, primary care, and early intervention, all of which is good, of course. But this shift in culture, along with price controls to slow spiraling health care costs, will also certainly mean limits on access to very expensive, specialized, and high-tech care, particularly at the end of life, as is now done in England.

The bottom line? We probably can't expect society to provide unlimited access to health care, long-term care, nursing home care, or in-home care at prices all of us can afford when we grow old and our bad habits begin to catch up with us; and if we do expect such care, it seems inevitable it will be at the expense of others, particularly the young and future generations.

That's the bad news, and the bad news makes it more imperative than ever that each of us takes personal responsibility for our own health, including working up at least a light sweat on a regular basis. Not only does this have enormous personal benefits—improved health, appearance, vitality, even intelligence—working up a sweat is an act of social responsibility; working up a sweat frees money for future generations to make their lives better. And that's the good news.

YOU'RE IN CONTROL

You can take control of our own health. You can reduce your risk of chronic diseases, increase your longevity, and, perhaps more important, increase your vitality to remain vigorous, active, independent, and fit well into old age, so you don't have to depend on ever-dwindling health care resources later in life, so you don't become a burden on future generations. It's as simple as being up on your feet a bit more every day "puttering around" in activities of daily living. It's as simple as lacing on a pair of athletic shoes and going for a brisk walk or jog three times a week for 30 minutes or more, or swimming or cycling regularly, or taking aerobics classes or tennis lessons.

But the blunt economic benefits of changing to an active lifestyle are no more important than other, perhaps less easily measured benefits such as improved zest for life. True, whether one's quality of life is high or low is to a degree a matter of personal perspective; one person may look forward eagerly to a brisk evening walk, whereas another might view that same walk with dread. But overall, it's fair to say that a life free of disease, a life that is lived with vigor and enthusiasm, a life that is productive, creative, and joyful, is a good life. It's also clear that an active and fit way of life contributes to a good life.

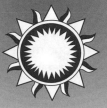

chapter 2

IT'S NEVER TOO LATE

To motivate yourself to take up an active life, or to stick with one, equip yourself with information about what to do, what the benefits are, and how to overcome the many roadblocks you'll encounter on the path to an active life, including what is perhaps the most pernicious roadblock of all—the notion that it's too late to become more active.

For 65-year-old Clyde Henry, the invitation to change came in the form of severe pain in his arms one morning in August 1990. "I knew right away what it was," he recalls. "It was bound to happen, considering the way I'd been living."

A football player in college and later in the Army, Clyde was lean and active until he entered the world of big business as a sales manager for a major West Coast steel manufacturer, where 14-hour days, steak dinners with clients, "with plenty of butter and at least one bottle of wine with dinner each night, followed by cigars, of course," were routine. "It was your basic 10,000-calorie-a-day diet," Clyde says, "a very comfortable life."

But a deadly life. His weight ballooned from 190 to 235. His blood pressure and cholesterol rose to dangerous levels, and he started taking medication for his hypertension as well as for high cholesterol. "I knew I should do something about the way I was living," he says. "But you know how it is. 'I'll start tomorrow,' I'd say. It was always tomorrow."

At least it was "always tomorrow" until the heart attack, when for the first time Clyde was forced to consider the possibility that there might be no "tomorrow." In a sense, the heart attack was the best thing that could have happened to him.

Clyde called his cardiologist, but it being August, the doctor was on vacation, so Clyde was referred to another cardiologist nearby.

"My wife drove me to the office," Clyde recalls. "The nurse there hooked me up to an electrocardiogram, took one look at the readout, and ran from the room. A moment later the physician came running in. 'We think you're having a heart attack,' she said, and dialed 911."

Minutes later, Clyde was surrounded by paramedics, firemen, cops, other physicians. "The funny thing was, the hospital was right across the street," Clyde recalls. "I could have walked, but they charged me $400 for an ambulance ride of about a hundred yards. But I did manage to get off one good line while they wheeled me out of the doctor's office. I told the nurse this wasn't how it was supposed to be: You're supposed to arrive in an ambulance and leave standing up."

A week later, Clyde was on his way to becoming a new man, his sense of humor still intact. Fortunately, Clyde's heart attack had been minor, if any heart attack can be considered minor, and the quick response kept damage to a minimum, as did three doses—at several hundred dollars a dose—of TPA, an anticlotting drug. An angiogram revealed that two arteries in Clyde's heart were 95 percent blocked by fatty deposits, so he underwent coronary angioplasty, a procedure in which a tiny balloon is inserted into the artery and inflated against the deposits, pressing them back and opening up the artery.

"By then," Clyde says, "my physician was back from vacation and working with me. He's a runner, a marathoner. In fact, all the physicians in his group are fitness nuts, skinny little guys and great believers in exercise. They told me to start getting some exercise."

On and off over the years, Clyde had jogged occasionally, but he'd never stayed with it; he didn't have the time. Besides, in the corporate culture of big steel, nine holes of golf from a cart was more acceptable, followed by several Scotch and sodas, then steak for dinner. Now, a week after his heart attack, Clyde went for a walk, a single mile. "That first mile was murder," he recalls, almost fondly. "But I realized by then I had a simple choice: I could go back to my old habits and maybe I'd have two or three years left, if I was lucky. Or I could change my life and have maybe 25 or 30 extra years. I figured those two or three years will go by awfully fast. Not that 25 or 30 won't, but I'll take 30 years over 2 any day."

Now Clyde walks briskly about five miles a day on tough, hilly courses around his home. He's made significant changes in his diet, cutting back on eggs, butter, red meat, and wine. "Now I'm up to 25 miles a week and feel great," he says. "My cholesterol is down to 185, and I'm off medication for that. I'm also off medication for high blood pressure. I don't feel like the changes I've made are a sacrifice at all, especially when you consider the alternative. Besides, life is more fun now. All I could think about before the heart attack was retiring. I was tired of work and of life. Now I love life again. It's like I've been given a second chance."

WHAT'S IN IT FOR THE REST OF US?

It's clear why Clyde Henry changed; he really had no choice, and unfortunately for too many of us, the impetus to change likewise comes in the form of something sudden and compelling like Clyde's heart attack, or the death of a friend or loved one, or our own brush with death, often in the form of early symptoms of coronary heart disease (CHD). And even more unfortunately, for about one-third of those with CHD, the first and only symptom is sudden death. Clyde was lucky.

What is truly puzzling is why the millions of us who, like Clyde, know very well that our sedentary habits are killing us don't change sooner, before the chest pains or other emergencies. Why don't we take up activity even when we know that such a change would be good for us, even when we know that change might be essential to our survival and to the well-being of our families, even when we know that if we become active now we can enjoy much longer the health benefits and added zest for life that are the gifts of an active life?

CLYDE'S TRAINING

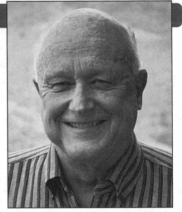

Clyde Henry, 66, sales manager for a major West Coast steel company

Training

"My goal," Clyde says, "is to put in 25 miles a week walking. I've found that's enough to keep my weight down and keep me feeling fit, and it fits in well with my work and other activities. I used to run now and then, but I find I get just as good a workout and walking is easier on my knees."

Clyde's 25 miles a week of walking typically includes two-hour walks twice a week (Sundays and Wednesdays, usually) down the hill on which he lives to the "flatlands," a distance of about 1.5 miles and a drop of nearly 1,000 feet. "That route takes me through a cemetery," Clyde notes, "which is always a good reminder of why I'm walking. I really believe if I don't walk, that's where I'll end up sooner rather than later." Once on the flatlands, Clyde buys a lottery ticket at a corner market, then makes his way about two miles north, then back up the hill and two miles south to his home. It's a distance of about seven miles and takes Clyde a bit more than two hours. "The hills are pretty grueling," Clyde notes. "I'm sweating and panting when I'm done." The other days, Clyde walks various shorter routes of three or four miles, two or three times a week.

Clyde also plays golf twice a week. The course is 7,000 yards, "But I'm all over the place," Clyde notes, "so for me, it's probably a lot more." Clyde carries his own bags and tries to walk at a brisk pace between holes.

Impetus to change

A heart attack. "Like I say," quips Clyde, "it's stay active or end up with my friends in the cemetery."

What he likes most about an active life

"I like life again," Clyde says. "Before my heart attack, I was tired all the time. All I could think about was retiring. Now I have more energy."

Advice

"Start slowly, then when you've become used to being active, start to push yourself, but gently. And try lots of different activities. I like to walk. You might like something else."

INFORMATION: THE VITAL INGREDIENT FOR CHANGE

Change can be difficult, even change from sedentary to active living, without question one of the most rewarding changes any of us can make. Such a change takes time and energy, things most of us are short of these days. When we've been sedentary for years, we simply don't feel like getting up and getting active; too often a sedentary life seems to create the demand for still more sedentary living, a vicious cycle in which lack of activity leads to lowered vitality, frailty, disease, and a depressive mind-set, which together make it all the more difficult to get out of the easy chair and get active.

Some are put off by physical activity because it can cause a bit of discomfort at first. It might make your feet hurt at the outset. It might

LIFEFIT PRINCIPLES

- To achieve a longer, healthier, more vigorous life, the least amount of activity for the greatest benefits should include two types of activities: (1) being up on your feet "puttering about" in daily activities for a total of an hour a day, and (2) three 30-minute bouts of moderately vigorous activity each week that brings a bit of sweat to your brow and elevates the heart rate.

- Any activity is better than none, but intensity of effort matters; for the most benefit, it's a good idea to work up a sweat regularly.

- Taking up and sticking with an active way of life is the single most important change you can make for improved longevity (except not smoking).

- For every year of added life conferred by physical activity, you can expect many additional years of improved health and zest for life, improved sleep, improved mood, improved vitality, improved attitude, clearer thinking, and more creativity.

- For those contemplating change from sedentary to active, the message is clear: It's never too late to benefit from such a change at any age.

- The sooner you make the change from sedentary to active, the more you'll gain both in added years of life and in better years.

- For those who have already made the change from sedentary to active, you've done exactly the right thing and should keep at it.

make your muscles sore. Unfortunately, too many don't stick with activity long enough to realize that these are minor impediments, and that in time—if you give it time—all the discomforts are replaced with improved health, increased energy, a growing sense of well-being and accomplishment, a new zest for life, and finally, a genuine love of an active life.

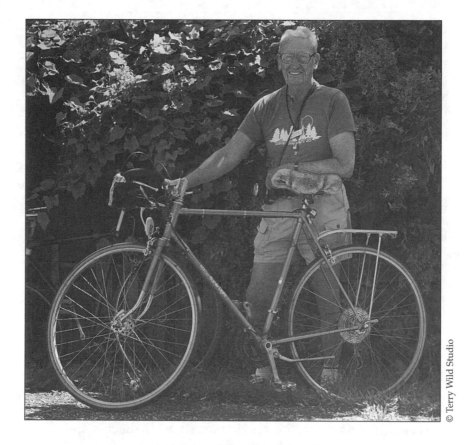

© Terry Wild Studio

NO MORE EXCUSES

More troubling are all the impediments put in our way by our culture and our cultural expectations. Society does not make it particularly easy to be physically active. Most of the messages we receive from the culture around us continually reinforce our addiction to sedentary living, particularly as we grow older—all those urgings to "take it easy" and to buy more and more labor-saving devices. At the same time, tight budgets have forced cities nationwide to cut funding for recreation facilities, and our devotion to the automobile has created urban and suburban environments that are decidedly hostile to walkers, joggers, cyclists, and other active types, while the distribution of services and lack of mass transit make our dependence on automobiles virtually unavoidable.

Taken together, all of these barriers to a more vigorous life can be truly daunting. Thus it's no surprise that most sedentary men and women in America never embark on the fulfilling journey to an active life, and of those who do begin, a disturbing number give up after a short time, discouraged, perhaps injured, certainly frustrated, all to the continuing consternation of public health educators and scientists.

The problem many of us face when trying to get started in an active life, or to stick with it once we start, is that it's often too easy to come up with excuses for not changing, even a few excuses that at first glance seem reasonably valid; in these sedentary times, excuses abound. Overcoming the tendency to make excuses and all the other barriers to successful change depends on four factors:

- the desire to change,
- the belief you can change,
- knowledge of the benefits, and
- knowledge of what specific changes to make and how to make them.

The fact that you're reading *LifeFit* means you probably already want to change, or at least you're giving it some thought, so you've taken a big first step. In part II, we'll talk in much more detail about the benefits of an active life, and in part III, we'll discuss specifically what changes to make and how to make them. For now, we'd like to concentrate on the issue of belief in all its various forms: all the beliefs you may have about what changes you can or can't achieve, or what you might gain from change. To make purposeful change in your life, you have to believe you can change and that change will produce the results you want.

MOVING BEYOND SEVEN COMMON MISCONCEPTIONS

Any belief is based on information—and sometimes misinformation—so you'll need to equip yourself with all the best information you can to help identify those mistaken beliefs that may be impediments to change and then move beyond them.

Misconceptions about exercise abound, but these can be overcome with the right information.

"I JUST DON'T HAVE TIME"

If you're busy with career and family, you may think you don't have the time for activity. Or maybe you believe that given these uncertain economic times, taking a half hour for a brisk walk when you could be taking a business lunch instead—or working late or coming in early—is fiscally irresponsible.

But taking time out from a busy day for a brisk walk or a few laps in a pool isn't time away from getting the job done; in fact, most active people find the time they spend exercising is fertile, productive time, a time to think, to work out problems, to reflect on the day past or the day to come, and most important, a time to feel better. In part III, we'll offer specific strategies you can employ to overcome the barrier of lack of time and turn almost any activity—mowing the lawn, cleaning the garage, raking leaves, doing housework—into an exercise opportunity.

"THERE'S NO PLACE TO WORK OUT"

Our culture's dependence on the automobile and the design of our cities and suburbs around the needs of drivers, not walkers or joggers or cyclists, makes it tough for some of us to pursue physical activity in safety and comfort; no one can be blamed for not going for a walk each evening if the streets are dark, if the sidewalks are broken, and if the traffic is roaring past at 60 miles an hour, belching noise and noxious fumes. Likewise, lack of community recreation facilities, community pools, or lighted tracks and jogging trails makes it logistically difficult for many of us to get active. But there are specific strategies you can employ to overcome these barriers or excuses, and we'll discuss these strategies in more detail in part III as well.

"UNCLE PHIL DIDN'T EXERCISE"

Again and again, we hear that we should get more exercise, cut back on saturated fats in our diets, eat more vegetables, lose weight, stop smoking, and so on, but then we consider the case of Uncle Phil, who smoked two packs a day, lived off steak, butter, and eggs, never di a lick of exercise in his life, drank a fifth of sour mash a day, and lived happily and vigorously until he died peacefully in his sleep at 95.

But Uncle Phil is a rare exception, and one can't—or shouldn't—make predictions based on a few isolated cases like Uncle Phil. What happens on average in modern-day society is a much better reflection of what is most likely to happen to each of us than what a handful of acquaintances—or even relatives—may have experienced in past years. And what's happening today to most of us is heart disease, cancer, stroke, depression, chronic stress, diabetes, arthritis, osteoporosis, and a host of other diseases of civilization, all of which can be delayed or prevented through even a modest amount of physical activity.

"LOOK WHAT HAPPENED TO JIM FIXX"

Others will point to the case of Jim Fixx, the noted author and runner who died of a heart attack during a jog in 1984. Even over a decade later, Fixx remains something of an icon for the "why sweat it?" crowd. "What's the use?" say those who continue to take a dim view of exercise. "Look what happened to Fixx."

Jim Fixx took up an active life at 36, the same age his father suffered his first heart attack. Jim lived to be 52, nine years older than his father, despite the fact he had several strikes against him from the start; aside from a bad family history, suggesting a genetic predisposition to heart disease, Jim had been overweight, an injudicious eater, and a heavy smoker for years—years during which plaque had been building up in his coronary arteries.

Most important for Jim, the years he lived after he took up exercise were better years. He described his own quality of life as much improved after he took up running. He looked better, felt better, and was essentially asymptomatic up to his demise. In other words, he achieved what we should all hope to realize—an active, vigorous, fulfilling life, our minds sharp, unhampered by debilitating illness, not dependent on anyone for care, active until the end of life.

"MEDICAL TECHNOLOGY WILL BAIL ME OUT"

Another hindrance to the adoption of a physically active lifestyle is the notion that we have excellent treatment for many major diseases now, so why worry about going out for a brisk walk to preserve good health? Although it is true that treatments for heart disease, for example, are sometimes effective, remember that as mentioned earlier, in fully one-third of CHD cases, the first and only symptom is sudden death, thus the availability of advanced medical treatment is irrelevant. Nor do effective treatments for heart disease have much impact on the effects on quality of life of years of "subclinical" heart disease—excessive fatigue, chest pains or pains in the limbs, depression and perhaps even mental decline—long before symptoms become severe enough to be recognized and treated.

Nor do treatments for a host of other diseases, from cancer to diabetes to arthritis, however effective, have much favorable impact on quality of life. Indeed, in some cases, the treatments are nearly as bad as the disease. Effective medical care can delay death and perhaps even alleviate suffering. And in some cases, effective medical care can work seeming miracles in saving life and restoring function. But even the most effective medical care is no substitute for prevention.

"THERE'S NO POINT"

One of the most powerful motivators for becoming and staying active is knowledge about the benefits of physical activity. Getting up out of the easy chair to go for a brisk walk around the neighborhood on a chill, damp winter evening can seem like the height of folly, but if you can arm yourself with knowledge about the specific benefits of that brisk walk, chill and damp though it may be, it will be much easier to take that first step and then the next.

Fortunately, we now know a great deal about the health benefits of changing to a more active way of life; we also know that an active life contributes to improved mood, increased creativity, productivity, mental alertness, and perhaps even intelligence. Anecdotal evidence also suggests that regular exercise even helps many men and women in their relations with others, on the job and at home.

As you begin and then stick with your new active life, however, you'll be confronted now and again—and then still again—by headlines in the popular press telling you that "less is more" or "easy does it." And then the writer will explain how only the very lightest exercise imaginable—or better yet, none at all—is "all you need" to remain healthy. This is a common theme in the media's treatment of exercise, and it derives in part from the concern of quite thoughtful individuals that the cause-and-effect relation between exercise and health hasn't been proven (or at least not to their satisfaction). The possibility of selection does complicate these studies, and it goes something like this: The more active individuals in these studies may be healthier and live longer, not because they exercise, but they have both the energy and inclination to be active and are also healthier because they have the "right genes." We'll have more to say in the appendix about how we know that the relation between exercise and health is one of cause and effect.

The bottom line here? Ignore the pundits. Try exercise. You'll like it. You'll benefit. It works.

"IT'S TOO LATE"

This is a variation on the previous misconception, and for those of us over 40 who've been sedentary for a while, even most of our adult lives, it's perhaps the most pernicious one of all—this notion that it's too late, that we've been sedentary too long, that we're too old or too "out of shape" for exercise to do any good, that we've missed our chance. But the College Study and the work of many others clearly demonstrate that nothing could be further from the truth. In the remainder of this chapter, we'll discuss these findings and what they mean to you.

TAKE UP ACTIVITY FOR A LONGER, BETTER LIFE

In 1986, College Study investigators published a paper entitled "Physical Activity, All-Cause Mortality, and Longevity of College Alumni," in which they noted that the College Study findings suggest "a considerable gain in man-years of life for the resolutely energetic"—that is, about 2 years of added life for the average alumnus aged between 35 to 79 years who expended 2,000 kilocalories[1] or more each week measured in walking, stair climbing, and sports play, compared with the less active[2] (see figure 2.1).

More recent analyses of data from the College Study considered specifically subjects who changed from a sedentary to an active life in middle age and even at advanced age, and these findings show just as compellingly that it's never too late to take up physical activity. If you become more active now and stay active consistently, you'll live longer and more vigorously. You'll have more vitality. You'll feel better about yourself. Your mind will work more quickly

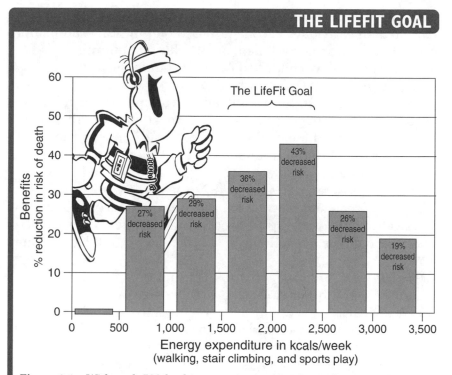

THE LIFEFIT GOAL

Figure 2.1   With each 500-kcal increase in weekly physical activity, the risk of death decreased and longevity increased, to a point. The greatest decreases in risk, that is the most benefit for energy expended, occur when the sedentary become just a little more active. Those who expended just 500 to 1,000 kcals a week had a 29 percent reduction in risk compared with the very sedentary. At the 2,000-kcal-per-week breakpoint, the risk of death was close to half that of the sedentary.

At about 2,000 kcals, though, the health benefits tend to level off, for most. You won't know how your body responds to higher levels of activity until you've tried it, being aware that for most, higher levels do seem to be "too much of a good thing."

and efficiently. And you'll reduce your risk of CHD, cancer, diabetes and a variety of other life-threatening diseases[3].

Sound too good to be true? The findings speak for themselves.

THE COLLEGE STUDY OF PHYSICAL ACTIVITY, HEALTH, AND LONGEVITY

The College Study is based on the analysis of information supplied on periodic questionnaires sent out to Harvard and University of Pennsylvania alumni who entered college between 1916 and 1950. It also analyzes information about the health status of alumni going back to their early days in college, based on physical examinations given to all entering freshmen, and additional information about such things as early childhood diseases, family history of disease, and participation in college athletics.

The first College Study questionnaires were mailed out in 1962 and 1966 to some 27,000 alumni, and 71 percent, or more than 19,000 alumni, responded. Since then, College Study investigators have continued to follow the alumni with periodic questionnaires as the alumni have moved from youth through middle age and into old age (the alumni now range in age from 62 to nearly 100), for the first time affording researchers the opportunity to gather data on the effects of physical activity on the aging process among a very large group of older individuals, something that has been largely lacking until now.

On these periodic questionnaires, the alumni report on a variety of health habits and activities, the existence of specific physician-diagnosed diseases, weight and height, smoking habits, alcohol consumption, history of parental disease and parental death, and their physical activities, including how many city blocks they walk each day and how many stairs they climb. The alumni also provide information about the type, frequency, timing, and duration of their sports or recreational activities, if any.

RATING THE ACTIVITIES

Next, the investigators rate all of these physical activities—all the stair climbing, walking, tennis, jogging, and so on—in terms of kilocalories expended: Walking one mile, for example, is rated at 100 kilocalories. That is, if you walk one mile, you'll burn about 100 kilocalories, about the number of calories in half an apple, a slice of bread, or a pat of butter. That figure of 100 kilocalories per mile of walking is for a man or woman of roughly average build, about 155 pounds, or 70 kilograms. If you are lighter or heavier than this average, you'll burn off somewhat fewer or more than 100 kilocalories in a mile of walking, but you'll receive the same benefit. Nor does it matter significantly how fast you walk that mile, or even if you jog it; you'll still burn roughly the same number of calories, and you can read more about this in chapters 4 and 10.

In addition, for purposes of the study, climbing and descending 100 stairs (five flights) is rated at 40 kilocalories. Sports and recre-

ENERGY VALUES IN KILOCALORIES PER HOUR OF SELECTED ACTIVITIES

	Weight (pounds)					
	95	125	155	185	215	245
Slow walking	86	114	140	168	196	222
Walking, moderate pace	172	228	280	336	392	555
Hiking	258	342	420	504	588	666
Jogging	430	570	700	840	980	1,110
Running	480	770	945	1,134	1,323	1,499
Heavy housework	194	256	315	378	441	500
Sweeping	108	142	175	210	245	278
Scrubbing	237	313	385	462	539	611
Tennis	301	399	490	588	686	777
Golf (carrying clubs)	237	313	385	462	539	611
Golf (in a cart)	151	200	245	294	343	389
Swimming (light laps)	344	456	560	672	784	888
Swimming (hard laps)	430	570	700	840	980	1,110

* The College Study's 2,000-kilocalorie benchmark for optimal health benefits is an average figure for people of about 155 pounds, and it represents the amount of energy that person will expend in physical activities during a week. Your own benchmark will vary, depending on your weight. The more you weigh, the more kilocalories you'll expend at any given activity. During an hour of brisk walking, for example, a 215-pounder will expend nearly twice the kilocalories of a 125-pounder. However, and this is very important, both will have achieved the same health benefits provided by that hour of brisk walking. What's important is how much time you spend being active. Totaling up kilocalories expended becomes a more important issue once weight loss is a concern; the larger or heavier person will lose more weight during any given activity (of course, he or she probably also has more weight to lose).

Reprinted, by permission, from B. Ainsworth et al., 1993, "Compendium of physical activities: Classification of energy costs of human physical activities," *Medicine and Science in Sports and Exercise* 25: 71-80.

ational activities are likewise classified in terms of kilocalories expended, as well as whether the activities are light, mixed, or moderately vigorous. This doesn't mean the alumni don't do other things as well, or that other activities don't contribute to health. For example, doing housework, mowing the lawn, gardening, and playing with the kids are all physical activities, and they all contribute to health, but the investigators use walking, stair climbing, and recreational sports as indicators of an individual's general tendency to be active or inactive.

From all of these reports about physical activity, a physical activity index (PAI) is computed for each individual, expressed in kilocalories per week, and each subject is then classified into one of several groups by PAI; for example, fewer than 500 kilocalories per week, 500 to 1,999 kilocalories per week, or 2,000 or more.

With this information on file, the investigators can then "sit back," pen and notepad in hand, and wait to see what happens to the alumni over the course of years. What they are hoping to see is who, in this huge population, becomes ill and of what, and also who dies and of what, allowing investigators to compare the experiences of those alumni who expend more energy with those who are relatively sedentary.

DRAWING CONCLUSIONS

The power of an epidemiological study such as the College Study depends on accurate and meaningful data collected on large numbers of subjects and long periods of follow-up. Getting the numbers can be a challenge in itself, but the greater challenge is the time involved. Researchers have to wait years for enough "events"—disease, death, or whatever end point they're concerned with—to occur so they can begin to draw meaningful conclusions. The problem is that the researchers themselves might pass on in the meantime, or lose their funding, which in the world of science is often worse than death. Because Harvard began giving standardized, comprehensive physicals to incoming students as early as 1916, and Penn a bit later, and because both schools preserved the records from these physical examinations, the schools had essentially begun collecting data for the College Study as much as 50 years before the study was even conceived, providing a big "leg up" on the data collection process. Thus very early in the study some conclusions could be drawn about the relations between the health status and activity patterns of the alumni when they were students and their health later in life as reported on the first questionnaires.

It became apparent, for example, that alumni who had been varsity athletes in their college years and then became sedentary as adults had no better health later in life than their less athletically inclined and now equally sedentary former classmates. This is a very important finding because it sheds some light on the thorny issue of cause and effect. Varsity athletes, who might be expected to have some genetic predispositions to good health and longevity, didn't seem to be protected from disease or premature death by good genes or past activity at all. Rather, only contemporary participation in physical activity protected their health. On the other hand, now-active alumni who weren't athletes in college had the same low risk of disease and early death as now equally active former college athletes. These findings provided the first solid evidence that the relation between physical activity and improved health was cause and effect, not selection. That is, one's good luck having the right parents and thus "good" genes doesn't provide as much protection from disease as does one's tendency to work up a sweat on a regular basis.

THE 1986 COLLEGE STUDY REPORT

Investigators have published their findings regularly, and among the reports was one in the New England Journal of Medicine in 1986 in which they drew the most definite conclusions to date about the benefits of activity. The College Study findings reported then were based on observations of the 17,000 alumni, aged 35 to 74, who returned questionnaires in 1962 or 1966 and who were followed through 1978. The findings were unequivocal:

- The more active alumni lived longer and had a lower risk of death from heart disease and other causes.

- The benefits of an active life in terms of added years of life began with "step one," and the benefits continued to increase in a gradient fashion as physical activity increased, to a point.

- The greatest benefits occurred when the most sedentary became even somewhat more active.

- The most active alumni in the study, those who reported themselves to be habitually active by expending 2,000 kilocalories a week or more in walking, stair climbing, and recreational sports, had the lowest risk—and most added years of life—of all.

Most of the increased longevity enjoyed by active men and women results from a decreased risk of cardiovascular disease, including CHD, heart failure, and stroke. Additional gains in longevity resulted from a reduced risk of diabetes, some cancers, and other chronic ailments. Unfortunately, the statistics on added years of life can't show the improved quality of life enjoyed by active men and women—the improved zest for life, energy, mood, and productivity.

THE 1993 COLLEGE STUDY REPORT—CONTINUITIES AND CHANGE

Because the 1986 College Study analyses looked at the experiences of all alumni—those who had been active for long periods, those who had been just as habitually inactive, those who had changed from sedentary to active, and those who had changed from active to sedentary—two important questions arose:

Question 1: Would those like Clyde Henry and many others of us who had been resolutely sedentary for years also benefit in terms of added years and improved pleasures of living if they took up exercise relatively late in life?

Question 2: The second and more troubling question concerned, again, cause and effect. The fact that former college athletes weren't protected later in life by their college athleticism sheds some light on this matter, but not enough light by the rigorous standards of science. Does exercise literally protect us from disease and add years to our lives? Exactly what role do our genes play in our health and longevity? Are there other factors we know nothing about that can select out those who were healthy and who also happen to be physically more active?

To help answer these questions, the College Study investigators began a long-term observation of a large number of individuals who changed their habits. Investigators noted which alumni adopted an active life during an 11- to 15-year period between the 1962/1966 questionnaires and a second questionnaire sent out in 1977, which alumni dropped activity, and which alumni stayed unchanged. Then the investigators again sat back, notebooks and pens in hand, and waited to see what would happen by the end of the follow-up period 12 years later, in 1988, this time to compare the experiences of those who changed from sedentary to active, or who stayed active, with those who remained or became sedentary.

Those who increased or decreased their activity levels by 250 kilocalories or less were classified as "unchanged" for purposes of analysis, and investigators looked at change in activity patterns in increments or decrements of 250 kilocalories. Based on data about who among the alumni got sick, who died, and the cause of death in each case, it was then possible to relate risk of disease and mortality to change or to lack of change (see table 2.1).

The subjects in the College Study (aged 45 to 84 in 1977) who increased their physical activity (measured as kilocalories of energy

Table 2.1 Added years of life to age 90						
	Age in 1977 (yr)					
Changed lifeway pattern	35-44	45-54	55-64	65-74	75-84	45-84
Physical activity increased from <1,500 to ≥1,500 kcal/wk	1.79	1.78	1.60	1.28	0.78	1.57
Walking increased from <15 to ≥15 km/wk	0.30	0.30	0.28	0.23	0.14	0.27
Stair climbing increased from <20 to ≥20 stories/wk	1.39	1.39	1.27	1.02	0.64	1.23
Took up moderately vigorous sports play ≥4.5 METs	1.81	1.77	1,60	1.25	0.79	1.54
Physical activity increased by 750 kcal/wk	1.17	1.70	1.54	1.23	0.77	1.51
Quit cigarette smoking	2.15	2.06	1.84	1.45	0.95	1.84
Remained normotensive	1.25	1.21	1.08	0.85	0.54	1.07
Body mass index remained <26	0.52	0.51	0.46	0.37	0.24	0.46
Physical activity increased from <1,500 kcal/wk and quit cigarette smoking	4.31	4.17	3.74	2.95	1.90	3.72

Adapted, by permission, from R.S. Paffenbarger et al., 1994, "Chronic diseases in former college students: LII. Changes in physical activity and other lifeway patterns influencing longevity," *Medicine and Science in Sports and Exercise* 26: 857-865.

expended in exercise) to more than 1,500 kilocalories each week in light and moderate exercise enjoyed an average of nearly two years of added life compared with those who stayed sedentary or changed from active to sedentary. Even the oldest individuals in the study, those aged 75 to 84, who took up physical activity at that advanced age gained an average of 0.78 years, demonstrating eloquently just how adaptable and capable of self-development the human organism can be, even an old human organism. Nine additional months of life may not sound like much, but coming near the end of life, this is not insignificant. Looking at this figure another way, it's almost a 10 percent increase in survival to age 90.[4]

The actual gains in added years of life you achieve depend on the age at which you change your health habits. The sooner you make the change, the more years you gain. Note that those who had smoked and then quit significantly improved their prospects compared with those who continued the nasty habit. Smokers who not only quit smoking but took up activity made huge gains in longevity.

Overall, the reduction in risk of death—and thus added years—for those who changed from a sedentary to an active life was comparable to the years gained by those who had always been active, at least through the duration of the observation (see figure 2.2).

PROOF THAT IT'S NEVER TOO LATE

Nor did it matter how resolutely sedentary the alumni may have been (at least to age 90, the current limit of the continuities and change study). These benefits of change seemed to occur regardless of past history of bad habits or a family history that might suggest a

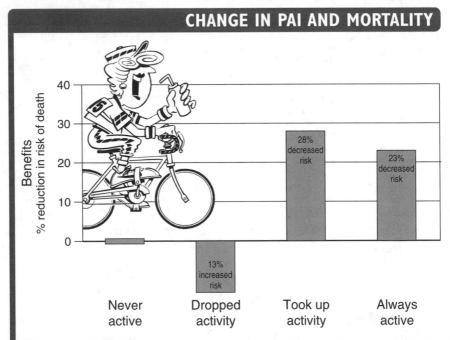

Figure 2.2   Taking the always sedentary as the starting point for comparison, the habitually active have a 23 percent lower relative risk of death; men who *changed* from inactive to active had a 28 percent lower risk. This isn't a particularly meaningful difference, though it is a clear *trend*, an indication of possibilities.

And what do we make of the fact that those who *dropped* physical activity seem to be worse off than those who were always sedentary? Most likely, among those who were active and then became sedentary were those who became ill with eventually fatal diseases.

hereditary predisposition to heart disease and other health problems; men who changed from sedentary to active, who took up sports play and changed other habits such as quitting smoking, simply reduced their risk of certain diseases, particularly cardiovascular disease (CVD), and added years to their lives. The message here for the rest of us? The 45-year-old or even the 75-year-old who becomes active even after years of sedentary living experiences the same lower risk of death and the same added years of life as the man or woman who remains habitually active all along.

In other words, it's never too late to change. This is remarkably encouraging news. Perhaps you've been sedentary all your life; perhaps you're overweight, continue to smoke, and have high blood pressure and all the other risk factors for early death from heart disease; perhaps you've wondered "What's the use? It's too late for me." But you can benefit from change; increased physical activity will add years to your life and more life to your years.

Of course, if you happen to be a procrastinator, the obvious question arises: If all of this is so, why not just put off making that decision to take up an active life until next week, or next year, or maybe 10 or 20 years from now? First, the longer you wait, the longer it will be before you can enjoy all of the many benefits of activity. Next, the sooner you make activity a habit, the more added years of life you gain; the youngest alumni who took up and stuck with an active life gained the most years. Finally, and most important, when you are sedentary, your risk of disease and premature death from a variety of causes goes up, thus increasing the chances you won't last long enough to stop procrastinating.

THE LIFEFIT PROGRAM FOR OPTIMAL HEALTH

Is there an exercise prescription for optimal health? All of the available evidence from more recent analyses of the College Study data and data from a number of other studies indicate that there is. To fully achieve a longer, healthier, more vigorous life, the least amount of activity for the greatest benefits should include two types of activities, which we call Stage One and Stage Two activities, for a total of about 2,000 kilocalories of energy expended per week.

STAGE ONE: GET MOVING

Every day, you should be on your feet for at least one hour moving around, using the large muscles of the legs while walking, climbing stairs, working in the garden, shuttling about the kitchen, playing with the children, pushing a shopping cart through the supermarket, walking from the train station to your office, purposefully strolling about on your lunch hour, or just about anything but sitting quietly in front of a TV. This need not be continuous activity, nor is it necessary to work up a sweat. What's important is that you are up on your feet moving about every day and, through the course of a day, accumulate at least 60 minutes of activity.

At first glance, this doesn't sound like all that much, and for some, it's not, but in our sedentary society, it can take some planning and determination to achieve even that amount of activity. Certainly if you've had problems in the past sticking with activity, you may need

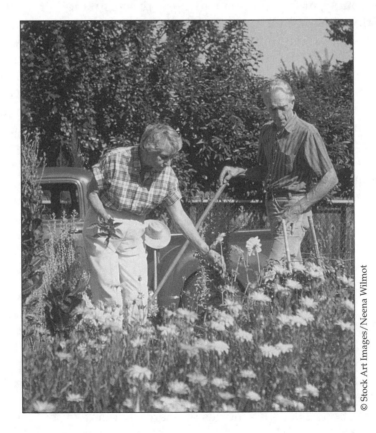

© Stock Art Images/Neena Wilmot

to employ some specific strategies for increasing your Stage One level of activity. In chapter 10, we'll discuss in more detail how you can tell if you are achieving your Stage One goal and how to get there if you're not.

STAGE TWO: BREAK A SWEAT

Once you've become accustomed to being up and "puttering about" at least an hour a day, you should gradually begin to add moderate activities to your weekly routine that eventually total at least 30 additional minutes, three times a week. Unlike Stage One activities, which you'll be able to achieve by simply getting through the day, Stage Two activities typically are deliberate and planned. These activities are primarily what we think of as recreational activities such as brisk walking, jogging, cycling, swimming, aerobic dance, or court sports. These activities should be sustained for 30 minutes or longer, they should be continuous, and they should be done at an intensity that brings a bit of sweat to your brow, raises your heart rate, and has you breathing more deeply.

Approximately half of the health benefits derived from physical activity occur during the one hour a day of Stage One puttering about, a total of seven hours each week for a weekly energy expenditure of about 1,400 kilocalories for someone of average weight, more or fewer kilocalories if you are heavier or lighter. The other half of the benefits, however, derive from the mere 30 minutes, three times a week, of sustained Stage Two activities, a total of 90 minutes during a week for an energy expenditure of roughly 500 kilocalories. Together, Stage One and Stage Two activities total about 2,000 kilocalories per week. This, we believe, is the least amount of physical activity to achieve the most health benefits, your long-term LifeFit goal.

If you adhere to your LifeFit program for about six months, combining Stage One and Stage Two activities into a weekly program, you will realize significant reductions in your risk for a number of life-threatening diseases and add years to your life. You will have more energy, lose weight, and look better. You will also realize a number of benefits in terms of psychological health and cognitive functioning. And you will become much more fit than you were before becoming active, within the bounds of your genetic endowment.

APPROXIMATE KILOCALORIES EXPENDED IN ONE WEEK OF THE LIFEFIT PROGRAM ACTIVITIES

Weight			Kcal/week	
kg	lb	to age 59	age 60-74	age 75+
43	95	1,200	930	600
47	105	1,330	1,000	665
52	115	1,440	1,110	720
57	125	1,580	1,190	780
61	135	1,680	1,300	840
66	145	1,810	1,410	905
70	**155**	**1,940** (average)	**1,500**	**1,000**
75	165	2,080	1,600	1,040
80	175	2,220	1,710	1,110
84	185	2,330	1,800	1,165
89	195	2,470	1,900	1,235
93	205	2,580	1,990	1,290
98	215	2,720	2,100	1,360
102	225	2,830	2,180	1,415

The above figures were calculated this way:

Age 59 and under: kg × 7 hrs × 3 METs* (Stage One) + kg × 1.5 hrs × 4.5 METs (Stage Two) = total weekly kcal

Age 60-74: kg × 5.25 hrs × 3 METs + kg × 1.125 hrs × 4.5 METs = total weekly kcal

Age 75+: kg × 3.5 hrs × 3 METs + kg × 0.75 hrs × 4.5 METs = total weekly kcal

If you know how much time you spend in both Stage One and Stage Two activities, you can calculate your exact caloric expenditure using the same formula: kg × time × 3 METs + kg × time × 4.5 METs.

* A MET is a unit of measurement used to represent the metabolic equivalent of work for a particular activity (see page 39 for a thorough discussion).

WHY SWEAT IT?

In terms of providing health benefits, there is a qualitative difference between simply puttering about (Stage One) and engaging in activities that raise the heart rate (Stage Two). Most studies, including the College Study, demonstrate that the greatest health benefits come from moderately vigorous or more intense activities—that is, Stage Two activities that elevate the heart rate, increase breathing, and bring some sweat to the brow. Of course, most of us have to participate in Stage One activities consistently before we can begin to participate in Stage Two activities.

As figure 2.3 shows, moderate sports play is the single most important thing you can do to lower your risk of disease and add healthy and happy years to your life.[5] For this analysis, the College Study uses the term sports play to refer to any deliberate recreational activities as distinct from getting about during daily activities. The

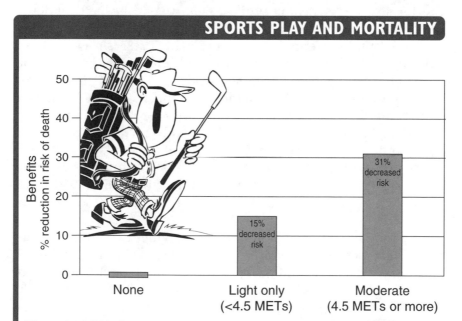

Figure 2.3 This figure compares the experiences of active alumni based on the intensity of activity. Those who were active, but not intensely, that is, those who engaged in Stage One but no Stage Two activity, were assigned a relative risk of 1.00 for purposes of comparison (please keep in mind that this group has a much lower risk than the totally sedentary). Those who indulged in some sports activities but not at levels of intensity sufficient to elevate the heart rate 30 minutes or longer had a 15 percent lower risk compared with the first group. Those who worked up a sweat at least once a week had a 31 percent reduced risk compared with the first group. Again, keep in mind that *all* of these alumni enjoyed much better health than the totally sedentary.

most common light sports reported by the alumni were golf, walking for pleasure, and a combination of gardening, housework (yes, for some, apparently, housework is recreational), and carpentry; moderately vigorous—or simply moderate or more intense—sports most often reported were swimming, tennis, squash, racquetball, handball, jogging and running, cycling, cross-country hiking, downhill and cross-country skiing, rowing, heavy yard work, and the like.[6]

Investigators also assigned a metabolic equivalent (MET) score to each activity. A MET is the ratio of work metabolism to resting metabolism, or active to sedentary metabolism. Metabolism refers to all of the physical and chemical changes taking place within a living organism, the ongoing process of building cells and breaking them down, the process of taking in and using energy to remain alive, in other words, of digesting food, of breathing, of pumping blood, of the tiny muscular movements such as squirming around in our theater seats or twitching while asleep (we're never completely motionless, even when at rest).

The amount of energy it takes to remain at rest is classified as 1 MET, and other activities are rated as multiples of this. For example, a leisurely walk of about two miles an hour—the speed at which you might stroll from one gallery of the Museum of Modern Art in New York to another—is classified at about 2 METs, or twice as vigorous as resting or sitting in front of a Picasso abstract while you try to figure out what it means; carrying a bag of groceries up a flight of stairs, however, is rated at about 5 METs, or five times as vigorous as resting; running a 10-minute mile is rated at 10 METs, or 10 times as vigorous as sitting quietly trying to figure out what Picasso was up to.[7]

Investigators classified as light those activities that ranged from 1 to 4.4 METs (less likely to elevate the heart rate, breathing, and so on, sufficiently for significant health benefits); moderately vigorous or simply moderate activities as those from 4.5 to 5.9 METs (within the target level of effort); and heavy or vigorous activities as those rated at 6.0 METs or greater.

CHANGE (ADDING OR DROPPING MODERATELY VIGOROUS ACTIVITY)

In comparing alumni who changed their exercise habits and either took up or quit moderately vigorous sports play, it becomes very apparent that current physical activity is what counts; you can't

SUSTAINED ACTIVITY BY METABOLIC EQUIVALENTS (METS)

Stage One

METs	Description	Type of activity
1	Sitting	Eating, reading, desk work, watching TV, driving on the highway
2	Very light exertion	Office work, driving in the city, personal care, standing in line, strolling in the park
3	Light exertion with normal breathing	Mopping, slow walking (e.g., shopping), bowling, sweeping, golfing with a cart, gardening with power tools, table tennis, tai chi chuan, yoga
4	Moderate exertion with deeper breathing	Normal walking, golfing on foot, slow hiking, raking leaves, cleaning windows, hanging wallpaper, interior painting, slow dancing, housework

Stage Two

METs	Description	Type of activity
4.5	Moderately vigorous activity with deeper breathing, some sweat on the brow	Calisthenics, hunting, baseball, recreational volleyball, downhill skiing
5	Vigorous exertion with panting and sweating	Slow jogging, fast walking (5 mph or more), golf carrying clubs, cross-country skiing, cycling (10 mph or more), heavy gardening, splitting wood, lap swimming, backpacking, judo, karate

(continued)

SUSTAINED ACTIVITY BY METABOLIC EQUIVALENTS (METS) *(continued)*		
6	Heavy exertion with gasping, heavy sweating	Running, fast jogging, competitive field and court sports, singles tennis, rowing machine, fast dancing, heavy calisthenics
7+	Extreme or peak exertion	Sprinting, fast running, jogging uphill, aggressive sports with frequent sprinting and no rest, pushing or pulling with all one's might, unusually heavy work

Adapted, by permission, from I-M Lee, C-C. Hsieh, and R.S. Paffenbarger, 1995, "Exercise intensity and longevity in men," *Journal of the American Medical Association* 273(15): 1179-1184. Copyright 1995, American Medical Association.

"rest on your laurels," or on your sweatsuit either, in other words. Figure 2.4 charts the experiences of four groups of active alumni. These alumni were assessed for intensity of their activities in 1962/1966 and again in 1977. Then they were watched for the next 12 years to see what sorts of health problems they developed.

- Those who were resolute in their commitment not to engage in moderate sports of any sort were assigned a relative risk of 1.0 for purposes of comparison.

- Those who changed their sports habits and took up moderate activity sometime between 1962/1966 and 1977 had a 27 percent reduced risk (a relative risk of 0.73) of death during the follow-up through 1988 compared with the resolutely nonvigorous. Their experience, in fact, was nearly identical to that of alumni who had always engaged in moderate sports (relative risk of 0.72).

- Surprisingly, those who were moderately vigorous at the time of the first assessment but then dropped the habit by the time of the second assessment in 1977 had a 12 percent rise in risk (relative risk of 1.12) compared with the persistently nonvigorous contingent, most likely because among those who dropped moderate activities were those who were forced to give them up by the onset of eventually fatal conditions such as cancer.[8]

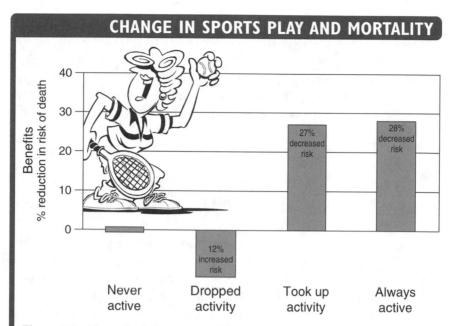

Figure 2.4   Not only did moderately vigorous sports play decrease the risk of death for the alumni, it also added years to their lives. At each age level, from 45 to 84 years, alumni who continued in or took up moderate activity (4.5 METs or more) gained years of life.

LESS IS NOT MORE

Puttering around an hour a day will help specifically in reducing the risk of heart disease and will contribute to some reductions in many other diseases. But it also appears that only moderately vigorous activity at an intensity high enough to elevate the heart rate and increase breathing will elicit other physiological changes that lead to further reductions in the risk of heart attack. Only moderately vigorous activity appears to significantly reduce the risk of other diseases, including non-insulin-dependent diabetes mellitus (NIDDM), hypertension, and perhaps some cancers, while also providing significant benefits in cognitive performance and mood.

The conclusions?

- Again, moderate physical activity is vitally important to increasing longevity, reducing risk of disease, and improving quality of life.
- For the very sedentary, any activity at all, and certainly Stage One of the LifeFit program, will provide enormous benefit.

- But contrary to the recent "less is more" trend in exercise recommendations, it's apparent that intensity of physical activity also matters.
- Simply put, men and women who regularly break a sweat live longer and have still less disease than those less intensely active (and both groups will live longer and better than those who are sedentary).

"JUST" TWO YEARS?

When the conclusions about the association between physical activity and increased longevity came out in 1986, stating a "considerable gain" of two years or more for the most active, the popular media had a field day. Two years? You call that a "considerable gain"? Besides, look how you have to spend those two years: jogging, working up a sweat . . . how awful. And what's worse, aren't these additional years tacked onto the end of life? Who wants two more years of being old and miserable?

But some missed the point both arithmetically and conceptually, and as you set out to become and remain physically active, it's important that you keep in mind what "just two years" really means to you:

- First, an average gain of two years may not seem like that much at first glance, but two additional years of life is nothing at all to scoff at, considering the alternative.

- Given the current level of medical knowledge, it appears that of all the changes you might make in your life, taking up and sticking with activity is the single most important change you can make for improved longevity (other than quitting smoking if you smoke), which means, of course, that these two added years are enormously significant. It now appears that short of major and so far unforeseen breakthroughs in genetic engineering, pharmacology, or medicine, there are not many other changes we can make, aside from becoming more active, to add more years to our lives and more vitality to our years.

- The additional years of life that result from activity are simply an average of the experiences of a large population observed over many years; among the population of active alumni were, of course, some who exercised regularly and nonetheless suffered a fatal disease. But also among the active alumni were even more who were active and fit and thus avoided a fatal heart attack at 45 or 55 or 65 and may have gained a decade or two of added years, and who are still going strong. By working with a large population over a long period, the extremes tend to cancel each other, and what's left is a meaningful picture of what most of us can expect to gain by taking up and sticking with an active life.

• More important, these added years of life are in a sense a by-product of many better years. The College Study measured the relation between physical activity and added years of life through the reduction of death from a variety of causes. But there are many very debilitating diseases that don't necessarily result in death, or at least not immediately. For example, before someone dies of a heart attack, he or she may have suffered for years from the debilitating effects of cardiac insufficiency, chest pains, shortness of breath, and even anxiety about such symptoms. For every year of added life conferred by physical activity, in other words, you can expect many additional years of improved vigor and zest for life, improved sleep, improved mood, improved vitality, improved attitude, clearer thinking, and more creativity. Indeed, these less easily measured benefits are available from the first day you lace on those walking or running shoes, dust off the 10-speed, or take up tennis and have at it.

SOME IS BETTER THAN NONE

Is the 2,000-kilocalorie-per-week level of activity for optimal health a threshold of physical activity we all must strive for? Not at all. Rather, there is a gradient of increasing health benefits that occurs with the very first step and an optimal level of physical activity for the greatest health benefits possible for which we should all strive. Most important for those of us who have been sedentary or only sometimes active, physical activity of any kind, even the most leisurely stroll, is much better than no activity at all and offers significant health benefits. Moderately vigorous Stage Two activity is not absolutely necessary for improved health and longevity, but for optimal health, a combination of Stage One and Stage Two activities totaling 1,500 to 2,000 kilocalories a week is best.

Unfortunately, the figure of 2,000 kilocalories came to be seen originally as a threshold level of activity that everyone had to achieve. One of the greatest dangers in the concept of an exercise threshold is that people will get the idea that if they do anything less than that amount, they're wasting their time, so they may opt to do nothing at all.

Some have misinterpreted the 2,000-kilocalorie break point discussed in the College Study to mean about 20 miles a week of walking or jogging, or the equivalent in swimming, cycling, or other recreational activities. Although it's true that the 1,500- to 2,000-kilocalorie-per-week goal for optimal health is roughly equivalent to walking or jogging 20 miles each week, you don't literally need to put in 20 miles a week on the roads to enjoy improved health and longevity. Remember, Stage One and Stage Two activities together total about 1,500 to 2,000 kilocalories per week. This is an accumulation of a variety of physical activities through a week, from walking to the corner grocery, mowing the lawn, or taking the stairs to the office each morning instead of the elevator, as well as brisk walking, jogging, a few laps of swimming, a bit of tennis, some weight training, aerobic dance, or what have you (see figure 2.5).

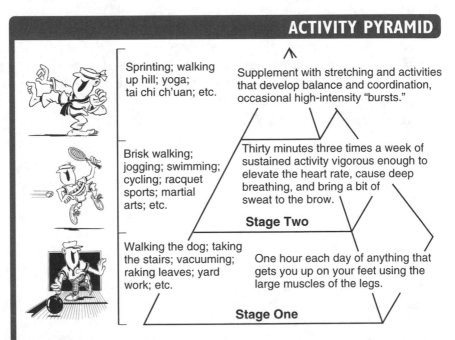

Figure 2.5   You can combine Stage One and Stage Two activities in any number of ways to reach the weekly 1,500- to 2,000-kilocalorie energy expenditure goal for improved health and longevity.

Of course, in these sedentary times, it's not easy to expend 2,000 kilocalories a week in physical activity without deliberately going out for a brisk walk, a jog, a bike ride, or whatever, and as we've seen, this type of activity is an important feature of your LifeFit program for longevity: To gain the most benefits from physical activity, it is a good idea to deliberately go out and sweat at least a little on a regular basis.

As you begin and maintain an active life, keep in mind that all additional physical activity will be beneficial: A little exercise is much better than none at all, more is better than a little, and somewhere around 1,500 to 2,000 kilocalories of physical activity per week seems to be the point at which most of us will have achieved most of the health benefits possible through exercise.

The gains in added years of life increase sharply from sedentary to about 1,500 to 2,000 kilocalories per week. At this point, these benefits level off and there's no additional lowering of disease risk with increasing physical effort. In other words, you've gotten all you can out of physical activity in terms of improved physical health and longevity. But we want to emphasize that many of us will derive great pleasure and emotional benefits from additional activity well beyond this level, including continuing improvements in appearance or personal satisfaction, improvements in physical fitness for specific activities such as beating your neighbor at tennis, and the simple fun of being active, no matter what the long-term health benefits. At about 3,500 kilocalories per week, the health benefits definitely level off.

THE LAW OF DIMINISHING RETURNS

What all of this suggests is a law of diminishing returns—the very sedentary man or woman who increases his or her activity level even slightly will realize significant benefits by becoming even a little more active. As we become still more active, however, additional benefits come only with greater effort. Thus the LifeFit program describes the least amount of activity for the most health benefits.

Most of the increased longevity enjoyed by active men and women results from a decreased risk of cardiovascular diseases, including heart failure and stroke. To a lesser extent, additional gains in longevity result from a reduced risk of diabetes, colon cancer, and perhaps other chronic ailments.

This trend in benefits gained per effort expended has been noted in a variety of other studies as well. For example, in a "study of the studies," Ken Powel, Carl Caspersen, and colleagues[9] reviewed a large number of studies of fatal and nonfatal heart disease and physical activity, including the College Study, noting the points on which these studies agreed.[10-18] Investigators found that in each of these studies, risk of fatal and nonfatal heart disease declined most sharply as activity increased from the lowest levels, and that this declining risk tended to flatten out as activity increased. This has important implications for those of us trying to fit physical activity into our busy lives; there comes a point at which more time spent working up a sweat fails to provide additional gains in terms of reduced risk of disease and added years of life.

Also, as we grow older, there seems to be an inevitable but very slow decline in cardiac output, strength, and ability to perform work; thus the amount of effort required to maintain optimal health also decreases. The available evidence seems to indicate that to fully achieve the goal of optimal health and vitality, you need to strive for a total weekly energy expenditure of about 2,000 kilocalories to age 59, 1,500 kilocalories if you're between ages 60 and 74, or 1,000 kilocalories if you are 75 or over in combined Stage One and Stage Two activities.[19] (See the table on page 36 for more information.) This doesn't mean you shouldn't do more if you choose to, of course.

THE TRICKY RELATION BETWEEN FITNESS AND HEALTH

The health benefits of physical activity may level off at about 2,000 kilocalories per week, but does this mean there's no point going further? Although it's true that at this level you will have achieved most of the health benefits possible in terms of added years of life and reduced risk of disease, by no means does this suggest that the mental, emotional, philosophical, or even spiritual benefits of being active also level off at the 2,000-kilocalorie point.

Indeed, it's for the less tangible consolations of activity, such as improved self-image, improved confidence and mood, and even improved cognitive functioning, that many of us push ourselves well beyond the 2,000-kilocalorie level, about which much more in part II.

If you train more and more, even beyond the 2,000-kilocalorie level, you'll become more fit; that is, you'll be faster, stronger, and have more endurance. And if that is your goal, you'll certainly want to train more. But LifeFit is a program for the development of optimal health and longevity. Stage One and Stage Two together represent the least amount of activity needed for the most health benefits. Your fitness will improve as your health improves, to a point, because fitness and health are closely linked, but there are limits to their relation. Fitness is not quite the same thing as health.

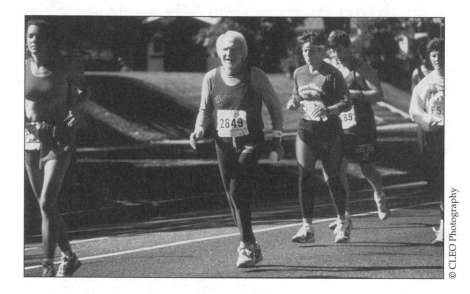

© CLEO Photography

FITNESS AND HEALTH DEFINED

Fitness is a measurable state or condition partially determined by genetics. Health is also a condition but is not nearly as easily measured or defined in precise terms as fitness. Health is not merely the presence or absence of disease; rather, it's a complete state of physical, mental, and social well-being, a complex of factors that represents all levels of vitality from the highest to the lowest (or death, to put it bluntly).[20] On the other hand, the World Health Organization defines fitness as "the ability to perform work satisfactorily"[21,22] thus making the definition of who is fit and who isn't somewhat dependent on personal inclination and social context. One's ability to perform work satisfactorily depends on the type of work involved and on how one defines satisfactorily. To a competitive runner, for example, fitness is measured in faster times and longer distances; fitness means fit or conditioned for beating the other guy, the clock, or one's previous best. To the Olympic athlete, fitness is ultimately measured in terms of gold medals and world records. To the plodder, fitness is measured perhaps in simply getting through the next mile.

A hundred thousand years ago, the fit man or woman might have been someone who could hunt for dinner all day long and then spend the night in a tree or cave to keep from becoming dinner. A hundred years ago, the fit man might have been someone who could plow the back 40 from sunup to sundown, then still have energy left to shoe the horses or mend the harnesses by lantern light; the fit woman of that era might have been someone who could cook all day; knead four loaves of bread; wash a week's worth of clothing by hand; take care of the baby, the two-year-old, and the four-year-old; tend the chickens; can the peaches; and still have energy left at the end of the day to work on a quilt. Fifty years ago, the fit man or woman might have been someone who could work 12 hours a day on an assembly line, doing the same job over and over again.

These days, one's ability to perform work satisfactorily typically depends on one's ability to get up every morning, brave rush-hour traffic on the way to work, put in at least eight hours sitting at a desk, often in some high-pressure job with an ill-tempered supervisor, then brave rush-hour traffic coming home and still have the energy to mow the lawn, play with the kids, and in general remain productive and vital long enough to retire, collect a pension, and enjoy his or her remaining years free of disease.

No one these days is dying of not being able to throw a spear at a potential dinner, or not being able to climb a tree quickly enough, or even of not being able to plow the back 40. These days, people are dying from diseases our more active hunter-gatherer or farmer ancestors probably never had to worry about, the diseases of civilization—coronary heart disease, stroke, diabetes, cancer, depression, mental decline, and so on—all the chronic ailments that result directly from adverse lifestyle habits, including an imprudent diet, sedentary living, smoking, and chronic, unrelieved stress. And this is where fitness and health merge; these days, being healthy does mean being fit—fit for life in these times.

FIT DOESN'T NECESSARILY MEAN HEALTHY

But can there be good health without a high level of fitness? Or fitness without health? Does one cause the other? All of these issues are still open to debate, yet it appears that, to an extent, one can be fit without necessarily being healthy. For example, fitness is generally measured in the lab as maximum oxygen uptake, or $\dot{V}O_2$max, as it's called. This is a measure of the body's ability to take in and use oxygen. If you have a higher $\dot{V}O_2$max, this means you use more oxygen, so you can perform more work before fatigue sets in. As such, $\dot{V}O_2$max also functions as a reasonable measure of the health of an individual's cardiovascular system, because a cardiovascular system that has been compromised by atherosclerosis (clogged arteries), for example, or lung disease from smoking won't be able to deliver oxygen to the working muscles as effectively. Beyond this point, though, fitness and health tend to part company.

An elite professional athlete, for example, will likely test as very fit in terms of $\dot{V}O_2$max, but is he healthy? Very likely, but not necessarily; he might be exquisitely fit, but if he's under stress from trying to perform at his best in game after game, or from worrying about his contract or endorsement deals, as are so many elite athletes these days, or if he's taking steroids to build his strength or using illicit drugs or abusing alcohol, he may not be all that healthy. Elite athletes—the very fittest of the fittest—are often on the verge of physical breakdown from overuse injuries; professional football players, in particular, are typically walking textbooks of sport-related injuries. Are they healthy?

Likewise, the average man or woman might be quite healthy in terms of mental, physical, and social well-being but without being particularly fit, or at least fit in terms of cardiopulmonary capacity as measured in the lab. In a recent Danish study, four researchers looked at highly fit subjects (as measured on a treadmill) who were either sedentary or active and at unfit subjects who were likewise either sedentary or active. Surprisingly, the study found that the active though unfit subjects had nearly the same low risk of heart disease as the active fit subjects. Likewise, it didn't matter if the sedentary subjects were fit or unfit; both groups had the same high risk of heart disease.[23]

In other words, fitness doesn't seem to be as important a factor in one's risk of disease as one's current level of physical activity. But how can someone be active and healthy and still remain unfit? Or how can someone be inactive, unhealthy, and nonetheless fit? Genetics, apparently.

GENETICS' ROLE IN HEALTH AND FITNESS

Just how much of one's fitness or one's health is genetically determined is open to considerable debate. Estimates range from 20 percent to as much as 90 percent. Claude Bouchard, the internationally renowned Canadian exercise physiologist, estimates that 25 to 40 percent of one's fitness is genetically determined, a figure achieving a certain respectability these days.[24] Which leaves an estimated 60 to 75 percent within our control through regular exercise and a healthful diet—we become more active, eat healthfully, lose excess weight, and become more fit—and of course more healthy as well.

Certainly some men and women are born with hearts and lungs that work more efficiently, with reflexes that are a bit quicker, with muscles that are stronger. If they become active and train sufficiently, some can fully realize that genetic potential. And if that potential is high enough and they train sufficiently, they can become elite athletes and make lots of money, get endorsement contracts, and play golf in Arizona with retired presidents. Likewise, no matter what their genetic makeup, if they're couch spuds, their genetic gifts have little effect on their risk of disease and provide little protection from their bad habits.

If you are sedentary and then take up an active life, even a modestly active one, you'll certainly improve your health, and almost as certainly you'll also improve your fitness—within the bounds of your genetic potential. And you won't know what that potential is until you do become more active. With aging, one's fitness level, as measured in terms of cardiopulmonary fitness, at least, seems inevitably to decline. Even so, if you take up or maintain physical activity, you'll continue to be much healthier and remain more fit for a longer period than if you are sedentary.

The health benefits of exercise level off for most of us at about 2,000 kilocalories per week of physical activity, but because fitness and health are to some extent independent of one another, gains in fitness for specific sports activities may continue well beyond that level. Thus dedicated athletes striving for their best in a given sport train for hours and hours every day, well beyond what they need for optimal health and often up to and sometimes beyond their physical limits. And as anyone who has trained hard to become fit for a given sport knows all too well, at the highest levels, improvements in performance, like health benefits, come increasingly slowly and only after more and more physical effort.

COMING FULL CIRCLE

Let's get back to the cases of Clyde Henry and Jim Fixx. Clyde Henry has already had one heart attack; Jim Fixx died of a heart attack while jogging. How do they fit into the College Study findings? By taking up activity, losing weight, quitting smoking, and making other favorable changes in his habits, Jim Fixx probably added well over two years to his life (he lived nine more years than his father), and as noted above, these additional years were better years. Thus he probably lived as long as he was able, given his genetic predisposition to heart disease and the damage already done to his heart by years of imprudent health habits before he took up a physically active way of life.

An active life does not guarantee perfect health, nor does it guarantee 8, 9, 10, or even more years of life. Rather, an active life will significantly improve your chances of living more years and, more important, better, more vital years.

As for Clyde Henry, it's impossible to say at this point how many extra years he can expect to live thanks to his new way of living. Statistically, by becoming more active, he is reducing his risk of a second, perhaps fatal, heart attack. Thus he's increasing his chances of gaining not just a few years of added life but perhaps several decades. But that's of little concern to Clyde. What's important to him today is how much better he feels and how much more energy and zest for life he has.

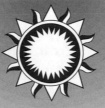

chapter 3

NOT JUST MORE YEARS, BUT BETTER YEARS

Society imposes on us many preconceived notions about how we are supposed to be and act when we grow older, many of which are wrong. Fortunately, a growing number of men and women are pushing back the boundaries of what is considered old and challenging our notions about aging. And they're helping to redefine what we think of as normal aging, even as they lead the way toward defining a new stage or phase of life, one characterized by vitality and zest.

There is something about Shirley Dietderich that suggests athlete—a certain youthfulness in her carriage, in her straight, head-up posture, a jauntiness in her step that reminds one of an exuberant teenager. The only clues to her age—she's 69—are her graying hair and the creases around her eyes and mouth. At an age when many Americans are considering the rocking chair, Shirley is among the best javelin throwers in the world in her age group.

Shirley became an athlete at 48, when her marathoner husband was planning to compete in the 26-miler in a masters contest in Sweden. He suggested to Shirley that she train for something and go with him to compete. "There wasn't time for me to get in shape for something like the marathon," Shirley recalls. "But Rex, my husband, had heard stories about how I was always fast as a kid, so he suggested the sprints."

Shirley competed in the 100, 200, and 400 meters in Sweden and even won a gold medal in the 100-meter relay. Over the next several years, she competed in masters competitions all over the world, including Rome, Moscow, and Melbourne, Australia. "It's great fun," she says. "Anyone can compete. You meet all kinds of interesting people from all over."

While recovering from an injury that prevented her from running, Shirley started looking for something else to do. "I was going nuts," she recalls. "I had to do something. Fortunately, there was a young guy who worked out at the track I trained on. He was training for the javelin, so I asked him to teach me. Turns out I have a knack for it."

SHIRLEY'S TRAINING

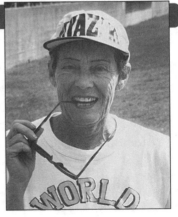

Shirley Dietderich, 69, interior designer

Training

- Sunday: to the track; warm up with a one-mile jog, then six throws each of the discus and javelin; run intervals of 100, 200, and 400 meters for time.

- Monday: a recovery day; 30 minutes to one hour of jogging; two or three "easy" 400s.

- Tuesday: a one-mile jog, then a couple of moderate 100s and two or three 600s, each faster than the other ("If I can't go faster with each, I quit for the day.").

- Wednesday: a one-mile jog, a couple of moderate 100s, then two 800s, and finish with some 150s.

- Thursday: a one-mile jog, then a variety of 800s, 600s, and 400s; a few 150s at the end.

- Friday: a one-mile warm-up, then some 300s or 200s with starts.

- Saturday: a day off; rest for Sunday's time trials again.

Shirley tries to swim about a quarter mile once a week. She also lifts weights two or three times a week; her weight routine involves a mix of upper and lower body work, with emphasis on movements that mimic throwing a javelin.

Impetus to change

Shirley was 48 when she took up track. "My husband and I had just returned from a visit with friends on the East Coast, and I'd put on some weight. Rex suggested I start training to compete in the World Masters Competition coming up in Sweden."

What she likes most about an active life

"It's a quality of life thing for me," she says. "I have lots more energy, and it teaches me to budget my time more effectively. Also, it gives me something different to think about, a real break in my day. When I go out at noon to train, I have an hour or two of freedom when I'm out in the sun running around with others of like mind; I've met some very interesting people on the track. Most of my friends are athletes."

Advice

"I always advise people first to try lots of different sporting activities. Find something you think you'll enjoy and that suits your abilities. Then stick with it long enough to really find out if you do like it. I also advise people to learn as much about the sport as possible. I find that motivating. Also, I think it's a good idea to join a group. There's a real motivation knowing there are others expecting me to be there training with them."

Thirty years ago, Paul Reese never would have guessed he would, as he puts it, "be out running around in my BVDs at 79." Paul, a retired Marine Corps officer and school administrator, figured he'd be dead by now. "Certainly I'd never have guessed I'd feel so young or have such zest for life," he says.

In 1990, at the age of 73, Paul was not only feeling young and zestful, he ran across the United States. He started in April, standing knee-deep in the Pacific Ocean just outside the town of Jenner on California's craggy north coast, and ran 26 miles a day for 124 consecutive days—through the hottest part of the summer, through deserts, over mountains, through the steamy South, through waist-deep roadside grasses. He was nibbled at by blackflies the size of small birds, frightened occasionally by snakes, and buzzed by oblivious drivers. And he finished up 3,192 miles later, on August 22, knee-deep in the warm Atlantic Ocean off Hilton Head Island, South Carolina, having loved every minute of the run, despite the flies.

Except for feeling justifiably tired at the end, and a bit of tenderness in his knees, he was none the worse for wear. "There were some old injuries that would flicker now and then during the run and send up distress signals," he concedes, "so I'd stop and walk a few hundred yards, but throughout the run, everything worked pretty well. Through it all, there was a real sense of enjoyment and accomplishment."

PAUL'S TRAINING

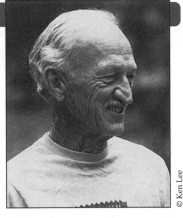

© Ken Lee

Paul Reese, 79, retired school administrator and Marine Corps lieutenant colonel

Training

Right now, Paul is averaging five miles a day, seven days a week. Twice a week, he trains with friends on a track and runs a few mile intervals or quarter-miles. The rest of the time, he runs by himself. "I like running alone," he says. "It gives me time to think."

Impetus to change

"When my son started high school, I decided to run with him. We'd go three miles and think we had just climbed Mt. Everest. Back then that seemed like a huge achievement."

What he likes most about an active life

"I think the thing I like best is the people I meet and associate with. I don't think I ever met an athlete I didn't like. Another thing I like about being active is that I have more zest for life. I go to reunions with my contemporaries, and some of them are in pretty bad shape. I think as we get older, it becomes *more* important that we stay physically active."

Advice

"First, be very patient. Then do lots of different things. I think you're more likely to stick with activity if you mix in lots of activities like running, walking, swimming, and cycling. Other things that help, I think, are changes of scene; don't run or walk the same route every day. I have five different routes, and I never run the same route two days in a row. Set some realistic goals for yourself to keep yourself motivated. Practice preventive maintenance; take care of yourself so you don't get hurt, and build your activities around a lifetime, not just one race or competition."

RETHINKING "NORMAL" AGING

Paul Reese, Shirley Dietderich, and the new, leaner, healthier Clyde Henry are just three of a growing number of men and women who are forcing us to rethink what we mean by "normal" aging and leading the way toward defining a new stage or segment of life offering new opportunities for personal freedom, growth, and self-development. This new phase of life beginning in the early or mid-sixties—following retirement typically—is characterized, not by the decline that far too many of us assume is the inevitable result of aging, but rather by 10, 20, or 30 additional years of vitality, a zest for life.[1]

Of course, you don't have to run across the United States like Paul or take up the javelin at 60 like Shirley to achieve the gains in health and vitality that they have. In truth, Clyde's much more modest daily walks are more typical of what the rest of us can and should be doing. But the experiences of all three provide instructive examples for the rest of us about what is possible. And what is possible is that with even a relatively modest increase in physical activity each week, we can not only put more years into our lives but more life into our years.

LIFEFIT PRINCIPLES

- All the evidence points to the fact that there is enormous individual variation in length of life.
- Aging is inevitable.
- Aging is at least in part programmed by our very genes— those of us with long-lived parents likely will be relatively long-lived ourselves.
- As a species, we may also be approaching some actual "top end" in terms of length of life.
- A host of factors, from noxious environment to imprudent diet to adverse health habits, "chip away" at whatever may be our individual potential longevity.
- We are gradually eliminating or learning to control the factors that limit individual longevity, and thus more of us are living longer.
- More years aren't necessarily desirable unless they're also better years, filled with zest for life and engagement with others.

ADDING QUALITY YEARS THROUGH EXERCISE

We all want to live longer, but added years are more desirable when they are also better years, or quality years, if you will. As discussed earlier, the College Study finds that you'll enjoy an average gain of two or more years if you adopt an active way of life. And although this may not seem like all that much, it is preferable to the alternative. And as noted, these two additional years may be about the most we can expect in terms of additional length of life from any lifestyle change, other than quitting smoking. Yet although we might add a few more years of life by taking up physical activity, we actually gain much more than this.

Noticeable improvements in physical well-being come slowly and with much effort. Many of the health benefits such as a reduced risk of heart disease take months to develop and are rather abstract benefits anyway; it's impossible to measure something that doesn't happen, such as a prevented heart attack. But many other benefits of activity are much more immediate, and one way of motivating yourself to take up physical activity and stick with it is to concentrate on these benefits, which could be lumped into a category of benefits that "improve quality of life." What are these?

Most studies to date of physical activity look only at the physical benefits and seldom at the mental and emotional benefits, and we'll review many of these in the following chapters. The fuzzier issues such as improvements in quality of life are rarely discussed in the scientific literature because researchers have a hard time deciding what to study and how to measure it. Quality is a nonspecific term, and whether or not your life has quality depends on how you define quality in light of your own likes, dislikes, and attitudes. What makes you happy might make the next person sad and a third quite desperate. For some of us, getting up at dawn no matter what the weather to go for a jog will be the height of pleasure, but for others it is a dreadful chore.

It's a bit presumptuous of any outside observer to judge whether or not another's life has quality, although it seems safe to say that a life free of disease likely has more quality than one plagued by aches and pains. But quality-of-life issues may ultimately prove to be the most important issues. Indeed, most of us go for a walk or swim, not with the conscious thought that this walk or this swim will reduce our risk of heart disease, but because the activity makes us feel better in a variety of ways and improves the quality of our lives. Having more energy would improve quality of life, and so would looking better and feeling better about yourself and having a more positive outlook, all of which can result from being more active. Likewise, the simple pleasure of doing something you enjoy, such as a brisk

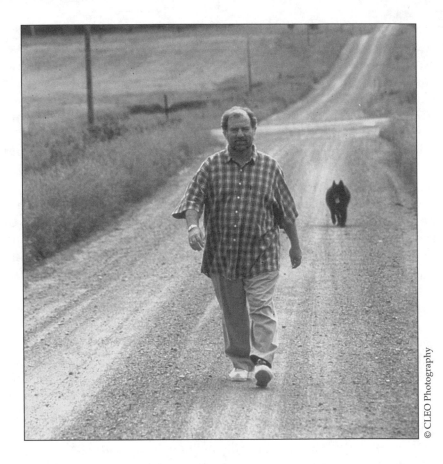

© CLEO Photography

evening walk or 30 minutes of lap swimming, can contribute directly to quality of life.

STRAIGHTENING THE LIFE CURVE

In *Vitality and Aging,* James Fries and Lawrence Crapo[2] discuss the notion of the "rectangularization of the life curve" charting an individual's vitality over time. By *vitality* they mean physical and mental energy, zest for or enjoyment of life, and the absence of disease, or what we'd call quality of life. Too often, they point out, the vitality curve looks like a ski slope, a steady decline in vitality year after year, ending in death, often after a long, debilitating, and usually expensive illness. Fries and Crapo believe that it's possible to compress morbidity—illness and disability—into a shorter and shorter period nearer the end of life, thus adding many years of what most of us would consider a higher quality of life (see figure 3.1). The ideal we should all aspire to looks more like a rectangle, with little or no decline in vitality, no decline in quality of life, and no lingering illnesses at the end of life, with death coming quickly, preferably after seven, eight, or nine decades (or even more) of vital life.[3] Certainly it's an ideal to which Shirley Dietderich, Paul Reese, and Clyde Henry aspire.

Some demographers, epidemiologists, and public health policy makers suggest a less rosy picture, however. They believe that for the vast majority of men and women living in "advanced"

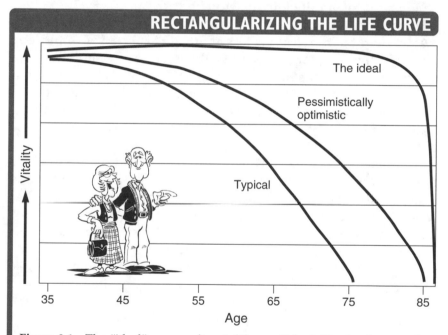

Figure 3.1 The "ideal" course of one's life would look like the "rectangular" curve Fries and Crapo describe: vitality and good health throughout life, with a very brief and precipitious decline near the end. The typical curve looks more like a ski slope, with declining health and vitality beginning early, and premature death, typically from CVD, cancer, or NIDDM.

The "pessimistically optimistic" view holds that it's possible to delay the onset of decline, and perhaps even add years to one's life, but the *slope* of decline, once it begins, is more like that of the "typical" slope, with a period of disease and fraility coming later, but lasting just as long.

industrialized nations, exactly the opposite of a "compression of morbidity" is occurring; that is, an "expansion of morbidity" during which the time we are debilitated by disease increases. Good medicine, these experts suggest, preserves life while it prolongs ill health. Before there were truly effective treatments for cancer or heart disease, for example, many victims would die quickly after the onset of disease. Improved medical care can now keep some of these patients alive for years, although not necessarily healthy. Demographer S. Jay Olshansky, with the Center on Aging, Health and Society and the Population Research Center of the University of Chicago, suggests that "an inadvertent consequence of the decline in old-age mortality may be a proportional rise in the untreatable disabilities now common among the very old. This is," Olshansky suggests, "trading off longer life for worsening health."[4]

Tony Smith, associate editor of the *British Medical Journal*, writes that we ought to be worrying less about life expectancy—how long we might live—and more about health expectancy—how long we might live, as he puts it, "firing on all six cylinders," or putting it another way, how long we might live enjoying a high quality of life. Smith notes that male life expectancy in the United States rose by 2.2 years through the 1970s, but that disability-free life expectancy rose by only 0.6 years in the same period.[5]

Pessimists even question the ability of healthy habits such as physical activity to compress morbidity. Although Fries and Crapo believe that we can make changes in our habits to compress the time we're debilitated by disease into a short period at the very end of a long, healthy life, the pessimists think that the best we can do is simply delay the time when the debilitation sets in, but that we can still expect the period of decline to last as long, if not longer, thanks to more effective medicines. Thus, they suggest, the best we can hope for is to get heart disease at 70 or 80 years of age rather than 50 or 60, for example, but once disease sets in, we'll still be sick the same length of time.

This less than hopeful view of things is only a theory, however. And for that matter, so is the more positive view of Fries and Crapo. The fact is, no one really knows for certain at this point what is likely to happen when men and women remain vigorously active well into the third phase of life because it's a subject that is just coming under scrutiny, as only now are there enough older, active men and women available for adequate study. It appears, though, from what data and anecdotes are available, that Fries and Crapo are right. Of course, even if the pessimists prove to be correct, and we sincerely hope they're not, most of us would probably prefer to develop heart disease at 70 rather than 50, if we have to develop it at all.

WHAT IS THE LIMIT OF THE HUMAN LIFE SPAN?

If the human "life curve" can be rectangularized, what is the point where the drop-off typically begins?

Paul Reese started running nearly 40 years ago, at an age when men of previous generations were considered "old," if they weren't already dead. Clyde Henry took up an active life at an age when most men a generation or two earlier really were dead. And Shirley Dietderich is traveling the world and throwing the javelin when some, if not most, her age are already dependent on others for the simplest tasks of daily living.

The average length of life has risen from 47 years at the turn of the century to the mid-70s today, thanks to improved sanitation, better living conditions, sufficient—often more than sufficient—food, a reduced risk of infectious diseases, and increasingly effective medical care.[6] We've steadily reduced or eliminated premature death from such causes as infections, malnutrition, accidents, wars (at least sometimes), and the exhaustion and complications of difficult births.

SOME STATISTICS ON LONGEVITY MISLEAD US

But gains in length of life seem to be leveling off; during the past century, for example, gains in average length of life could be measured by years or even decades from generation to generation. Now such gains are being measured by months or weeks, suggesting there is some upper limit to human longevity and that, as a population, we're approaching it.[7] It also appears that in some ethnic and social groups in this country, longevity is actually declining.

But the import of these figures can be misleading precisely because they include those who died at birth, in early childhood, or relatively early in life due to accident or violence. British scientist J.D. Montagu suggests that the ancient Greeks and Romans who survived the perils of birth and childhood, for example, and who were lucky enough to avoid accidents and violence, may have lived nearly as long as we do today.[8] Indeed, in an analysis of the quoted dates of birth and death among ancient Greeks and Romans, Montagu found that ancient Greeks born before 100 B.C. lived about 72 years, or about as long as we do now. Interestingly, Montagu also found that Romans born after 100 B.C. lived an average of 66 years, and he speculates that their shorter life span, compared with the Greeks, was due to the advent of lead plumbing. It may also reflect the Romans' richer diet and more sedentary lifestyles, which resulted from relative peace and prosperity.

Only in the last 50 years or so have advances in modern health care and early childhood care resulted in truly significant improvements in infant and child mortality, which account for most of the advances we've made in life expectancy in recent years.[9] In terms of adult health and life expectancy for those of us who make it past childhood, we actually haven't made very significant gains at all; we've cut the risk of death from accidents and violence and at least delayed the risk of infection, but we've replaced these causes of death with the so-called diseases of civilization, diseases caused by lack of exercise, a high-fat diet, obesity, chronic stress, dangerous habits such as smoking, and so on. These diseases—primarily heart disease, cancer, and diabetes—are debilitating, chronic, and often fatal only after the victim has suffered years of declining health, vitality, and quality of life. Likewise, we're living long enough to begin to suffer a host of nonfatal diseases such as arthritis that drain our energy and zest for life but don't necessarily kill us outright. We're living longer but not necessarily better.[10]

WE CAN'T LIVE FOREVER, EVEN IF WE DO EVERYTHING RIGHT

But what happens when we exercise regularly and eat healthfully and thus reduce our risk of heart disease, at least some types of cancer, and diabetes—the three most significant diseases of civilization? What happens when we also strengthen our immune systems through exercise and thus fight infection more effectively? Do we live forever?

Certainly not. The fact is, we still get old. In truth, none of these diseases can be prevented entirely, only delayed. Demographer S. Jay Olshansky calculates that if we completely eliminated cancer, life expectancy at birth would increase by 3.17 years for women and 3.2 years for men; completely eliminating heart disease would add another 3.0 and 3.55 years, respectively. Eliminating all circulatory diseases, diabetes, and cancer would mean an additional 15.82 years and 15.27 years, respectively, but alas not immortality. Something still gets us—infection, accident, or time simply runs out.[11]

WHAT IS THE THEORETICAL LIMIT?

Legends abound about individuals who've lived to incredible ages. These individuals have almost invariably been men, and often, it seems, they've been cave dwellers, eaters of rice or barley gruel, wearers of loincloths, and seekers of truth.[12] Individuals described in the early Old Testament were living 800 or 900 years, until the God of the Old Testament got fed up with their wanton lifestyles and put a cap on things, announcing in Genesis 6:1-3 that mankind's "days shall be a hundred and twenty years," an interesting figure which we'll return to shortly.

Legends are one thing, but reality is something else entirely, and as far as we know, all species have distinct limits on their life spans. The mouse's is about two years; elephants in the wild live about 35 years. And the cap on the human life span, Fries thinks, is around 85 years, plus or minus 15, assuming we haven't been killed earlier by infection, accident, or bad habits.[13] Whether or not this 85-year limit represents an absolute is open to debate, however, and there are researchers working in the areas of the biology and genetics of aging who expect—or at least sincerely hope—that someday a breakthrough of some sort will greatly expand this cap. In any case, keep in mind that a figure of 85 years as an upper limit for the human life span is simply an average for a huge population. There is wide individual variation. However, some researchers have come up with theoretical limits as high as 120 years, a figure that possesses a certain theological validity, and we certainly hope they're right.[14-18]

HOW LONG CAN WE REALLY EXPECT TO LIVE?

If this 120-year cap is correct, it's probably an ideal, and for most of us perhaps an unapproachable ideal at that, assuming an ideal diet, ideal living conditions, an ideal outlook. No one knows for sure what effect environmental pollution has on longevity, or what effect childhood diseases will have, or noxious stress, a negative attitude, or all the other insults and injuries that befall each of us through a lifetime, but in all likelihood, dozens of factors are chipping away at the years we ought to have.

Granted, a few individuals in recent history have lived to be 110 or even slightly beyond, and they've done it in the same world we're living in, facing the same challenges to life and limb, but they're exceptional cases. We're talking here about what is likely for most of us, and what appears to be likely, at least for now, is that taking into account huge individual variation and all the variabilities in terms of what chips away at our longevity, 85 years or so is what most of us can expect.

CAN WE CONTROL AGING?

Aging is an unavoidable process leading to the same end for all of us, no matter how favorable our circumstances, and aging seems to affect each of us differently. But despite this wide variability, we will all grow old and die. Is it possible to take control of the aging process in our own lives? To slow it down? Or even reverse that process, for a time at least? We believe it is.

FOUR THEORIES ABOUT HOW WE AGE

Aging is almost certainly not the result of any one cause, but rather results from a variety of interacting processes, some of which are probably genetic or internal in origin, and some of which result from wear and tear caused by environmental or external factors. Thus an individual's genetic or internal makeup, for example, may make him or her more or less vulnerable to certain environmental or external factors such as dietary fats, stress, carcinogens, or perhaps even a tendency to be distracted while driving. Any or all of these factors working together or independently may tend to shorten life.[19]

Gerontogenes

Before about 1960, many scientists studying aging thought that the body itself somehow imposed a death sentence on the cell, and that freed from the body, cells in a dish on a lab bench, under ideal conditions, might live forever. And of course there was the underlying hope that if we could isolate whatever it was in the body that imposed this cellular death sentence, maybe we could one day get our sentences commuted.

But 30 years ago gerontologist Leonard Hayflick pulled the plug on this hopeful vision.[20] He showed that cells growing in a lab under precise conditions divided a finite number of times, then died (some cancer cells, however, don't seem to have such a limit). Apparently, DNA can only reproduce itself a specific number of times within a cell before it stops, as if a switch has been turned off.

Further, Hayflick found there is a species-specific limit on the number of doublings a population of cells can go through, the "Hayflick limit," as it has become known. Populations of human cells taken from embryos seem to divide about 50 times, then stop. Likewise, populations of cells taken from older subjects divide fewer times before shutting down. Using a bit of not-so-simple arithmetic, it's possible to calculate that, based on the Hayflick limit for human cells, the theoretical maximum life of a population of cultured human cells is about 120 years.[21,22]

This may indicate that the human organism actually is "designed" to live that long, and again, we hope so. But Hayflick's studies were conducted in a lab under carefully controlled conditions. Hayflick's cultured cells didn't overeat or drink too much; they didn't have to put up with the insults of air pollution, toxins in their food, or the aggravations of a rush-hour commute, the prime-time news, and income taxes, like we do, all of which are unavoidable and all of which, in various ways, may tend to increase the speed at which cells wear out.

Exactly what lies behind this limit is not fully understood. In fact, a fixed and species-specific limit on cell divisions is only one of many changes in the cells that are associated with aging, but the limit suggests that the cells of each species contain "gerontogenes." No one's found one yet, or even a hint of one in humans, but certainly there appears to be one or, more likely, a great many that program into each cell a limit on how many times, and how accurately, its genetic material can divide and pass on its information. The gerontogene literally seems to turn off the genetic switch at a predetermined time, like switching off the lights.

The question, of course, is why would living organisms of any kind have evolved gerontogenes that turn off the switch?

Planned Obsolescence?

In fact, there might be a very good reason for this switch, or what might be viewed as a sort of planned obsolescence, although from the individual's standpoint, a very harsh reason. Back in the 1950s, biologist George C. Williams proposed that an individual's evolutionary fitness was a matter of the genetic contribution he or she makes to later generations.[23] Thus evolution favors traits that make it more likely an individual will grow to sexual maturity, reproduce, and then stick around long enough to nurture the young. But once we've fulfilled our reproductive potential, selection pressures would diminish; from the viewpoint of our genes, there's simply no point in working to evolve long life or immortality after reproduction, thus damaging traits that tend to limit life after breeding and nurturing wouldn't be eliminated.

Further, Williams suggested, some traits that were destructive later in life would be adopted if, in some way, they improved fitness for reproduction earlier in life. An example of this would be estrogen, a hormone required for fertility early in life, but one that also increases the risk of breast cancer later in life. Why should evolution select for protection from the harmful effects of estrogen later in life? From the evolutionary perspective, there's no point.

From the harsh perspective of genetic utility, then, a 40-year human survival would seem to make sense, as it typically takes about 40 years to grow, reach maturity, breed, and then support the young until they can grow, support themselves, breed, and support their young, and so on. If too many individuals lived much beyond that 40-year point—beyond their useful period, that is—they'd compete with younger generations for limited resources (as seems to be happening now in this country), and the overall result might be limited genetic diversity.

But if that's so, why do most of us live well beyond that 40-year limit? We'll get to that in a bit.

Death: The Price We Pay for Sex?

T.B.L. Kirkwood of the National Institute for Medical Research in London suggests what he calls the "disposable soma theory."[24] The theory states that organisms divide their energy between sexual reproduction and maintenance of the body, or the "soma." The best strategy for survival of the species, according to this theory, is the allocation of energy for maintenance that is less than required for complete, ongoing repair, or immortality, leaving some energy left for reproduction. Aging, then, is simply the consequence of unrepaired defects in cells and tissues; in other words, aging is the price we pay for reproduction.

This theory also suggests a more likely explanation for what appears in the lab to be gerontogenes that switch off cells at a certain point, causing cell death, aging, and then death of the organism, once enough cells have died. Instead, the switching off occurs when enough unrepaired defects build up within a cell, disrupting the normal regulation of cell activity. What seems to be a fixed limit of cell reproduction for each species is instead the point at which cells from a given species can no longer tolerate unrepaired defects. Perhaps there's no preprogrammed switch, but simply a species-specific average tolerance for mistakes.

Cell Failure and "Free Radicals"

Alex Comfort, in "Theories of Aging," suggests that aging is a result of "information loss" expressed as the death of individual cells, the failure of cells to reproduce, or the failure of cells to perform their proper functions.[25,26] Consider a string of DNA in the nucleus of an individual cell and the individual genes on that string. The DNA is essentially coded information telling the cell when and how to divide, and so on. The DNA represents ordered information. The cell's life and functioning depend on the integrity of that order, the accuracy of the information provided by the DNA. With time, however, the information encoded in the DNA becomes increasingly disordered. "Noise" enters the system and the information becomes vague, or mistakes occur with increasing frequency.

Such a notion is in keeping with Hayflick's findings, as well as with the notion that aging is an accumulation of mistakes in cells; the "Hayflick limit" may be the point at which so much "noise"—or so many mistakes—have entered the typical cell's system that it can no longer pass on enough accurate, useful information and divide. And when enough cells in the human body have reached that point, senescence—aging—sets in; in other words, all the physical and mental changes and symptoms we generally associate with getting old, with death the end of the process.

One of the more intriguing theories of aging focuses on what are called "free radicals." Free radicals are highly charged or energetic particles produced by radiation from outside the body, by the body's own metabolism in the normal course of living, or taken into the body in the air we breathe and the food we eat. Free radicals, primarily highly energized molecules of oxygen, can attack the body's tissues by causing mistakes in DNA, thus disrupting the normal gene structure and producing mistakes in the information the genes carry. Free radicals also cause damage to the body by interacting with unsaturated fatty acids in the membranes of cells; these highly energized molecules are oxidants that cause the body to "rust," as it were, literally turning the body's fats rancid.

Genes in which DNA is damaged by free radicals can no longer make proteins properly. Also, proteins themselves can be damaged by free radicals. The net result of all this damage is a decline in cell functioning, a decline in the body's ability to produce energy, an increased risk of disease, and ultimately aging and death. Anything that increases the production of or exposure to free radicals will accelerate aging; in lab experiments, for example, animals exposed to above-normal radiation, which produced free radicals, showed all the normal effects of aging but at a faster pace.[27-29]

SIX WAYS TO CONTROL THE AGING PROCESS

In the young, damage to DNA by free radicals is repaired by special enzymes called antioxidants that look for and repair unnatural breaks in the DNA. Over time, however, this repair system can't keep up with the accumulating damage. Thus anything we can do to reduce the number of free radicals produced in our bodies or consumed in our food and air, or anything we can do to enhance the body's natural repair systems, should, in theory, slow aging. These repair systems can be strengthened and aided through changes in health habits.

• Exercise: Exercise may combat the effects of free radicals by stimulating the body to produce more natural antioxidants.

• Stress reduction: The stress-reducing effects of exercise and meditation may also help reduce the harmful effects of free radicals. Japanese researchers have found oxidative damage to DNA produced by psychological stress.[30]

• A smokeless lifestyle: Each puff of a cigarette contains billions of free radicals, and so does each inhalation of second-hand smoke.

• Vitamin supplementation: Vitamins C, E, and beta carotene may also help. These vitamins act as antioxidants and "scavenge" free radicals.[31,32]

• Diet: Some research suggests that caloric restriction—what researchers somewhat euphemistically call "controlled undernutrition"—may also slow the ravaging of free radicals. Cutting caloric intake to 60 percent of normal (but not nutritional intake) seems to increase longevity by as much as 50 percent in lab animals.

• Turn down the heat: Along the same lines as controlled undernutrition, research with fruit flies and fish suggests that living in a cold

BASIC HEALTH HABITS

Studies of nearly 7,000 adults followed for five and one-half years[a] showed that life expectancy and health are significantly related to the following basic health habits, all of which are in our control:

1. Three prudent meals a day at regular times and no snacking
2. Breakfast every day
3. Regular, moderate exercise
4. Adequate sleep (seven or eight hours a night)
5. No smoking
6. Maintain moderate weight
7. No alcohol or only in moderation

We'll add these other life-extending habits:

- Food supplementation with modest levels of vitamins A, C, E, and beta carotene
- Stress reduction
- Social involvements

A 45-year-old man who practices zero to three of the first seven habits has a remaining life expectancy of 21.6 years (to age 67), whereas one with six to seven of these habits has a life expectancy of 33.1 years (to age 78). In other words, 11 years could be added to life expectancy by relatively simple changes in living habits, recalling that only 2.7 years were added to the life expectancy at age 65 between 1900 and 1966. The authors of the study also found that the health status of those who practiced all seven habits was similar to those 30 years younger who observed none.

Note. [a] Beloc, N.B., & Breslow, L. 1973. Relationship of health practices and mortality *Preventive Medicine* 2:67-81.

Reprinted, by permission, from J. Knowles, 1987, The responsibility of the individual. In *Doing better and feeling worse*, edited by J. Knowles (New York: W.W. Norton & Company, Inc.), 61-62.

environment may promote longevity, perhaps by slowing the rate at which free radicals introduce "noise" or mistakes into the cell's DNA-based information system. Attempts to reproduce the effect in the lab haven't been as successful, however, and it's perhaps too soon to recommend that we all turn our thermostats down in the winter and our air conditioners up in the summer.

What we see here, in any case, is a curious trend—recommendations all pointing toward a lifestyle not all that different from that of the 200-year-old legends meditating in caves, likely cold ones at that, and subsisting on the occasional bowl of rice gruel, which is definitely undernutrition, if not controlled. The obvious question is, "What kind of life is it when one is chronically shivering and hungry?" After all, most advances in what we think of as civilization have tended toward improved and more reliable food supplies and an increasingly pleasant, secure, comfortable environment, complete with central heating and air conditioning.

TWO VIEWS OF AGING

In any case, the apparently inevitable result of complex interactions between wear and tear, genetics, increasing "noise" in the system, and so on—even when we do everything possible to limit such interactions—is senescence and an ever-increasing likelihood of dying.

AGING AS LOSS OF ADAPTABILITY

An intriguing discussion of how we might ultimately define aging comes from Roy J. Shephard.[33] Referring to the work of two other researchers, Shephard defines senescence as a progressive loss of physiological adaptability to the environment, culminating in death.

Older adults are progressively more vulnerable to changes in the environment. Thus a "cold snap" or "heat wave" might be life-threatening for an older man or woman and a mere inconvenience for a younger person. This is because the aging body is less able to sense changes in the environment and to regulate its own internal temperature—to increase its metabolism to maintain temperature in the cold or to sweat and dissipate heat on a hot day. Likewise, a fall or a relatively minor case of the flu that would be merely inconvenient for a younger person might be fatal for an older man or woman less able to adapt to and accommodate the new stress.

We're living longer today at least in part because we have the ability to regulate and control our external environments; thus, although our aging bodies are less able to sense and adapt to changes in the environment, the environment itself is less changeable and less threatening.

AGING AS LOSS OF MENTAL FLEXIBILITY

Although none of these researchers comments on the mental, psychological, or even spiritual side of aging, in fact, a loss of mental flexibility or adaptability seems to occur all too often with aging.

That the mind seems to "stiffen" with age is something we've known for millennia. Two thousand years ago, Virgil wrote that "time bears away all things, even our wits."[34] Whether or not this is inevitable is open to considerable debate. In any case, anything we can do to maintain our physical and mental adaptability and flexibility should help slow the aging process, and it may be that one of the chief ways exercise slows the aging process is by helping the body maintain its adaptability. Regular exercise helps the living organism remain accustomed to change, keeping the organism's ability to adapt to change functioning smoothly. After all, the essence of exercise is change: You change from a sedentary to an active state whenever you get up out of the easy chair. During a walk, for example, or a jog, a tennis game, or an aerobics class, your body and mind are constantly being called on to change and adapt to continually altering conditions, some of them internal, some external. Weather, terrain, a tricky opponent—all of these call for adaptation. Over time—a period of weeks, months, or years—your body is called on to make further adaptations as you become fitter, as you increase your pace, distance, and intensity of effort. Altogether, these changes provide us with practice in adaptation, helping to keep our adaptive skills honed to a fine and effective edge.

WHY DO WE LIVE AS LONG AS WE DO?

If there are gerontogenes and some sort of genetic limit on life span, or processes at work such as accumulating damage caused by free radicals or evolutionary processes that limit life span, then why do we live as long as we do? After all, assuming there is a limit, as a species we appear to live 40, 50, or even 60 years beyond the period during which we are necessary for reproduction and thus necessary for the species.

OUR BODY OVERCOMPENSATES FOR OUR EXCESSES

One explanation is that these extra years are simply the normal redundancy the human organism has built into all its systems, reserves to help us cope with the wear and tear of daily living in a tough world: nutritional abuses, smoking, drinking, disease, or accident.

Most of our organs and organ systems have huge operational reserves; they're capable of functioning normally even when severely compromised by disease or injury. Thus we have two kidneys when one is sufficient (but why not two hearts?), and this may be the reason much of the brain supposedly is not used; the extra gray matter is a sort of cognitive or neurological "spare parts warehouse."

Only when the reserves of any organ or organ system are depleted does noticeable aging occur, disease become clinically manifest, and death threaten. Smoking begins to destroy the lungs with the very first puff, but only after many months or years of smoking does this damage affect enough of the lung's tissues that the smoker finally becomes short of breath. Likewise, what may be our extra years could be thought of as reserves, and as a population we're living longer now because more and more of us are using up fewer of these reserves, thanks to comparatively more comfortable environments, fewer infections and more effective treatments when they occur, less physical trauma, and so on.

WE GAIN WISDOM THAT MUST BE PASSED ON

All these notions about who or what is necessary can get pretty depressing. Perhaps we need to expand our notion of what is useful from the standpoint of a given species' needs. In fact, the wide variability in the human life span may actually be programmed into the species, and a life span well beyond 40 years may in fact be necessary to the survival of the human race.

In primitive times, although many people may have died in childhood and many adults didn't make it past their forties due to external factors such as famine, exposure, infection, or being eaten by hyenas, a very few would live much longer, and these long-lived people would of necessity become the source of a society's accumulated experience and knowledge. They provided the community with information and insights. They provided wisdom, if you will, that all too rare ability, based on experience and intelligence, not to make the same dumb mistake twice. It was that wisdom, which only the oldest possessed, that helped the community survive. By passing on information, as well as insights about how to use that information, these individuals would help the community avoid such life-threatening and life-shortening factors as famine, war, or being eaten alive; thus it's not inconceivable that the evolutionary processes did in fact select for long life and, better yet, such mental qualities as wisdom, or even values such as sympathy, duty, responsibility, and selflessness.[35]

Today's social, economic, and environmental problems are so seemingly intractable that it may be up to mentally and physically

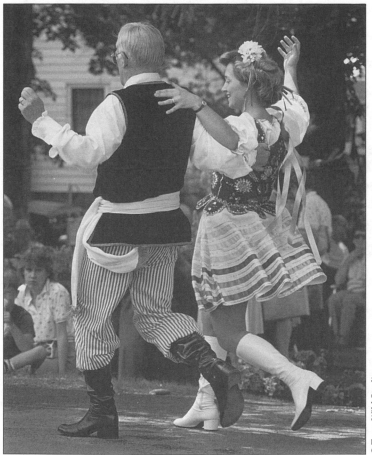

© Terry Wild Studio

vigorous, socially engaged older men and women, possessed of the wisdom that comes from learning and experience, to find solutions. Thus a very long life is essential to our species' survival and continued evolution.

In any case, perhaps one's sense of his or her own usefulness to the family or society in general thus plays a role in how long that individual lives; because we're steadily eliminating many of the external factors that limit life, gains in longevity beyond those provided by exercise, good diet, and so on will come from attitudinal factors. To live long, we need the conviction that we need to live long, that we have something to contribute—that is, wisdom—if not to society then to our families or to ourselves, perhaps through continuing education, a second career, or volunteer work in the community. We need to stay engaged.

WHAT DOES ALL THIS THEORIZING MEAN, ANYWAY?

For all the tentativeness of our knowledge about the aging process and how to slow it, we can say a few things about aging with

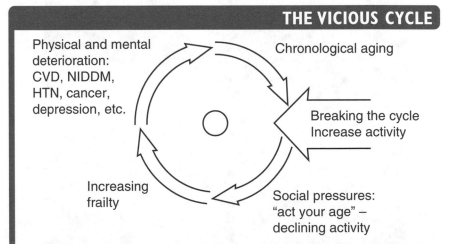

Figure 3.2   Assumptions about aging lead to behaviors that lead to conditions that reinforce the assumptions in a vicious cycle of declining activity. It's possible to break the cycle at one point, however, and that's where aging leads to declining activity. *Take up* an active life and the chain of relations comes apart.

Adapted from originals by Dr. Greg Payne, San Jose State University, and Dr. Bonnie Berger, University of Wyoming.

reasonable certainty.

Perhaps the two most important things we're learning about aging are, first, how to distinguish between changes which may be inevitable and inescapable causes or results of aging, and changes that may be merely associated with aging but which can be delayed, prevented, or perhaps exchanged for other changes later in life. Second, and of paramount importance here, we're learning how an active life can delay or prevent many of those changes.

It is becoming increasingly clear that many of the physical and mental changes we've long assumed or feared were the inevitable results of aging are not unavoidable. Many of the aches and pains, the forgetfulness, trembling, stiffness, faltering, the shortness of breath, and finally, the sudden onslaughts of heart attack or stroke are really the results of chronic illnesses that are themselves often the result of genetic predispositions complicated by poor health habits accumulating over time, habits that can be changed (see figure 3.2).

WE SOMETIMES CONFUSE WHAT IS TYPICAL AND WHAT IS NORMAL

Certainly heart disease and all the other diseases we commonly think of as the unavoidable results of getting old—an increasing likelihood of diabetes, cancer, arthritis, gall bladder disease, hypertension, emphysema, mental decline, and so on—have a profound impact on the quality of our lives, making us feel old.[36] But are they the inevitable legacy of added years? Here we face the cause-and-effect quandary again: Are we more likely to suffer from heart disease—or for that matter arthritis, diabetes, hypertension, or even cancer—because we're getting older, or are we in fact older (or older than we should be) because we have heart disease, arthritis, or whatever?

Most of us 40 and over probably have some atherosclerosis if we've lived all our lives in the West and enjoyed all the dubious benefits of Western living, including such things as fast-food and TV. The challenge facing us is to distinguish what is normal or inevitable in aging from what is truly preventable disease. Here we all live roughly similar lives in terms of diet, exercise, smoking, and other factors, and what is typical begins to appear normal and what is normal begins to appear inevitable. When we see that most adults have at least some atherosclerosis, it begins to look as if it can't be avoided.

RECONSIDERING WHAT IS NORMAL

But what if Shirley Dietderich, Paul Reese, or even a newly fit Clyde

Henry are in fact normal and the other 90 percent or so of American adults who don't exercise sufficiently are abnormal? Perhaps Shirley's vitality, zest for life, and even javelin throwing at the age of 69 should not be viewed as exceptional. Rather, perhaps the fatigue, discomfort, and disability suffered by so many men and women her age should be considered the aberration.

The fact is, we simply don't know for sure what is normal aging because, until now, no one has paid much attention to physically active men and women in the third phase of life and asked whether these individuals are normal or exceptional. Indeed, we make plenty of assumptions—usually grim ones—about what is typical or normal for older adults, but it's almost impossible to lump older adults into categories. Young children develop in neat stages that are reasonably easy to identify and define—we know when children normally sit up and when they normally begin to crawl and walk and say their first words. However, as we grow older and mature, we become increasingly diverse, idiosyncratic, and eccentric, so that by the time we're in our fifties or sixties, it's very difficult to generalize about what is the norm.

It may be that men and women like Shirley, Paul, and Clyde are providing us with the real markers of healthy aging, not the exhausted oldsters who fill our rest homes, and who, in the conventional thinking of the modern American medical establishment, are normal. For all the uncertainty, we have steadily chipped away at the list of conditions that conventional wisdom has said were the inescapable effects of aging, and it may be that too many of us may "think" ourselves into rocking chairs when we grow older assuming that the rocking chair is the unavoidable result of added years. Men and women like Clyde Henry, Paul Reese, and Shirley Dietderich are showing that many of the changes we associate with aging can be avoided or at least delayed through physical activity, a healthy diet, smoking cessation, stress reduction, and other conscious choices.[37,38]

In the next chapters, we'll look specifically at how physical activity can delay, alter, or entirely prevent many of the seemingly inevitable results of aging for improved longevity and zest for life.

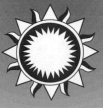

part II

BENEFITS OF CHANGE

Those who think they have not time for bodily exercise will sooner or later have to find time for illness.

—Edward Stanley, Earl of Derby
The Conduct of Life, address at Liverpool College,
December 20, 1873

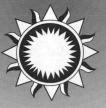

chapter 4

FORM AND FUNCTION

A reduced risk of disease and the possibility of a few additional years of life are rather abstract reasons for taking up and sticking with an active life. After all, it's hard to prove that your exercise habits have prevented the heart attack or cancer you never have. For many of us, then, what becomes very certain once we become more active is that we begin to look better and feel better; we begin to move with more vigor and certainty as we go about our daily lives; we're better able to engage in life in myriad ways; and these positive changes begin with the very first step on the walking path or the first lap in the local pool.

In the two previous chapters, we've discussed in general the added years of life you'll gain through taking up and maintaining activity. And we've briefly discussed what aging is and the general distinctions between the unavoidable effects of growing older and those effects that can be delayed, prevented, or even reversed. We can live longer and better, adding years to our lives and compressing—we hope—those months or years when we are truly old into a smaller and smaller period, nearer and nearer the end of life.

In the following chapters, we'll discuss in more detail the specific benefits you will enjoy if you adopt and stick with an active life. Some of these benefits, such as improved energy and mood and increased mental acuity, seem to be almost immediate, or what might be called "acute" effects of physical activity. Other benefits develop more slowly, over a period of weeks or months. These include improved appearance and carriage, weight loss, increased muscle tone, a stronger heart muscle—one less vulnerable to disease and heart attack—and a reduced risk of some cancers, diabetes, hypertension, and many of the other so-called diseases of civilization.

In this chapter, we focus on form and function. The added pounds that seem to appear inevitably with added years, the stooping posture, the weakened muscles, and the aches of arthritis are some of the changes that conventional wisdom tells us make aging synonymous with frailty, loss of independence, and a diminished quality of life. But many of these conditions can be prevented outright, delayed, and in some cases at least temporarily reversed when we become and stay more active. As we grow older, for example, our posture often changes and we become stooped. The reasons for this are complex and varied, having to do with metabolic changes, changes in the composition of our bones, changes in our muscles, and even changes in our attitudes. With aging, we are also more prone to lose muscle and bone mass, even as we gain fat, so we become physically weaker and less able to perform the tasks of daily living, even as we have more weight to lug around. Balance becomes less certain, and for many older adults, poor balance and the fear of falling become major impediments to a normal, independent, and fulfilling life.

Although none of these changes are in themselves directly associated with an increased risk of mortality, some, such as reduced sense of balance, physical weakness, or reduced ability to respond quickly in novel situations, can contribute to an increased risk of potentially fatal falls or accidents. And most important, all of these changes can

LIFEFIT PRINCIPLES

- Know the benefits of exercise and confirm them through your own experience. This is perhaps the most powerful motivation there is to take up and stick with an active life.

- Don't pay too much attention to what the conventional wisdom says you can expect with aging. Most of the changes we assume are inevitable, such as diminished strength, a stooped posture, and increasing weight, are not the results of aging but of *disuse*.

- Be flexible and even circumspect in your pursuit of a healthier life, including your endeavor to trim down. There's more to life than dogged devotion to health, if that devotion excludes other activities that also add enjoyment—double-fudge walnut brownies, for example, or going to the opera rather than for a jog around the block. Quality of life is as important as quantity of life.

- Dieting alone for weight loss is largely futile; most dieters eventually regain the weight they lost and then some. The only effective method of weight control involves exercise and prudent eating habits.

- More intense Stage Two activities, especially resistance training, contribute most to weight loss.

- Contrary to what seems like common sense, it may be that as we get older, strength training becomes increasingly important.

- Regular physical activity can delay or prevent entirely the onset of osteoporosis, arthritis, and weight and posture changes that characterize aging, or reverse their effects when already present.

impact our quality of life. At any age, our physical capacity sets the bounds of our experiences—whether we end up sitting quietly in front of the TV or are out in the world engaged with life. Gerontologist Waneen Spirduso notes that the loss of mobility and increasing frailty common among older adults is more than the "inability to transport our brain from one place to another." These losses, she suggests, involve diminished communication, changes in self-identity, deteriorated mood states, and "limitations in self-actualization."[1] But none of these changes are inevitable. Each of us has considerable control over how and how fast we age.

A WEIGHTY MATTER

Very likely the most common reason most of us take up activity, or at least think about taking it up, is the desire to lose weight, and that's a good thing. We do seem to be obsessed with our weight in this country, perhaps because so many of us are overweight. And exercise with prudent eating—not dieting necessarily, but eating sensibly—is the only truly effective means of taking off excess weight and keeping it off.

THE SHAPE OF AMERICA

According to the National Center for Health Statistics, 28.4 percent of American adults today aged 25 to 74 years are obese or overweight (the terms are generally used interchangeably); that is, 20 percent or more are above "desirable" weight.[2] This represents a 39 percent increase in the prevalence of obesity when compared with similar data gathered between 1966 and 1970. Just as alarming, considering implications for the health of future generations, obesity among children 6 to 11 years old has increased 54 percent.

The average American will gain about one pound of additional weight each year from age 25, or 35 additional pounds by the age of 60; because we typically also lose about a half pound of bone and muscle mass each year—unless we're physically active, of course—then our body fat is increasing by 1.5 pounds each year from the age of 25 to 60, or over 50 pounds of fat over 35 years. Sometime later in life, after the age of 70 or 80, our weight typically begins a slow decline. However, this decline in weight doesn't mean loss of all the fat we gained through middle age; rather, as we age, we tend to lose still more muscle tissue and bone density while the amount of fat on our bodies remains the same or even increases.

These long-term weight fluctuations and changes in body composition have long been viewed as inevitable results of the aging process, but in fact they are the result of lifestyle choices. As we age, we tend to become less active; thus the muscles atrophy, the bones lose mineral density, and because we tend to become more sedentary, our bodies don't burn the excess calories we've consumed; thus we become fatter, and then fatter still.

Paradoxically, even as our passion for leanness and a preoccupation with dieting consumes our national psyche, our collective waistlines have continued to expand. All this weight gain comes despite the fact that about 40 percent of women and 24 percent of men in this country are trying to lose weight at any given time, a number that is actually somewhat higher than the number of people who really should lose weight.[3] Writing in the President's Council on Physical Fitness *Physical Activity and Fitness Research Digest*, Jack Wilmore, of the University of Texas, notes that the irony in all of this is that while so many millions are dying worldwide from lack of food, many of us here in the United States are dying from an overabundance of food, and we're spending billions of dollars each year overfeeding ourselves and then treating the health problems that result.[4]

CONSEQUENCES OF OBESITY

Excess body weight simply makes it hard to get around. We feel continually sluggish and fatigued. Life becomes a burden. Excess weight also puts an extra burden on the back and legs, increasing the risk of degenerative diseases such as arthritis and low-back pain Excess weight strains the heart and circulatory system, increases blood pressure, and vastly increases the risk of stroke and heart attack, as we'll discuss in the next chapter. Obesity increases the risk of insulin resistance, diabetes, and gallstones, and probably at least some cancers, including prostate, breast, and colon cancer. In cases of severe obesity, fat crowds the spaces between organs, making it difficult to breathe, which makes it even more difficult to be active, leading to still more obesity.

Figure 4.1 charts the experiences of college alumni by body mass index (BMI), looking at their risk of premature death. (Body mass index is the relationship of weight to height. We'll talk more about this measure later in this discussion.) The shaded bars represent the risk of premature death from all causes, including cardiovascular diseases, cancer, diabetes, accidents, and other causes. The white bars represent the risk of premature death from cardiovascular diseases alone. Among the college alumni, for example, the heaviest individuals had a hefty 67 percent higher risk of death from all causes, including NIDDM, heart disease, stroke, and so on, compared with the leanest.[5,6]

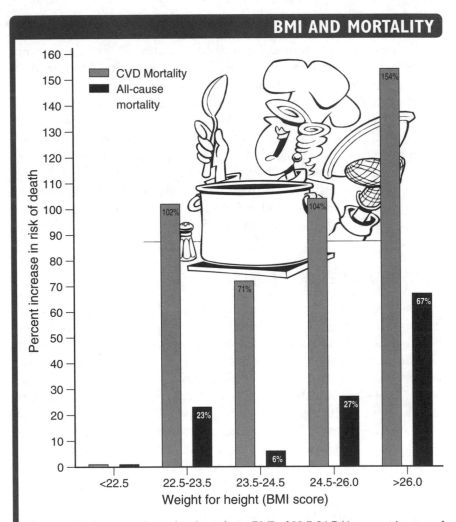

Figure 4.1 It *appears* from the chart that a BMI of 23.5-24.5 (6 percent increased risk) is much less hazardous than the next lightest category (22.5-23.5, 23 percent increased risk), and only slightly more hazardous than being very lean (<22.5). However, statistically, the differences in risk between a BMI of 22.5-23.5 and 23.5-24.5 are not significant; what is significant is a steady trend of increasing risk from the leannest to the most overweight.

Adapted, by permission, from R.S. Paffenbarger, Jr., 1988, "Contributions of epidemiology to exercise science and cardiovascular health," *Medicine and Science in Sports and Exercise* 20: 426-438.

But there's still more bad news for the overweight. Aside from the health hazards of being overweight, leanness has also become a mark of superior social or cultural status, plus a quality essential to achieving such status. The social pressures to be thin in this country are enormous. Icons of male and particularly female beauty are almost impossibly gaunt. And there's even ample evidence to suggest a link between body weight and financial success. One study of business school graduates found that men who were at least 20 percent above their "desirable" weights made $4,000 less per year compared with their leaner colleagues, and the earnings gap widened over the years.[7] An analysis of income and attractiveness found that men and women rated as unattractive suffered a 10 and 5 percent income deficit, respectively, compared with those of average looks. Those rated as attractive, on the other hand, enjoyed a 5 and 4 percent premium, respectively.[8] Of course, beauty is at least somewhat in the eye of the beholder, but the authors of the income

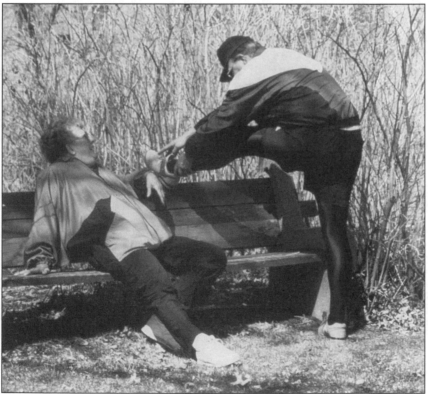

© CLEO Photography

and attractiveness study note there is broad consensus about what is attractive in our culture today, and among the qualities is leanness.

If you're contemplating exercise as a means of losing or maintaining weight, you definitely have the right idea. But there are several things to keep in mind if weight loss is a motivation.

DO YOU NEED TO LOSE WEIGHT?

Before you join the millions of men and women on diets today, you need to determine if you actually need to lose weight.

Weight for Height and BMI

In deciding what to tell you about your weight and health, your physician probably relies on the standard height/weight charts for desirable weights put out by the U.S. Department of Agriculture (USDA) or Metropolitan Life Insurance Company, keepers of the most common such charts (see table 4.1).

In the health professions and sciences, however, the body mass index (Quetelet's index, or BMI) is used more often for its precision and convenience. BMI represents the relationship of height to weight, yielding a single number; the more you weigh in relation to your height, the higher your BMI. Using BMI as the measure, "obese" or "overweight" are defined as a body mass index of 27 or higher.[9] A desirable BMI is anything less, and the lower the better.

You can calculate your own body mass index using the following formula:

$$BMI = \frac{\text{your weight in kilograms}}{\text{your height in meters, squared}}$$

This formula is less daunting than it appears. To figure your BMI, follow these steps:

1. Weigh yourself without your clothes. Divide your weight in pounds by 2.2 to get your weight in kilograms. If you weigh 190 pounds:

   $$190 \div 2.2 = 86 \text{ kilograms.}$$

2. Measure yourself without your shoes. Then divide your height in inches by 39.4 to determine your height in meters. For example, if you are 5 feet 10 inches tall, you are 70 inches tall and your height in meters is

   $$70 \div 39.4 = 1.78 \text{ meters.}$$

Table 4.1   1983 Metropolitan Height and Weight Tables for Men and Women (According to Frame, Ages 25-59)

Height (in shoes)*		Weight in Pounds (in indoor clothing)†		
Feet	Inches	Small frame	Medium frame	Large frame
Men				
5	2	128-134	131-141	138-150
5	3	130-136	133-143	140-153
5	4	132-138	135-145	142-156
5	5	134-140	137-148	144-160
5	6	136-142	139-151	146-164
5	7	138-145	142-154	149-168
5	8	140-148	145-157	152-172
5	9	142-151	148-160	155-176
5	10	144-154	151-163	158-180
5	11	146-157	154-166	161-184
6	0	149-160	157-170	164-188
6	1	152-164	160-174	168-192
6	2	155-168	164-178	172-197
6	3	158-172	167-182	176-202
6	4	162-176	171-187	181-207
Women				
4	10	102-111	109-121	118-131
4	11	103-113	111-123	120-134
5	0	104-115	113-126	122-137
5	1	106-118	115-129	125-140
5	2	108-121	118-132	128-143
5	3	111-124	121-135	131-147
5	4	114-127	124-138	134-151
5	5	117-130	127-141	137-155
5	6	120-133	130-144	140-159
5	7	123-136	133-147	143-163
5	8	126-139	136-150	146-167
5	9	129-142	139-153	149-170
5	10	132-145	142-156	152-173
5	11	135-148	145-159	155-176
6	0	138-151	148-162	158-179

* Shoes with 1-inch heels
† Indoor clothing weighing 5 pounds for men and 3 pounds for women
Source of basic data: *Build Study*, 1979, Society of Actuaries and Association of Life Insurance Medical Directors of America, 1980.

Reprinted, by permission, from Metropolitan Life Insurance Company, 1983, *Statistical Bulletin.* Copyright 1983, Metropolitan Life Insurance Company.

To find the square of your height in meters, multiply this figure by itself:

$$1.78 \times 1.78 = 3.2.$$

3. Finally, divide the answer to No. 1 by the answer to No. 2:

$$86 \div 3.2 = 26.8.$$

Your BMI is thus 26.8, or rather too close for comfort to the danger zone.

There's a much simpler way to determine your approximate BMI, however: Consult the chart in table 4.2.

But do you really need to lose weight if your BMI is 27 or higher? In fact, you may want to consider losing weight even if your BMI is lower than that, for reasons we'll discuss shortly. On the other hand, for reasons we'll also discuss later, you may be perfectly healthy even if your BMI is well above 27.

Leaner Is Usually Better

Unfortunately, the official standards of what is a desirable weight appear to be overly generous. Both the College Study and a 14-year study of nearly 116,000 women conducted by the Harvard School of Public Health find that even if you're within the bounds of what the charts say is healthy or desirable (under a BMI of 27), you can still be at much greater risk for heart disease and a host of other obesity-related health problems. For example, if you are a man, 35 years of age or older, stand 5 feet 10 inches, and weigh 179 pounds (BMI of 25.4), you're within the bounds of desirable according to the current Met Life tables and well within the healthful range (under 188 pounds) for men your age according to the USDA standards. But it appears your risk of heart disease is still significantly higher, over twice as high, in fact, as the risk experienced by your leanest peers, those with a BMI of about 21. The bottom line? Leaner is better.

For optimal health, in general, it seems you should weigh about 20 percent less than the standard height/weight charts indicate is within the desirable range for you; that is, you should strive for a BMI of about 22 if you're a man or 21 if you're a woman.[10,11] If you're a woman and stand 5 feet 4 inches, for example, then for optimal health you should weigh no more than about 122 pounds; if you're a man and stand 5 feet 10 inches, you should weigh no more than about 157 pounds, or about 170 pounds if you stand 6 feet 2 inches.

Table 4.2   Calculating Body Mass Index (BMI)

Height	Healthiest (Women)			Healthiest (Men)				Less healthy							
BMI →	**19**	**20**	**21**	**22**	**23**	**24**	**25**	**26**	**27**	**28**	**29**	**30**	**35**	**40**
4' 10"	91	96	100	105	110	115	119	124	129	134	138	143	167	191
4' 11"	94	99	104	109	114	119	124	128	133	138	143	148	173	198
5' 0"	97	102	107	112	118	123	128	133	138	143	148	153	179	204
5' 1"	100	106	111	116	122	127	132	137	143	148	153	158	185	211
5' 2"	104	109	115	120	126	131	136	142	147	153	158	164	191	218
5' 3"	107	113	118	124	130	135	141	146	152	158	163	169	197	225
5' 4"	110	116	122	128	134	140	145	151	157	163	169	174	204	232
5' 5"	114	120	126	132	138	144	150	156	162	168	174	180	210	240
5' 6"	118	124	130	136	142	148	155	161	167	173	179	186	216	247
5' 7"	121	127	134	140	146	153	159	166	172	178	185	191	223	255
5' 8"	125	131	138	144	151	158	164	171	177	184	190	197	230	262
5' 9"	128	135	142	149	155	162	169	176	182	189	196	203	236	270
5' 10"	132	139	146	153	160	167	174	181	188	195	202	207	243	278
5' 11"	136	143	150	157	165	172	179	186	193	200	208	215	250	286
6' 0"	140	147	154	162	169	177	184	191	199	206	213	221	258	294
6' 1"	144	151	159	166	174	182	189	197	204	212	219	227	265	302
6' 2"	148	155	163	171	179	186	194	202	210	218	225	233	272	311
6' 3"	152	160	168	176	184	192	200	208	216	224	232	240	279	319
6' 4"	156	164	172	180	189	197	205	213	221	230	238	246	287	328

Body weight in pounds

To find your BMI, locate the row that corresponds to your height and read across to the number that is close to your weight. The number at the bottom of that column is your BMI. For example, a person who is 5'8" and weighs 164 pounds has a BMI of 25. A cautionary note: This table will incorrectly label very muscular people as overweight. Reprinted by permission of the *Western Journal of Medicine* (G.A. Gray, 1989, vol. 149, pp. 429-441).

For many of us, of course, a BMI of 21 or 22 is probably an unrealistic, perhaps impossible, goal. But don't get discouraged. These are only general guidelines, and several other factors come into play when deciding how much an individual should weigh. Although for optimal health, it appears that leaner is better, regular physical activity offers substantial protection for those who are heavier than desirable, as we'll discuss shortly.

Why this discrepancy between what the charts say is desirable and what seems to be healthiest? The definition of desirable has been revised steadily upward over the years. Until 1983, the Metropolitan Life Insurance Company listed desirable weights that were considerably lower than today's. For example, before 1983, the Met Life charts recommended that a 35-year-old man who is 5 feet 10 inches tall weigh no more than about 172 pounds (BMI of 24+). (For women, according to these charts, desirable was about six pounds less at any given height.) Then in 1983, Met Life essentially said that a 5-foot 10-inch man can weigh as much as 179 pounds and still be considered a good risk (BMI of 25+). In 1990, the USDA issued another weight/ height table that said this same 5-foot 10-inch 35-year-old could weigh as much as 188 pounds (BMI of about 27). The USDA's standards also suggested it's okay to gain a few pounds as we enter middle age.

These ever more generous definitions of desirable were based in part on studies indicating that very lean individuals, along with the obese, had an elevated risk of premature mortality. But some of these studies failed to account for the fact that some individuals were lean because they smoked; smokers are typically leaner than nonsmokers, and significantly less healthy and more likely to die young, thus increasing the association between leanness and poor health. Some of the leaner men and women in these studies also had undiagnosed wasting diseases such as cancer, and as a result, it looked as if being very lean was itself a health risk, good news for those of us who wanted to feel good about ourselves, even if we were a bit plump. When the biases of smoking and disease were removed from the analyses, however, it turned out that the thinnest individuals have the lowest risk (look for the standard height/weight charts to be revised downward soon in recognition of these new data). [12]

These upward trends in what the conventional wisdom says is acceptable may also reflect our national tendency to define what is normal and healthy in terms of what is typical. Thus, as we have become fatter as a nation, and as most of us have gained weight as we grew older, we've simply redefined upward the definition of what is "too fat," so that more of us seem to be healthfully lean. Certainly this is easier than losing weight.

But your weight-to-height ratio, or BMI, are only crude indicators of what you should weigh or whether or not you should lose weight.

Overweight Versus Overfat

We often use terms such as overweight and obese indiscriminately, but when it comes to your health, the important issue is not really what you weigh but the amount of body fat you have. You need some body fat to maintain good health. Fat is the body's primary source of stored energy, and you need at least some energy reserves to get you through tough times—periods of physical stress such as pregnancy, growth, or an illness that prevents you from taking in sufficient calories. As you grow older and the risk of wasting diseases such as cancer rises, stores of body fat play a role in improving survival through treatment or the course of the disease. Body fat also plays an important role in the metabolism of some hormones; thus women with too little body fat have low estrogen levels, interfering with fertility and increasing their risk of osteoporosis and fractures.

Although a little body fat is good for your health too much body fat is not. Acceptable levels of body fat range from about 15 to 20 percent of total body weight for men and 20 to 25 percent for women. More than this is thought to be unhealthy, although given the recent findings about the importance of leanness, these percentages may be somewhat overgenerous. But stepping on a scale and then studying BMI or height/weight charts won't tell you much about your health risks; your weight in relation to your height is only a very crude indicator of your body fat and thus only a crude indicator of risk.

Suppose you're 5 feet 10 inches tall and weigh 190 pounds. According to the standard height/weight charts, you are slightly overweight and presumably at greater risk of obesity-related diseases, and your doctor will probably tell you that you "ought to lose a few pounds." But these standards are based on the assumption that if you are heavier for your height, it's because you are also fatter than you should be. And usually this assumption is correct; if you are overweight, you are likely overfat.

But you could in fact be overweight (according to the charts) and still quite lean—and thus healthy—if you're very active and muscular, with large bones. Muscle tissue and bone are much denser than fat. Indeed, you may well weigh exactly as much as your 5-foot 10-inch sedentary neighbor, yet his body might contain twice as much fat as yours. Although your weights are identical, only your neighbor is truly overfat and presumably at greater risk (actually, very little attention has been paid to the health consequences of being "overweight" but lean and muscular; thus we have to assume, for a variety of good reasons, that the consequences are good).

Some Other Considerations

You probably already have a good idea if you're overfat or not. Certainly, you need to lose fat if you're overweight according to the height/weight tables, with these additional considerations:

- If you are sedentary
- If you know you are not particularly muscular
- If the bulges over your belt are unmistakable
- If you have a health condition that's associated with obesity: hypertension, diabetes, high cholesterol, arthritis or other joint problems, or any symptom associated with cardiovascular disease
- If you have a family history of any of the chronic diseases mentioned above
- If you smoke, drink more than two alcoholic drinks a day, or spend much of your time under stressful conditions. A system already stressed by cigarette smoking, drinking, or chronic aggravations will do better if it's not under the added stress of excess body weight.[13]

Even if you don't have any of the risk factors mentioned here, obesity in itself may be a health hazard, although the data on this matter are somewhat unclear. A recent study of 115,886 U.S. women showed a strong relationship between obesity alone and heart attack risk. Women with a BMI of under 21 had the lowest risk. Those with a BMI of 21 to 25 had a 30 percent higher risk; women with a BMI of 25 to 29 had an 80 percent higher risk; and women with a BMI over 29 had a frightening 230 percent higher risk.[14]

The College Study data suggest that obesity in itself is not nearly as serious a health risk as a sedentary life. In other words, if you are fat and active, you'll be much, much better off than if you're fat and sedentary. Among the alumni, for example, the most active at any level of BMI have a significantly lower risk of premature mortality from all causes compared with their sedentary peers; compared with the sedentary and overweight, even the heaviest have only half the risk of premature mortality if they regularly engage in Stage One and Stage Two activities.[15]

The overweight who are not only active but also have normal blood pressure, don't smoke, have no parental history of early death from heart disease, and don't have diabetes appear to have virtually no higher risk of early mortality than their thinner counterparts, although this is rather speculative. The findings do suggest the protective power of physical activity, but it's no small task being both overweight and active or being overweight with normal blood pressure. Although perhaps less of a risk in itself, being overweight is typically a marker of other unhealthy habits that usually increase the likelihood of disease.

THE REAL "SKINNY" ON WEIGHT LOSS

If you've decided to take up physical activity to lose weight, the first thing to do is to stop thinking about losing weight. Instead, resolve to lose fat and understand that you might very well gain weight if, through exercise, you lose fat and layer on muscle. Next, understand that such changes come rather slowly and require much resolve and conscious effort.

Alas, it's much easier to become fat than it is to lose fat or become muscular. But by employing a few simple diet and exercise strategies, you can meet your weight- or fat-loss goals relatively painlessly and keep the weight off without feeling deprived, so you look and feel better and feel better about yourself.

Before you set out to lose your excess fat, it will help to know what you're up against, which is primarily your own physiology. Our bodies contain tens of billions of fat cells—adipose tissue—each of which is nothing more than an expandable sack that readily, even eagerly, stores as fat any calories you've taken in but don't immediately need for energy. These cells can expand several times and, when full, divide to produce more fat cells waiting to store still more fat. It's a remarkably efficient and effective system.

But there's another problem facing us as well: Much of what we think we understand about obesity is probably wrong or at least questionable, thus many of our weight-loss strategies are also questionable. As a nation, we not only need a dietary and lifestyle overhaul, we need a conceptual overhaul.

ROLE OF WILLPOWER

Obesity is not simply the result of lack of willpower. More willpower can't hurt when it comes to making a choice between a carrot and a chocolate chip cookie, or between a cookie and nothing at all, but more willpower won't absolutely guarantee weight loss and a new, leaner you.

It may help to think of obesity as a chronic disease like diabetes or hypertension, not a failure of willpower, and thus it should be treated as one. The overweight or formerly overweight man or woman must maintain a lifelong campaign against obesity, with daily attention to all those habits of living such as diet and activity that impact on weight, just as a diabetic must be continually vigilant about those habits that affect his or her insulin sensitivity. And above all, the chronic disease of obesity is best treated with regular, ongoing exercise and prudent eating.

This disease probably also has a genetic component. Some individuals have naturally higher metabolisms; they burn more calories just sitting around watching TV or reading the paper. We all know people like this—they munch on potato chips and cheese Danish with impunity, while the rest of us nibble disconsolately on lettuce leaves, thanks to our genetically determined ability to store fat with ease. Life is not always fair.

But this doesn't mean you are destined to be fat if you have a family history of overweight, a genetic predisposition to hanging onto pounds. You can rev up a sluggish metabolism. No matter what your genetic tendencies, if you keep a balance between your energy consumption and energy expenditure, you won't get fat. But if you do have a tendency to be overweight, you have to be especially careful about your diet, exercise, and other health habits.

THE DIET TRAP

Dieting alone is usually futile. Despite the diet industry's regular proclamations of new secret formula nostrums or programs guaranteed to burn off pounds while you continue to eat your fill and never exercise, all the research indicates that dieting (restricting calories consumed) without exercise is usually a doomed endeavor.

First, when you go on a diet and start to restrict your caloric intake, the flesh assumes with a wisdom born of millennia of hard times that you're in the middle of still another famine, so it slows the metabolism and starts hanging on for dear life to every calorie it can get, at the same time sending out ever more desperate pleas for more food, and sending you to the kitchen again and again to stare longingly at the fridge. It's a very effective survival mechanism, and this metabolic slowdown can be significant, as much as 5 percent or more, which means as you diet and lose weight, your body could be hanging on to an extra 200 or more kilocalories every day, or close to half a pound a week; that is, if you don't also become more active.[16-20]

Next, even when a dieter does manage to lose weight despite the difficulties, most dieters gain it back. Harvard's JoAnn Manson, MD, notes that one-third to two-thirds of the weight most dieters lose is gained back within a year and nearly all of that weight is back within five years, at which point most dieters start all over again, if they aren't so discouraged they give up entirely.

But when dieters gain weight after losing it, they're not back where they started; in fact, they're often worse off than if they had never dieted and lost weight at all. When we slip off the diet and start eating the way we used to again, we regain weight more rapidly because our metabolisms have slowed as a result of the original food restrictions. More of the additional calories we take in are stored as fat. And when we restrict caloric intake, we lose not only fat, but muscle, so that when we start regaining weight, we replace that lost muscle tissue with still more fat. The end result is that once we've returned to our original weight after dieting, in fact, we're fatter than ever.

DANGERS OF "YO-YO" WEIGHT LOSS

Worse, it appears that weight changes, either loss or gain, are associated with an increased risk of heart disease and premature mortality. Whereas an increased risk from weight gain is perhaps understandable, given all the health hazards associated with being overweight, an increased risk from weight loss is more perplexing. After all, health experts have been telling us for decades that most of us need to lose weight to remain healthy. But the increased risk seen among those who lose weight appears to be the result of cycles of weight loss and gain, or "yo-yo" dieting, an inherently unhealthy process that seems to stress an often already overstressed system. Yo-yo dieting is probably also dangerous in part because when we lose weight through dieting and gain it back, we tend to regain more fat. It's likely that over time, any health risk associated with one-time weight loss is far outweighed, as it were, by the many health benefits of remaining lean.[21-23]

THE BEST WEIGHT-LOSS PLAN

The message here is that the only effective approach to weight loss or management combines regular exercise with a sensible low-fat diet (without great preoccupation with calorie counting).

If you adopt an active life to lose weight, your goal should be to lose it slowly (certainly no more than one percent of your body weight each week) and cautiously, not necessarily by eating less, but by increasing energy expenditure and making healthful changes in your diet so you're eating more foods rich in complex carbohydrates and fewer foods containing fats or simple sugars. And once you've lost weight, continue to exercise and eat sensibly to maintain your desired weight.

HOW EXERCISE WORKS

In theory, weight control is a simple enough proposition: To maintain body weight, the energy you consume in the form of calories must equal the total energy expended. If you consume more calories than you expend, you'll get fat, and there's no loophole through this grim biological fact of life. To lose that fat, you need a caloric deficit; you need to expend more energy than you're taking in, which you can do by reducing caloric intake, increasing caloric expenditure, or both. In practice, though, it's more complicated, as we'll see, but by employing the simple exercise and diet strategies outlined here, you can reach your weight- or fat-loss goals and keep the weight off so you look and feel better and feel better about yourself.

METABOLIC BASICS

The total energy each of us expends in a day is the sum of three broad categories of energy expenditure.

Resting Metabolic Rate (RMR)

Your RMR is the rate at which your body expends energy at rest—simply being alive and doing all the things a body does at rest, such as taking in and expelling air and pumping blood. At rest, a man or woman who weighs 155 pounds (70 kilograms) will expend about 1.2 kilocalories per minute, or about 72 kilocalories per hour, assuming he or she doesn't do anything else (your weight in kilograms roughly equals the number of kilocalories you'll expend in an hour at rest). Add or subtract 10 percent for every 15 pounds above or below 155; subtract 4 percent for every 10 years over age 25. Your RMR accounts for about 60 to 75 percent of the calories you expend in a day.[24] Thus even a slight increase in RMR will have significant benefits.

Thermic Effect of Feeding (TEF)

When you eat, your metabolic rate increases slightly as your body works to process the food. This TEF accounts for only about 10 percent of the calories you expend in a day, but it is possible to maximize the TEF through changes in diet and eating patterns. Proteins and complex carbohydrates have the greatest thermic effect; that is, perhaps as much as 25 percent of the energy in these foods is expended digesting them. Fats, on the other hand, have negligible thermic effect; almost all the energy in fat is used either for energy or, more likely, layered around the midsection or thighs.

Thermic Effect of Activity (TEA)

This is the key to weight loss and weight control. The TEA typically accounts for 15 to 30 percent of the energy you expend in a day, depending on how active you are. The 155-pounder who expends 72 kilocalories per hour at rest will expend about 120 kilocalories per hour sitting at a desk writing, or 150 kilocalories per hour puttering about the house, or about 350 kilocalories in 30 minutes running a six-minute mile. The heavier you are, the more kilocalories you'll expend at any given activity; the lighter you are, the fewer kilocalories you'll expend. Thus the larger person seems to have a distinct advantage when it comes to losing weight and keeping it off, but chances are he or she has more weight to lose. You can determine how many kilocalories you expend at any intensity of activity by referring to the activity characteristics chart on pages 240 through 243 .

Depending on the intensity and duration of the activity, the metabolic boost from the thermic effect of activity can linger for hours after exercise, even when you're at rest, and this is perhaps one of the most significant weight-loss benefits of exercise.

TAKING IT OFF

Suppose you're fairly typical, and your weight has been steadily creeping up over the years, so that now you would like to lose a few pounds. You can go on a diet and perhaps drop that weight, but as we've noted, the odds of long-term success are not good; chances are you will gain that lost weight back and then some.

Or you can become more active.

Some of the best information we have on the value of exercise for weight loss comes from the laboratory of Peter Wood at Stanford. In early studies, Wood and his associates demonstrated the necessity of exercise when they found lower relative weights or body fat content in exercisers as compared with nonexercisers, even though the exercisers had higher caloric energy intake. In an intervention trial, Wood and his colleagues showed that changes in body fat in the exercisers were inversely related to the amount of exercise; subjects who increased their exercise the most experienced the greatest reduction in percent body fat.[25]

Then, in a trial of exercise versus dieting in moderately obese men, Wood and company showed that substantial loss of body fat by increased exercise alone (no caloric restriction) could be accomplished and maintained using feasible endurance exercise programs.[26]

And most recently, Wood's group conducted a trial of weight loss with and without exercise in subjects on a prudent diet. They showed that the diet-plus-exercise group had become substantially more fit (improved lipoprotein status and decreased estimated risk of developing CHD) than either the control or the diet-only group (both men and women). Their findings indicated a 64 percent improvement in body fat loss as a result of adding an exercise program. Moreover, their findings suggested that physical activity may be a particularly valuable means of producing a more healthy body fat distribution.[27]

Where the Fats Are

Simply being overfat is bad for the health, but how bad it is depends somewhat on where the body has stored the fat. Fat stored around

BODY FAT DISTRIBUTION

Remember, the standard weight/height charts and BMI estimates are only crude indicators of potential health risk. Your body fat content is the real factor in your health, but dangers lie not only in the amount of body fat, but in its distribution. For example, an apple-shaped person with body fat stored around the midsection seems to be at a higher risk of heart disease, stroke, hypertension, and diabetes than a pear-shaped person with body fat around the hips and thighs. In his book *Staying Well*, Harvey Simon suggests a quick way to better assess your body fat and distribution of fat. To do so, measure your waist at the narrowest point and your hips at the widest. Then divide your waist measurement by your hip measurement:

$$\text{ratio} = \frac{\text{waist size in inches}}{\text{hip size in inches}}$$

Men with a ratio greater than 1.0 are at twice the risk of heart disease and probably NIDDM compared with men whose ratio is 0.85; women with a ratio greater than 0.85 are also at increased risk.

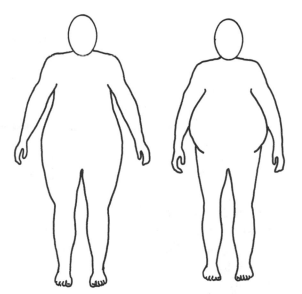

Body Mass Index, from *Staying Well*. Copyright © 1992 by Harvey B. Simon. Reprinted by permission of Houghton Mifflin Company. All rights reserved.

the midsection appears to be associated with the greatest health risks of all, including a significantly higher risk of heart disease and diabetes when compared with that associated with the same amount of fat distributed around the thighs and buttocks. This may be one of the reasons men—who are more likely than women to store fat around the midsection—usually tend to have more heart disease at a younger age and overall shorter life spans.[28-30]

Weight-Loss Strategies

Let's assume you stand about 5 feet 10 inches and weigh about 190 pounds (BMI close to 27), but you'd like to weigh 155 (BMI of 22). At rest, if you weigh 190 pounds, you'll expend about 90 kilocalories an hour; this is a measure of your RMR, and it's about the number of kilocalories in a piece of bread (remember, we're choosing the more accurate measure of kilocalories here; product labeling uses the term calorie to designate the same thing), just one tablespoon or pat of butter, a large apple, or better yet, four wedges of lettuce, which is probably more than enough to fill you up. In a 24-hour period, at 190 pounds, you'll expend about 2,100 kilocalories simply being alive.

But it's hard to get through the day being totally at rest. All of us, no matter how sedentary, are up and on our feet at least a few minutes a day, if to do nothing else than rummage through the fridge for some snacks, so let's add another 400 kilocalories to that original figure (your RMR, TEA, and TEF). If you weigh 190 pounds and you aren't particularly active, you probably expend about 2,500 kilocalories in a 24-hour period. If you don't consume more or less than that amount, you won't gain any weight, but you won't lose any either.

And that's the problem, of course. The typical American diet makes it awfully easy to consume 2,500 kilocalories in a day, if not in a few minutes, and then some. A typical American-style fast-food lunch of a double cheeseburger, fries, a chocolate shake, and a couple cookies accounts for close to that amount, and we haven't even begun figuring in breakfast, dinner, and an evening snack of, say, two small chocolate chip cookies and an eight-ounce glass of whole milk (which add up to a not insignificant 300 kilocalories).

Which is why, of course, you now weigh 190 pounds instead of the 155 you want to weigh.

As noted earlier, to lose weight (or better yet, to lose body fat), you need to expend more energy than you consume. You need a caloric

CALCULATING YOUR DAILY CALORIC NEEDS

1. Select your desired weight (DW) in pounds.

2. Determine your daily basal caloric requirements (the calories you need to consume to maintain the body's functions when inactive): DW × 10.

3. Add daily activity calories (needed for various levels of activity; choose one):

   For sedentary (almost no exercise),
   multiply DW × 3 = _____.

   For moderately active (20 minutes, three to five times a week), multiply DW × 5 = _____.

   For the very active (one hour, five to seven times a week), multiply DW × 10 = _____.

4. To find your total daily requirements, add your basal calories (No. 2) and your activity calories (No. 3): _____.

5. Subtract daily calories for weight loss. To lose one pound a week, you need to cut your caloric intake by an average of 500 kilocalories a day, or better yet, increase your energy expenditure by that amount.

- Daily calories for weight loss of one pound per week (answer to No. 4, minus 500).

- Additional weekly activity for weight loss of one pound (approximately 100 kilocalories for every 10 minutes of additional activity), add 50 minutes of activity per week.

Adapted, by permission, from "Losing weight: A new attitude emerges," *Harvard Health Letter* 4: 1-6. Copyright by the American Diabetes Association Inc.

deficit. One pound of fat contains about 3,500 kilocalories of energy; thus, if you can expend 3,500 kilocalories more than you consume, you'll lose a pound of fat. To lose a pound a week, then, you need a daily caloric deficit of 500 kilocalories, about the number of calories in just three cans of beer, or three eight-ounce glasses of whole milk, just two bagels with butter, or a couple pieces of toast with butter and jam and a glass of orange juice, two waffles, or, alas, just one hamburger with cheese. Obviously, the problem here is that it's much easier to consume 3,500 kilocalories than it is to expend them, particularly if the calories come in the form of something particularly tasty. That doesn't mean you still can't lose weight effectively. Here are some principles to keep in mind as you try.

- We use terms such as overweight and overfat indiscriminately; with regard to your health, it's not what you weigh that's important, but how much of you is fat. If you've decided to lose weight, stop thinking about losing weight; think about losing fat instead.

- Take the long view and set realistic short- and long-term weight-loss goals. Healthful weight loss is slow and steady. Too-rapid weight loss is bad for the health and almost always results in rebound and overall weight gain. Don't try to lose more than one percent of your body weight each week.

- Become more active. Although any activity will help you lose weight, for best results, try to include some moderately vigorous activity in your weekly routine.

- Don't diet by restricting calories; instead, shift your diet toward more healthful eating.

- Eat a variety of "nutritionally dense" foods, whole-grain products such as bread, pasta, and cereal, and vegetables and fruit.

- Protein is important, but as much as possible, opt for lean meats, including fish, poultry with the skin removed, and lean cuts of beef and pork with any fat trimmed off.

- As you limit fat in your diet, make sure you cut the most harmful fats. These are the saturated fats found in animal products and solid vegetable oils such as margarine or other hydrogenated vegetable oils.

- Use liquid vegetable oils whenever you need to use oil for cooking. Liquid vegetable oils, and olive oil in particular, contain vitamin E, an antioxidant that may help fight free radicals that accelerate aging.

- Vitamin and mineral supplementation may benefit the health, although there's some debate whether they're necessary when the diet is varied and nutritious. Important antioxidants are vitamins A (15 to 30 milligrams daily), C (250 to 1,000 milligrams daily), E (100 to 400 international units), and folic acid. Calcium (1,000 to 1,500 milligrams daily) is essential to prevent osteoporosis.

- Eat at least three meals a day—breakfast, lunch, and dinner—but more smaller meals throughout the day are even better than three larger meals.
- Drink six to eight glasses of water a day; water helps induce satiety and helps carry nutrients throughout your body.
- Plan your meals throughout the day.
- Keep plenty of low-calorie snacks on hand, such as carrot and celery sticks.
- Begin each meal with a salad; salads are low in calories and filling, so you're less likely to overindulge in more caloric foods throughout the meal.
- Eat slowly.
- Don't weigh yourself every day. Visit the scale only once a week, on the same day of the week and at the same time of day; it's the best way to get a clear idea of your true weight loss during the previous week.
- Keep a weight-loss record.
- Treat yourself now and then with some of your favorite foods (in moderation). It will be hard to stick with a weight-loss routine that's too strict.
- Identify the situations in your life that provoke you to overeat or to eat when you're not hungry. Most likely, these are stress-filled situations, and if you can work to relieve the sources of stress, it will help you control your eating. Use exercise as a stress-reduction technique and as a substitute for the candy bars or cookies you usually reach for when on edge.

Now let's suppose you don't want to cut out those bagels or hamburger, at least not right away (you should, of course, or at least skip the butter on the bagels and hold the mayo on that burger, and we'll get to that shortly). But that's okay, for now. Let's see how you can still eat what you have been eating and lose weight anyway by becoming more active:

Goal: Lose 35 pounds through a 3,500-kilocalorie-per-week deficit.

Strategy 1: Add 30 minutes of Stage One activities each day to expend 700 kilocalories each week.

Weight-loss benefit: Weekly weight loss of one-fifth of a pound, or four-fifths of a pound per month.

If you resolve to be up on your feet puttering about in Stage One activities for an additional 30 minutes every day, walking the dog, playing with the kids, helping more with housework, and so on, you'll expend an additional 100 kilocalories each day, or an additional 700 kilocalories in a week. Keep in mind that this is an additional energy expenditure beyond what you've been accustomed to. It may help if you know how much time you have usually spent on your feet, and in part III we discuss how you can assess your present activity levels, as well as effective strategies for increasing your level of activity through the day. In any case, by adding 30 minutes of Stage One activity to your usual routine and expending an additional 100 kilocalories a day, you now have 400 kilocalories a day to go to achieve your goal of a 500-kilocalorie daily deficit.

Strategy 2: Add another 30 minutes of Stage One activities each day to expend another 700 kilocalories.

Weight-loss benefit: Weekly weight loss of two-fifths of a pound; almost 1.5 pounds a month, or 18 a year, half your weight-loss goal.

If you can add another 30 minutes a day of puttering around—take up gardening, for example—you'll expend an additional 100 kilocalories a day for another 700 kilocalories a week. You now have 300 kilocalories a day to go, and you still get to eat as much as before.

Strategy 3: Add 30 minutes of Stage Two activities three times a week to expend another 600 kilocalories.

Weight-loss benefit: Weekly weight loss of nearly two-thirds of a pound; over 2.5 pounds a month, or 35 pounds in 14 months.

Let's suppose you have neither the time nor the inclination to add any more puttering around to your daily routine. No problem.

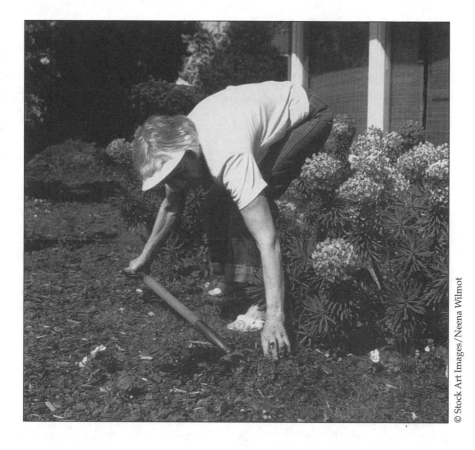

Instead, add some moderately vigorous exercise, say about 30 minutes of brisk walking three times a week. You'll expend about 200 kilocalories during each 30-minute walk (or more in more intense effort such as jogging or swimming laps). If you stick with it, you'll expend another 600 kilocalories in a week. Add that to the 1,400 additional kilocalories you're already expending puttering about and you're now expending 2,000 kilocalories a week in activity, representing a fat loss of two-thirds of a pound each week, or 2.5 pounds a month, or 35 pounds in 14 months.

And all of this is achieved without the miseries of dieting and the hazards of a slowing metabolism. In fact, as we'll see shortly, your overall metabolic rate, including your RMR, will increase thanks to all this activity, meaning a more rapid weight loss and more effective weight maintenance once you've met your goals. Along the way, you will also have cut your risk of heart disease, diabetes, some cancers, and a host of other diseases, as we'll see in later chapters, and you'll have improved your appearance, strength, balance, and ability to carry out the activities of daily life. Most likely, you will even have improved your cognitive efficiency, memory, mood, and overall vitality and zest for living. Assuming, of course, you don't start eating more.

Now, what happens if you make healthful changes in your eating habits?

SENSIBLE EATING

Although a healthful diet can provide significant health benefits, diet alone, contrary to what many self-proclaimed diet experts tell us, is not sufficient to provide optimal health. Diet alone won't protect us from the hazards of sedentary habits. Nor is exercise alone sufficient; regular physical activity can't offer complete protection from a steady diet of hamburgers, fries, and milk shakes. Eventually, and particularly as we grow older, a lifetime of bad eating habits will begin to take their toll in the form of disease, no matter how active we may be, just as sedentary living will take its toll, no matter how healthful our eating habits. The ideal combines plenty of exercise and a healthful diet.

Based on what is known with reasonable certainty about the interplay between diet and health, you should keep in mind a few fundamental concepts as you begin to plan your diet around an active life.

EAT A VARIETY OF NUTRITIONALLY "DENSE" FOODS

In fact, people who eat more apparently have lower rates of coronary artery disease, and if this sounds like a contradiction of everything the experts have been telling us for years, you're right; it is a contradiction. But Walter Willett, MD, professor of epidemiology and chair of the Department of Nutrition at the Harvard School of Public Health, has been reexamining many of the old assumptions we make about our diets, and one of his most consistent findings is that those with the highest caloric intakes have the lowest rates of coronary heart disease.[31] The reason? Those who are more active eat more; and those who are active, as we've seen, are healthier.

The overweight do not necessarily eat more than their leaner neighbors; rather, they eat too many of the wrong foods, calorically dense foods such as fatty meats or nutritionally empty yet caloric foods such as sweets, and more important, they don't get enough exercise to burn off any excess calories. The result, of course, is that the excess is stored, usually in the form of bulges over the belt. On the other hand, a variety and abundance of foods is the surest way of getting all of the nutrients our bodies need; and exercise is the surest way of protecting us from weight gain.

The USDA's new recommended food guide (see figure 4.2) emphasizes the complex carbohydrates found in whole grains—bread, cereal, rice, and pasta (6 to 11 servings daily)—and in fruits and vegetables (2 to 4 and 3 to 5 servings, respectively). The new guidelines recommend that we go easy on dairy products and meats (2 to 3 servings of these proteins each) and to keep the consumption of fats, especially animal fats, to a minimum.

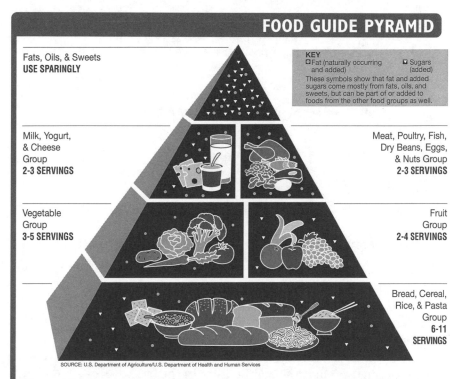

Figure 4.2 Each of these food groups provides some, but not all, of the nutrients you need. No one food group is more important than another—for good health you need them all. Go easy on fats, oils, and sweets, the foods in the small tip of the pyramid.

U.S. Department of Agriculture, Human Nutrition Information Service, August 1992, Leaflet No. 572.

So what's a serving?

Breads, cereals, rice, & pasta (about 80 calories)	• 1 slice of bread • 1/2 English muffin • 1 small roll • 1/2 cup cooked cereal • 1 ounce ready-to-eat cereal
Fruits (about 80 calories)	• 1 whole fruit such as an apple or banana • 1/2 grapefruit • 3/4 cup juice • 1/2 cup canned or cooked fruit
Vegetables (about 20 calories)	• 1/2 cooked or chopped raw vegetables • 1 cup of leafy raw vegetables such as spinach
Meat, poultry (about 200 calories)	• Amounts should total 5 to 7 ounces of cooked lean & fish meat, poultry or fish a day (about 3 ounces per serving).
Dry beans, eggs, nuts (about 150 calories)	• 1 egg • 1/2 cup cooked beans • 2 tablespoons peanut butter
Milk, cheese, & yogurt (about 150 calories)	• 1 cup of milk or yogurt • 1-1/2 ounces cheese

Carbohydrates

Carbohydrates are molecules of carbon, hydrogen, and oxygen in our foods that are broken down by the body and stored for energy as glycogen in the muscles. All carbohydrates—or "carbs," as they're known in the fitness game—contain the same amount of energy (that is, four kilocalories per gram), but not all carbs are created equal. What are called "simple" carbs—short chains of carbon, hydrogen, and oxygen (the sucrose of table sugar or the fructose that makes ripe fruits taste sweet)—are absorbed rapidly into the bloodstream; they raise the blood sugar rapidly, requiring the pancreas to produce large amounts of insulin. Simple sugars are good for a "rush" and quick energy but offer little sustenance, and diabetics need to be especially wary of simple carbs. And the simple sugars often come in refined foods such as candy which are calorically dense but nutritionally "empty," that is, devoid of most essential nutrients we need for good health.

The complex carbohydrates—longer molecules of carbon, hydrogen, and oxygen—take longer to break down in the digestive system and thus raise blood sugar levels more slowly to provide a steadier and longer-lasting source of energy. And the complex carbs have a higher TEF because they require more "processing" before they can be used by the body. This means less of the energy they contain is likely to end up stored around your midsection. Complex carbs are found abundantly in grains, breads, and cereals, and in starchy foods such as potatoes and beans. They're also found in fruits and vegetables, along with more simple sugars. And unlike foods containing simple carbohydrates, these foods are also rich in other essential nutrients, including protein, vitamins, and minerals. They're nutrient-dense. These foods also contain indigestible carbohydrates— bulk and fiber—which are important in reducing serum cholesterol and in preventing some types of cancer, especially colon cancer. And because complex carbs contain indigestible (read "no calories" here) bulk, you fill up sooner after taking in plenty of essential nutrients but fewer calories. Thus it will be much easier to lose weight on a diet rich in complex carbs.

Protein

Protein, made of small molecules called amino acids, is the basic building material of our cells and tissues, but it's not stored in the body like the glycogen from carbohydrates. Protein must be replenished daily. A general rule of thumb for estimating daily protein needs is that 0.8 grams of protein for each kilogram (2.2 pounds) of body weight is more than enough. For a 155-pound individual, that amounts to less than a quarter pound of protein a day, not all that much, and you don't have to get this protein from animal sources at all; beans and grains in combination, for example, provide adequate protein, with the added benefits of abundant complex carbs and fibers and little fat. Most of us eat much more protein than we need.

Does exercise increase the need for protein? This issue is still being debated. Many assume that because muscle is protein, the more protein they eat, the bigger their muscles will become, but it doesn't seem to work that way. The only way to make a muscle larger or stronger is through exercise. Very heavy exercise of long duration may increase the need for extra protein, although this is uncertain.

It is known that excess protein in the diet can be harmful, placing added stress on the liver and kidneys. Although there is little reliable data on the effects of protein consumption on longevity, lab studies with animals at least suggest that decreased protein intake increases length of life.[32]

Fats

Fat is the most densely caloric food—nine kilocalories per gram (more than twice the calories in a gram of carbohydrates or protein). Thus the more fat in your food, the more likely you are to take in more calories than you should. Fats are quickly and easily stored by the body, so most of the fat in your food tends to go directly to the waistline. And dietary fat contributes to the buildup of plaque deposits in your arteries.

Unfortunately, it's the fat in our foods that generally makes them taste good. Indeed, our bodies actually seem to crave fat from time to time. So why should something that's bad for us be so desirable? Again, it may have to do with the conditions under which our bodies evolved. Before agriculture, when our ancestors were scrambling hard for every calorie they could get and were lucky to get enough on any given day, calorically dense fats were prized finds. Indeed, some anthropologists suggest that our hominid ancestors were probably saved from extinction by the fat they scavenged from the marrow of bones. Forced from their trees by a changing climate, some think, these hominids had to find new sources of food. Without the speed or strength to hunt game, they probably turned to scrounging whatever other animals left behind. But after the lions and hyenas were through with their prey, about all that was left were the largest bones, which even the hyenas couldn't crack. However, by wielding rocks, our dexterous and hungry hominid ancestors could. They'd split the bones and eat the marrow, and it saved their lives. Thus our craving for fat is probably "hardwired" into our very flesh and psyches. Too bad.

But our ancestors had to work awfully hard for their fat, and they didn't get much of it at any one time. The problem we have with fat is not that it's inherently bad for us; it's just that we eat too much of it. Way too much.

But how much is too much? These days, there seems to be a rather polite furor in the halls of academe surrounding the topic of dietary intake of fats and their role in heart disease, cancer, and other health problems. The National Heart, Lung and Blood Institute and the

American Heart Association recommend that no more than 30 percent of calories in your diet come from fat. Some researchers think this is much too much. Dr. Dean Ornish, who has developed a program of exercise, diet, and meditation to treat heart patients, recommends no more than 10 percent of calories from fat.[33]

But a crucial issue is not how much fat is in your diet, but what types of fat. Indeed, the "right" fats may actually be good for your health, in moderation, and moderation is important. Based on data from the Nurses' Health Study Cohort and the Health Professionals Follow-up Study, Walter Willett suspects that there may be little health benefit, especially in terms of heart disease, to be gained by reducing fat intake to less than 30 percent.[34] More surprisingly, Willett thinks that reducing some types of fat such as olive oil could actually be bad for your health. Indeed, fat intake per se may not be related to heart disease at all, but rather to the type of fats we consume. Based on available data, Willett thinks that if we reduce fats in our diets, we should reduce saturated fat from meats and dairy products (for example, butter, whole milk, meat) and partially hydrogenated vegetable oil (solid oils such as margarine and shortening or tropical vegetable oils such as palm oil). When we have to use fat, we should substitute liquid vegetable oils, particularly olive oil and canola oil.

The principle holds that the saturated fats found in meats (particularly red meats) and dairy products such as butter are bad, lead to heart disease, and should be reduced, whereas the liquid, unsaturated fats in vegetable oils, although just as densely caloric, aren't as harmful to health (although too much of any fat will make you fat). The term *saturated* refers to the number of hydrogen atoms in fat molecules. Saturated fats in meats are loaded with hydrogen atoms; the unsaturated fats in most liquid vegetable oils are not. Products such as margarine and vegetable shortening start out as liquid vegetable oils, then manufacturers "saturate" them, loading them with hydrogen atoms, a process that converts the oils to soft solids, which makes them a bit more like the butter we once loved and thus more marketable.

CONQUER THE CHOLESTEROL CONFUSION

There's much confusion about fat and cholesterol—confusion that advertisers have exploited to sell low-cholesterol products based on the implication that these products are more healthful. Because a high level of serum cholesterol in the blood is strongly associated with an increased risk of cardiovascular disease, it is logical to conclude that if we can limit cholesterol in our diets—substituting olive oil for butter, for example—it will be good for our hearts. There's some truth to this, but the real situation is not so simple. Some foods advertised as low-cholesterol and thus healthy are really healthful, but not all of them, unfortunately, if they contain saturated fat, the real culprit.

Because cholesterol is found only in animal tissue, many people confuse cholesterol and animal fat; some assume that cholesterol is just another type of fat. Cholesterol is not a fat at all, but rather a waxy substance, a sterol. It's found only in foods that come from animal sources, but our own livers also manufacture cholesterol as an essential component of a well-functioning metabolism. Cholesterol is a precursor to several essential hormones, including sex hormones and adrenaline (interestingly, and perhaps not surprisingly, research with rats notes that those on severe low-cholesterol diets have very bad tempers, and any human who has also spent time on a low-cholesterol diet can probably sympathize).

Whereas dietary cholesterol has some impact on the cholesterol level in your bloodstream, saturated fat in the diet has a much greater impact; saturated fat, it seems, stimulates the liver to produce cholesterol. Eating foods that contain saturated fat, whether from animal products or hydrogenated vegetable oil, will elevate blood cholesterol. Thus that no-cholesterol cookie—the one touted as "heart healthy," might be just as bad for your heart as an equal amount of fried meat if the cookie has been made with hydrogenated vegetable oil.

And new research reveals that in the process of hydrogenation, still another dangerous substance is produced, a type of fat called "trans-fatty acid." It seems that not only are saturated fats in animal products or hydrogenated vegetable oils bad for health, so are these trans-fatty acids. The ongoing Nurses' Health Study of some 85,000 women found that subjects who consumed large amounts of margarine and shortening used in cookies, bread, and other baked goods had a 70 percent higher risk of heart disease than women who used little or none.[35] Another study of the dietary habits of 239 heart attack patients and 282 healthy people looked at the amount of trans-fatty acids in their diets and found that the risk of heart attack was twice as high among those who consumed the most trans-fatty acids compared with those who consumed the least.

On the other hand, monounsaturated fat (liquid vegetable oils, particularly olive oil) may be healthful; Willett notes that these vegetable oils are a primary source of vitamin E, an antioxidant that may fight free radicals and slow the aging process and perhaps help prevent cancer. Moreover, in a study of vitamin E intake and CHD, Willett and colleagues found a 40 percent reduced risk of CHD among those with the highest consumption of the vitamin. Reducing vegetable fats that are rich in vitamin E may in fact raise the risk of CHD.[36]

We also need to rethink the assumption that total serum cholesterol—measured by a simple blood test—is meaningful in predicting health risks. High serum cholesterol levels (above about 200 mg/deciliter) are believed to increase the risk of heart disease, but many experts are no longer convinced the data support this assumption. Rather, we need to pay more attention to the types of cholesterol in the blood. Low levels of high-density lipoproteins (HDLs) are more predictive of future heart disease than are high total serum cholesterol levels. And unfortunately, reducing certain types of fats in the diet to lower the more harmful LDLs (low-density lipoproteins) tends to lower HDLs as well (see table 4.3). When olive oil is substituted for saturated fats, however, total serum cholesterol

Table 4.3 Cholesterols	
Total Blood Cholesterol	
Less than 200 mg/deciliter	Desirable
200-239	Borderline high
240+	Too high
LDLs	
<130	Desirable
130-159	Borderline high
160+	Too high
HDLs	
40-50 (men)	Desirable
50-60 (women)	Desirable
<35	Too low

levels decline while HDLs are maintained. (And exercise, as we'll see, also raises HDLs.)

The message here? Minimize your intake of saturated fats and solid or semisolid vegetable oils and, wherever possible, substitute olive oil or canola oil for butter and hydrogenated vegetable oils. (Willett, incidentally, makes chocolate chip cookies using olive oil. He says they're delicious.)

REPLACE EXCESS DIETARY FAT

Now let's suppose you resolve not to butter your toast in the morning. Suppose, instead, you use jam. A teaspoon of jam contains about half the calories found in the same amount of butter. And the butter contains saturated fat and cholesterol, which are bad for the heart.

Strategy 4: Don't butter your toast, substitute nonfat for whole milk, and eliminate 1,400 kilocalories from your caloric intake each week.

Weight-loss benefit: Total weekly weight loss with exercise plus diet changes is 3,400 kilocalories, or about 1 pound a week, 4 pounds each month, or 35 pounds in nine months, your weight-loss goal.

Eliminate the butter on those two pieces of toast you have each morning and substitute jam and you've probably eliminated about 100 unnecessary kilocalories from your diet, or another 700 kilocalories in a week. And if you use skim milk on your cereal rather than the whole milk to which you've long been accustomed—not a terribly great sacrifice—you've just eliminated another 100 kilocalories a day (per eight-ounce glass) from your diet. These aren't major dietary changes. In fact, you're eating just as much in quantity as you did before, so you're not really dieting at all. But you are eating more sensibly and losing fat.

These relatively minor dietary changes add up to a weekly reduction of 1,400 kilocalories. Taking this into account with your physical activities—an hour a day of Stage One puttering about and three 30-minute sessions of Stage Two activities expending 2,000 kilocalories in a week—you'll enjoy a weekly caloric deficit of nearly 3,500 kilocalories, or the loss each week of one pound of body fat. In truth, though, you may not actually lose a pound a week on this regimen of exercise and diet because you'll be adding heavier muscle while losing fat, but that's exactly what you want. Indeed, depending on how fat and muscular you are to begin with, you may actually gain weight at the same time you lose fat and layer on muscle.

Better yet, this added muscle appears to be the single most important factor in weight loss and long-term weight maintenance.

MUSCLE MATTERS

For the most effective weight or fat loss, strive for moderately vigorous Stage Two exercise as much as possible. Of course, if you've been sedentary for years, and particularly if you're very overweight, you won't want to start out at Stage Two intensity. You'll need to work up to it, and part III lays out a step-by-step program for getting started and progressing through your LifeFit program. But your long-term goal for optimal weight loss should be Stage Two activities, and here's why.

INCREASE CALORIC EXPENDITURE DURING ACTIVITY

Any activity is better than none when it comes to weight loss, but if you walk a mile briskly, you'll probably burn a few more calories than if you walk the same mile more slowly, a fact that runs somewhat counter to the conventional thinking that a mile is a mile, no matter how fast you cover the distance. Why? As we increase the pace of walking, most of us tend to become less physiologically efficient, calling on more muscles to maintain the more rapid pace, which means expending more calories. When we walk briskly, most of us use our arms more, as well as the large muscles of our back. For instance, if you weigh 155 pounds, you may expend about 85 kilocalories if you walk a mile at about two miles an hour. If you cover the same mile at three miles an hour you may expend closer to 90 kilocalories. You may expend more than 100 kilocalories walking that same mile at a four-mile-an-hour pace, and perhaps as many as 125 kilocalories at five miles an hour. If you break into a jog, you may become a bit more efficient, so you could expend about the same number of calories jogging a mile at six miles an hour as you will walking it very briskly at a five-mile-an-hour pace. But as you increase your jogging pace, you may again begin to expend more calories each mile. The same effects tend to occur with any activity as intensity increases.[37]

DO MORE IN LESS TIME

Suppose you're getting your exercise during your lunch break or before you go to work, or you have to squeeze it in before dinner in the evening. If you're pressed for time, by exercising more intensely, you can expend more calories in the time you have. By walking, jogging, or swimming faster, not only will you expend more calories per mile or lap, but by increasing intensity, you'll be able to walk, jog, or swim farther in the time available to you.

GET A METABOLIC BOOST

While exercising at any intensity, your metabolic rate increases, of course, but when you stop exercising, your metabolic rate doesn't return to its normal resting rate immediately. In fact, your RMR remains elevated—and thus you continue expending calories at a faster than resting rate—from several minutes to several hours afterward, even though you're at rest. The more intense the activity, the greater this postactivity metabolic boost and the longer it takes for your metabolic rate to return to its resting level. Some studies have found that after 30 minutes of very vigorous activity, a postexercise metabolic boost lasts as long as 24 hours or more, providing a significant weight-loss advantage.[38,39]

Is there an ideal weight-loss activity, one that most effectively provides a postexercise metabolic boost? Perhaps. It may be that resistance training is the most effective exercise for weight loss because, more than any other type of activity, it appears to elevate the metabolism and keep it elevated longer, even at rest.[40] You may burn the same number of calories during 30 minutes of brisk walking or jogging as you will during 30 minutes of resistance training, but overall, thanks to the postexercise metabolic boost, you'll probably end up with a greater caloric deficit as a result of resistance work. Plus you will enjoy the important benefits of greater overall muscle gain, including improved strength, better posture, improved appearance, and more.

But any activity done more vigorously will contribute to a metabolic boost. Compared with walking at a three-mile-an-hour pace for an hour, running six miles an hour for 30 minutes will result in a greater overall caloric deficit. You'll cover the same distance either way (three miles), but the end result will be a greater caloric expenditure at the higher intensity, not only because you've likely expended a few more calories during the jog for reasons we discussed previously, but because your metabolism will remain elevated longer after exercise. Swimming, however, although an excellent form of exercise, doesn't seem to offer the same postexertion benefits because it doesn't tend to elevate the body temperature as much as other activities, unless you swim very hard in warm water.

BURN MORE FAT

A common notion expressed by diet gurus in their various books and on their TV shows and videos is that the best way to lose fat is through low-intensity exercise. So, the reasoning goes, because we're trying to lose fat when we go on a weight-loss program that includes diet changes, exercise, or both, we should exercise at low intensities for best results (by this reasoning, sleep would seem to be the best fat-loss activity of all).

The Physiology of Fat

This is a matter of some current controversy and confusion. First, remember that any physical activity of any intensity expends calories and contributes to weight (or fat) loss if the energy expenditure results in a caloric deficit, which assumes, again, that you don't start eating more as you exercise more. That's the bottom line when it comes to weight loss. But there are strategies you can employ to give yourself the best shot at a caloric deficit.

When we eat, carbohydrates, fats, and proteins in our foods are used or stored in different ways. The carbohydrates in fruits, grains, and vegetables are converted by the body into a substance called glycogen. Some of this glycogen is stored in the liver. Some is sent to the muscles and stored as muscle glycogen, if those stores have been reduced through exercise or fasting, typically at night while sleeping (thus a breakfast should be rich in carbohydrates to restore muscle glycogen for an energetic start to the day). And some of the carbohydrates become glucose (sugar) and remain in the bloodstream to be used by the brain, the kidneys, and the red blood cells, which all depend on blood glucose to function. Once the liver, blood, and muscle energy stores are filled, any extra carbohydrates are converted to fat—for storage around such locations as the thighs and midsection, in the form of fat, of course.

Fats in the diet are digested and converted into triglyceride molecules and quickly stored as (what else?) more fat, again usually around the thighs and midsection, whereas protein is converted to several amino acids that are used by the body's tissues for a host of purposes, including tissue growth and repair, and hormone synthesis. Most of any leftover protein the body doesn't need just then is converted to energy, and if the body has plenty of stored glycogen, then any leftover protein is converted to even more fat, and stored.

During physical activity of any sort, whether you're sleeping, or sitting watching TV, or walking the dog, or running 10 miles, the body calls on both muscle glycogen and fat for energy, though it "prefers" glycogen, since glycogen is readily available in the muscles, where it's needed, and because it's more easily converted to energy than stored fat, which must go through a variety of chemical transformations before it can be used for energy. For this reason, the more intense the activity, the greater the percentage of stored glycogen the body turns to for energy; when your body is working hard, it needs a quick source of energy, and that's glycogen. At rest, your body has the "leisure" to convert fats to energy, thus your body will use a greater percentage of fat at rest or in low-intensity activities than it will during more vigorous activities. At rest, perhaps two-thirds of the calories your body consumes come from stored fat. Sitting in a chair for an hour, you might expend about 70 kilocalories, about 45 of them fat, 25 from glycogen—and thus the notion that the best "fat-loss" activities are low-intensity activities such as leisurely strolls. As you increase the intensity of the activity, the percentage of fat the body uses for energy drops, to less than half the calories consumed during a brisk walk.

The problem with low-intensity activities, if fat-loss is your goal, is that you simply don't expend many calories, fat or carbs, while you're at it. The bottom line, again, is that to lose weight, you have to expend more calories than you take in, and the more you can expend, the better. Period. At rest, if you weigh 150 pounds, you'll expend about 70 kilocalories; during an hour of brisk walking, you might expend upwards of 300 kilocalories. Maybe you burn a slightly lower percentage of fat during that brisk walk, but you've still expended many more calories overall, and that's what counts if you're aiming to lose fat.

The Message

More intense Stage Two activities will be more effective if fat-loss is your goal. But if you're just starting out in your active life, Stage Two activities might be too intense. The ideal fat-loss routine balances intensity with duration; you want to exercise at the highest level of intensity you can that allows you to sustain the activity for at least 30 minutes. Thus you're better off walking at a leisurely pace for 30 minutes or an hour than trying to jog and ending up exhausted after 10 minutes. With habitual exercise, you'll be able to gradually increase the intensity, to expend more calories in a given time, for increased fat-loss. And better yet, with regular exercise at higher intensities, the body becomes more adept at using stored fats for energy at any level of intensity, in order to conserve glycogen stores, thus accelerating fat-loss.

BUILD MUSCLE FOR A HIGHER RMR

Finally, intensity of exercise offers still another key benefit to anyone trying to lose weight, and that's its effectiveness at building muscle. As noted earlier, when you lose weight by dieting, you lose both fat and muscle. Because fat just more or less sits there in your body storing energy and not doing much to expend energy, your resting

---

REV UP YOUR METABOLISM

Strategies for maximum metabolic boost:

- Add at least 30 minutes, three times a week, of sustained Stage Two activities to your routine.
- More intense activities provide more metabolic boost.
- Exercise in the morning; this keeps the metabolism higher throughout the day.
- If you have the time and energy, exercise twice a day. This elevates the metabolism and keeps it higher throughout the day. A workable routine might include 30 minutes of activity in the morning with a "miniboost" at noon and perhaps again in the evening.
- Do something every day to elevate your RMR.

metabolic rate is comparatively low if you are overfat. When you lose weight by exercise, however, you lose fat but gain muscle, and the more muscle you have, the higher your resting metabolic rate. Even at rest, muscle is consuming calories to maintain itself, and the more muscle you have, the more calories you'll expend at rest. Two individuals of the same height and weight, one of them fat and the other muscular, will have markedly different metabolisms, and the more muscular of the two will have a higher RMR and can eat much more without gaining weight. Indeed, when you replace 10 pounds of fat with 10 pounds of muscle, your weight remains the same but you can expect to expend 500 or more additional kilocalories each day at rest. And the more muscle you build, the more you'll increase your RMR, making weight loss or maintenance even easier to sustain.

KEEP WEIGHT LOSS IN PERSPECTIVE

A BMI of 21 or 22 is a good goal to strive for, but for many of us, it's perhaps an improbable goal. In terms of health, lean is preferable to plump and plump is better than obese, but if the effort to lose weight becomes overwhelming, supplanting other activities that give you pleasure or add meaning to your life—such as double-fudge walnut brownies or going to the opera instead jogging—it may help to remember that the quality of life is just as important as the quantity of life.

AGING AND STRENGTH

So much for form. Now let's move on to function. While you're losing fat and gaining muscle, several other important changes will be taking place to improve the way you look, the way you feel and feel about yourself, and the way you get about during the day. According to conventional thinking, a hunched back and stooped posture are emblematic of aging, suggesting the crushing, inevitable weight of years. It is widely held that we inevitably begin sliding down a very slippery slope along which increasing years cause declining strength, which leads to sedentary living, which leads to further declining strength, which leads to more sedentary living. Eventually we are unable to do any of the things we have to do to get through the day without help, increasing our dependence on others as well as our risk of all the diseases associated with sedentary living.

Certainly muscular weakness can lead to increased risk of falls and a decreasing ability to live independently. For example, about 40 percent of those 65 and older fall at least once a year.[41] For most, these falls are relatively minor, but for many they result in possibly life-threatening fractures. Even the fear of falling can begin to severely restrict an individual's activities, leading to social isolation and lack of activity that create a downward spiral to increasing disability and dependence on others.

In this scheme, the equation of cause-and-effect relations linking aging, frailty, and dependence looks something like this:

aging = loss of strength = declining activity = frailty = dependence

But it's not a one-way street, with aging causing dependence. Rather, it's a two-way street. Aging may contribute to loss of strength, but loss of strength also contributes to aging, and this decline in strength is not at all inevitable. The other side of the equation linking age with strength looks like this:

increased activity = improved strength = physical vigor = independence = slowed aging

Thus, whether or not we are old is a matter not just of chronology, but of our ability to function fully and independently. Much of what conventional wisdom calls aging is rather the complications of disuse.[42,43]

NORMAL DECLINE VERSUS DISEASE

At about the age of 30, on average, we typically reach a peak in terms of muscle strength, and from then on, assuming we don't do anything to slow or reverse the trend, strength begins to decline slowly, with as much as a 45 percent decline occurring by age 85.[44-46] Among women, incidentally, this decline in strength with age seems to be less marked, perhaps because of fundamental inequities in the way men and women tend to divide up housework; men often become significantly less active when they retire, taking to the recliner, TV remote in hand, while their wives continue to do the bulk of the household chores and thus are generally more physically active well into old age.

As with most of the other markers of age, whether loss of muscle strength is the inevitable or largely the result of inactivity remains to be determined. Is typical in a largely sedentary society truly normal? We probably do tend to lose some strength as a normal aspect of growing older, (even trained athletes seem to lose muscle strength after the age of 60 or 65, for reasons that aren't understood), but most older adults certainly lose much more strength than they need to, even when completely healthy, because they tend to reduce their activity levels.[47]

EVEN AGING MUSCLES RESPOND TO TRAINING

Countering the conventional wisdom that "old" muscles don't respond to training are numerous studies showing that older men and women who train for strength improve not only their muscular strength, but with it their ability to live more independent, fuller lives. Although physical activity of any type will improve strength, more intense Stage Two activities, and particularly resistance training, are most beneficial. When older men and women incorporate strength-training activities into their exercise routines, even those who have been sedentary for years can achieve significant gains in strength, reversing the trend toward extreme, even disabling, weakness and slowing the general decline in strength associated with age.

After one 12-week strength training program, for example, a group of adults aged 60 to 72 benefited from significant muscle strength increases: a 107 percent increase in the strength of the knee extensors and a 227 percent increase in the strength of the knee flexors. This increase in strength was accompanied by increased muscle size as well.[48]

The benefits of strength training for even the very old have been well-documented. Harvard's Maria Fiatarone, for example, found strength increases of 174 percent among a group of men aged 86 to 96 after eight weeks of strength training.[49] Several investigations at Tufts University in 1988-90 also documented the benefits of strength training, even for subjects in their nineties. More recently, at the University of Maryland, these findings have been extended to show still more clearly that there is no age barrier to strength training and that the health benefits may be broader than previously thought. In one segment of the study, subjects in their sixties increased their lower body strength by 41 percent after 14 weeks of total-body strength training. In another segment, subjects whose average age was 59 increased their strength by 45 percent and their bone density by 3.8 percent, significantly reducing their risk of osteoporosis.[50-52]

The message here? Contrary to what seems to be common sense, it may be that as we get older, strength training becomes increasingly important. In other words, it's never too late to benefit from an active life. However, don't wait until you're older to consider building some muscle. Strength training, in particular, as early as possible in adulthood or middle age, when the most strength gains can be made, will build a reserve of strength, muscle, and bone mass to help delay or prevent any frailty that might be an inevitable aspect of aging. We will discuss this topic in more detail in part III.

OSTEOPOROSIS

Muscular weakness and postural changes not only affect appearance, or our ability to live life fully at any age, they can also reflect the potential presence of serious health problems, particularly osteoporosis, a progressive loss of bone mineral density (BMD) and weakening of the bones.

Altogether, osteoporosis affects some 24 million Americans, costing over $10 billion annually in health care expenses, a figure that's expected to double in the next 25 years as the population ages. By some estimates, osteoporosis is responsible for 70 percent of fractures in adults over 45; each year, more than 1.3 million Americans suffer fractures because of osteoporosis, including 300,000 hip fractures. In severe cases, these fractures can become frequent and crippling, or even fatal. Hip fractures among the elderly, in particular, have a one-year mortality rate of 20 percent, and 30 percent of survivors require long-term nursing home care. Osteoporosis of the spine can cause pressure on the nerves, chronic pain, and disability.[53-56]

Even if osteoporosis doesn't result in fractures, it can take a fearsome toll on quality of life, causing chronic back pain and even gastrointestinal or other problems caused by postural changes. As the curvature increases, we have to work harder to support ourselves; thus the muscles around the spine have to work harder and fatigue more quickly, causing the spine to become more and more curved.[57] This decreases the ability of the lungs to expand and take in oxygen, which leads to fatigue, which leads to increased sedentariness, which leads to increased muscle weakness, increased slouching, decreased lung function, and so on and on.

AGE AND OSTEOPOROSIS

The process of bone mineral loss typically begins around the age of 30, and the incidence increases steadily with age, so that almost 90 percent of those over 75 show some evidence of loss. Osteoporosis occurs in both men and women, but women lose bone density and suffer fractures associated with osteoporosis at about twice the rate of men.[58,59] By about the age of 80, one-sixth of men will have had a hip fracture, compared with one-third of women.[60] Why women lose bone mass more rapidly than men isn't fully understood, but osteoporosis in women seems to be linked to hormonal changes that occur with aging, particularly after menopause, when the rate of bone loss increases sharply.[61] And since men generally reach adulthood with larger, denser bones, they have more bone to lose before it becomes a health problem, which suggests an important strategy for preventing osteoporosis, assuming you start soon enough: Build bone mineral density through childhood and young adulthood, when bone mineral density can be significantly increased through diet and exercise. Then you'll have more reserves of bone later.

The conventional thinking about osteoporosis, as with so many other aspects of growing older, is that the relation of aging to osteoporosis and frailty is one of inevitability; the equation might look something like this:

aging = osteoporosis = frailty = declining activity

But the real relation is a two-way street; the other side of the equation looks like this:

increasing activity = stronger bones = less frailty = slower aging

By increasing activity, we decrease osteoporosis and frailty and slow the aging process. How?

PHYSICAL ACTIVITY INCREASES BONE DENSITY

Bone mass is subject to mechanical factors; when bone is stressed regularly through movement, it responds by increasing mineral density. When bone is not stressed regularly, it loses density. Thus athletes have more bone mass than sedentary individuals, and the most bone mass in those areas most stressed (the bones in the preferred arm of a tennis player will show more density).

Studies of osteoporosis in older women have shown that the rate of bone tissue loss can be slowed, stopped, and to a limited extent reversed through regular exercise, suggesting once again that the supposed normal changes associated with aging aren't normal at all but merely typical of a sedentary population. In a limited study of postmenopausal women, Fiatarone and colleagues found that women who engaged in high-intensity strength training twice a week for a year averaged a two-gram increase in total body bone mineral content.[62] An equal number of women of the same age who didn't engage in such exercise lost 33 grams of bone tissue in the same period. The women who exercised also increased their strength and muscle mass and improved their balance.

The following are some principles to keep in mind about aging, exercise, and osteoporosis:

- Any exercise is better than none, but low-intensity Stage One activities probably aren't as effective as Stage Two activities, and of Stage Two activities, careful resistance training that builds strength will be most beneficial. Swimming and cycling, in which the weight is supported, probably won't be as effective.

- Bones respond to unaccustomed loads by adding mineral; because bones won't respond effectively to loads to which they've been accustomed, they must be carefully overloaded to stimulate bone growth. However, those with advanced osteoporosis need to approach any exercise, but particularly resistance training, with caution and should consult with a physician first.

- Exercise, and particularly strength-building activities, not only build bone mineral density, they also provide the muscular strength necessary for improved balance, reducing the risk of falls and thus of fractures. And added muscle mass, strength, and flexibility reduce the risk of injury, even when a fall occurs.

- Bones build density only where loads are applied. Thus jogging might increase BMD in the legs and, perhaps to a lesser extent, in the lower spine, but won't do much for the upper spine or arms. An effective exercise program to prevent osteoporosis should systematically work the entire body.

- Consistency is important. The bones begin to "dump" calcium, even during relatively short periods of inactivity. Take a vacation from work, if you want, but not from activity.

- Hormone replacement therapy in postmenopausal women has been shown to reduce the rate of bone mineral loss.

- Dietary calcium is also an important part of good bone health. The recommended dietary allowance for adults over 25 is 800 milligrams of calcium a day, although the National Osteoporosis Foundation recommends 1,000, and postmenopausal women not on estrogen replacement probably should up that to 1,500 milligrams. And contrary to what many think, that doesn't mean you have to drink glass after glass of milk. Dietary calcium is abundant not only in milk, but in yogurt, leafy green vegetables, tofu, and corn tortillas. A cup of 1% milk or a cup of low- or nonfat yogurt has about 300 milligrams of calcium; a three-ounce can of salmon has about 200 milligrams; six ounces of calcium-fortified orange juice has about 200 milligrams; one cup of cooked, chopped broccoli has about 350 milligrams.[63]

- Use calcium supplements with caution. Calcium supplements may be a good idea, particularly for women who have cut back on dairy products to lose weight. But Canadian researchers analyzed 70 brands of supplements and found that those made from natural sources such as bonemeal, dolomite (a type of limestone), and crushed oyster shells contained dangerously high levels of lead. This is of particular concern for pregnant women and young people who take supplements because they're allergic to milk products. The researchers found that supplements with laboratory-produced calcium carbonate (as in some antacids) were much lower in lead.[64]

- Dietary calcium or supplementation aren't effective unless the body also has sufficient vitamin D. The body manufactures vitamin D on exposure to sunlight, so those living in the South or Southwest probably get enough. Older adults who don't get out much or those living in northern climates may not get enough sunlight to manufacture sufficient vitamin D, in which case supplementation is important.

- It's not clear whether dietary calcium or supplementation is all that effective in the absence of physical activity. Think of calcium as the raw material and exercise as the work necessary to turn that raw material into something useful, such as increased bone mineral density and a lowered risk of osteoporosis. You can't build a brick wall without bricks; likewise, a pile of bricks is just a pile of bricks unless someone makes them into a wall. In the same way, you won't get the full benefit of calcium unless you take it along with the stimulus of exercise.

ARTHRITIS

Arthritis—inflammation of the joints accompanied by pain and sometimes structural changes—is epidemic in this country, and there seems to be a clear association between aging and arthritis. By the time we're 60, most of us have at least a "touch" of arthritis, most likely in the joints of the hands, feet, or knees, a bit of stiffness in the morning, or perhaps some swelling in the joints. It's an epidemic of pain and physical limitation that costs the national economy billions of dollars annually in lost productivity and medical expenses. But no dollars-and-cents figures can encompass the cost to arthritis sufferers in terms of diminished quality of life.

Worse, arthritis, like so many other diseases we associate with aging, creates a vicious cycle of pain, declining activity, increasing frailty, and accelerated aging. And unfortunately, people with arthritis have historically been discouraged by their physicians from regular activity, making the arthritis worse, not better. Meanwhile, this increased sedentariness is contributing to an increased risk of all the other life-threatening diseases that we associate with lack of exercise.

TYPES OF ARTHRITIS

Arthritis can be divided into two broad categories: rheumatoid arthritis and osteoarthritis. Rheumatoid arthritis is a metabolic disease and involves inflammation of membranes around the joints; it can afflict children and young adults, and it can be a serious, even crippling, disease.

The most common type of arthritis, and the type of concern to us here, is osteoarthritis or degenerative arthritis. This type of arthritis is the result of injuries or wear and tear on the joints. It is characterized by degeneration of the cartilage in joints, so it seems reasonable that the risk of osteoarthritis would go up with age; as we live longer,

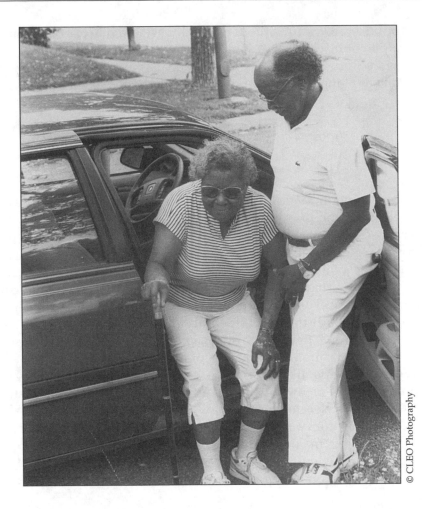

© CLEO Photography

there is simply more time for our joints to suffer wear and tear and eventually wear out, becoming inflamed, stiff, and painful.

But if osteoarthritis results from injury or wear and tear on the joints, wouldn't it also seem reasonable to assume that in our sedentary and relatively safe society, osteoarthritis would be less and less common than in more active, robust societies? After all, sitting in front of the TV all evening doesn't put much wear and tear on the joints. And wouldn't it also seem reasonable to assume that activities such as brisk walking, jogging, or swimming would increase the risk of osteoarthritis by increasing wear and tear on the joints? By becoming physically active, are we in fact trading a reduced risk of heart disease for an increased risk of arthritis pain and disability later in life?

Not at all. In fact, although all of these assumptions about arthritis and activity seem reasonable enough, they're also wrong.

JOINTS RESPOND TO PHYSICAL ACTIVITY

First, there's no evidence that sensible physical activity increases the risk of arthritis. We emphasize sensible physical activity here because inappropriate training habits can increase the risk of osteoarthritis—overtraining, training while injured, training through pain, or training despite underlying and uncorrected joint abnormalities can all add to the wear and tear on joints, and we'll have more to say on sensible training in part III.

Not only is there no evidence that sensible exercise causes arthritis, it also appears that using the joints during regular exercise actually seems to reduce the risk of joint problems, probably by increasing the flow of oxygen and nutrients to the tissues in the joints and by stimulating the growth of new tissue. And because being overweight adds significantly to the wear and tear on the weight-bearing joints of the feet, knees, and ankles, and thus to the risk of osteoarthritis, regular exercise also protects the joints by contributing to weight loss.

Thus more and more health professionals, as well as the Arthritis Foundation, are endorsing a new philosophy, encouraging regular physical activity both for those with arthritis and as a means of prevention.[65] The emphasis is on repetitive aerobic activities such as walking, cycling, and swimming. Gentle stretching to improve flexibility and range of motion is also recommended, and careful resistance training to build muscular strength is also important, as strong muscles help support the joints and protect them from injury or irritation. Indeed, resistance training for those with arthritis is proving particularly beneficial in building strength to protect affected joints before other types of activity such as walking are taken up.

Of course, regular physical activity won't eliminate the risk of osteoarthritis entirely; in truth, many of us, however active, can expect a bit of stiffness and pain in our joints as we get older. For most of us, though, this won't be a serious problem; the real danger we face is letting that stiffness or those nagging aches interfere with our active, vital, independent lives. When that happens, and we become more sedentary, the downward spiraling toward frailty and old age accelerates. Even when we are troubled by osteoarthritis, by remaining carefully active, we can help preserve a full range of motion in the affected joints and maintain muscle strength, and thus avoid the hazards of sedentariness. By exercising regularly and building strength, the added muscle will also help protect tender joints from the strain of daily use. If anything, then, as we grow older, and the first twinges of arthritis begin to nag at us, it's more important than ever to stay physically active.

We need to think of youth, young adulthood, and even middle age as a time to develop the mental and physical resources we need to preserve our health and vigor through a long, fulfilled third phase of life. Exercise builds the reserves of strength, endurance, and flexibility we need to carry us through our later years. Think of the first phases of life as the planning and preparation stage for the third phase. Consider, for example, the story of Flory Rodd.

DOES IT WORK IN REAL LIFE?

On an April day in 1966, Flory Rodd was sitting on a barstool in his favorite pub in Alameda, California, having a beer with drinking buddy John Brown, when the evening news came on. Flory wasn't paying much attention to the news, but around the soft edge of a couple of beers too many came something about a marathon in Boston, and it caught Flory's attention.

And at that moment, Flory's life changed.

Flory wasn't sure at the time what a marathon was, although as a native of the northeast United States, he knew it was an awfully long footrace of some sort. But nonetheless he turned to his buddy John Brown and said, "Next year, I'm going to run that thing," and John Brown allowed as how that sounded like a great idea, he'd run it too. Then they both announced to the bartender that they planned to run the Boston Marathon, and the bartender just grinned and said, "Yeah, sure. Have another beer, on me."

To say that Flory Rodd had a problem with his lifestyle at the time is putting it mildly. He was smoking two packs of cigarettes and downing as much as a fifth of vodka a day. "I was wasting my life," Flory says, "walking around in a fog all the time, hanging out in bars with borderline morons just like me. From that, I went to meeting a bunch of splendid, sober, interesting people."

Flory, now 72 and retired, was 43 when he resolved to run the

Boston Marathon. He was a flight navigator for a major airline at the time, on the San Francisco to Honolulu and Tokyo route. The day after he and John Brown decided to run the Boston Marathon, they measured out a mile-long section of roadway in front of the bar. Their plan? To run a mile that first day, two the next, three the next, and so on. In a month, they figured, the marathon would be a snap.

"We made it about a block on our first day before we were both sick to our stomachs," Flory recalls.

But they persisted. Flory isn't sure exactly what kept them motivated to stick with an activity that was so completely antithetical to their barhopping and smoking, plus made them sick to their stomachs.

"All I really wanted was to run the Boston Marathon once," Flory recalls, "so I could say I'd done it."

At first, training didn't put a crimp in Flory's drinking or smoking. He and John would plod through a block, then a couple of blocks, then three, until they were dead tired. Then they'd light up some cigs and head back to the bar for a few more beers.

"Unlikely as it seems, though," Flory recalls, "we slowly got better. It took us a month to work up to a mile. Then one evening we ran two miles around the local high school track, and we couldn't believe it. Afterward, back at the bar, John turned to me and said, 'You know, Flory, we ran two miles without stopping. That's a real accomplishment. But the really amazing thing is, we did it in only 22 minutes!' John and I still didn't know a thing about running."

During the next few months, Flory would run through the streets near his hotel in Honolulu during layovers and train with John when he was back on the mainland. Gradually, he built up his mileage to three, four, five miles, eventually making his way up to 18 miles that first year before Boston.

He was still smoking and drinking, but without really noticing it, he was gradually smoking and drinking less and less. Still, he'd carry a cigarette and a match rolled up in the sleeve of his T-shirt when he trained and light up when his workout was over. Obviously, health wasn't one of Flory's concerns; the idea of running—or doing anything at all—for his health was totally foreign to Flory at the time. "I remember just before the start of the Boston Marathon, I was so nervous I lit up right there in the middle of all those health nuts in the Hopkinton School gym and smoked the cigarette I had with me," Flory says, "the one I'd been saving for after."

FLORY RODD'S TRAINING

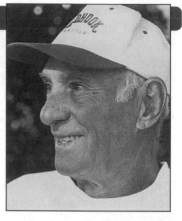

Flory Rodd, 72, retired airline navigator

Training

After several years during which Flory ran 100 or more miles a week, he had an operation on his left knee in 1978 to repair damaged cartilage. Later, he had additional operations, one on the right knee and a second on the left. After his third knee operation in 1991, Flory was forced to give up running. "I'd been putting in too many miles for too long," Flory says. "Now I walk between one and two hours a day, at a pretty good clip. I get my heart rate up, and when I come back after a walk, I'm sweating as heavily as I was when I ran. I think it's great exercise."

Impetus to change

Flory was sitting in a bar in California, drinking too much, smoking too much, and watching the evening news. When he saw a short item on the Boston Marathon, he resolved to run it.

What he likes most about an active life

"I always tell people the first thing they'll notice when they get active is they'll be more regular. You watch TV in the evening and half the commercials are for laxatives, so you have to figure constipation is a major problem in this country. But seriously, one of the things I like best is just the way I feel; there's a remarkable difference between how I felt in my drinking days and how I feel now. Now I feel awake and alive."

Advice

"Don't do what I did. Train prudently and pay attention to your aches and pains; don't try training through them. Another important thing, if you're going to walk or jog, is to get the best pair of shoes you can find. I trained too long in cheap shoes. And stay off concrete; do at least half of your walking or running on dirt trails if you can."

Flory completed that first Boston Marathon in 3:05:51 (an injury delayed his buddy John's ambitions), an amazing time considering his haphazard health habits. And that would have been that, but fate or whatever stepped in. After the race, Flory was sitting around with the few hundred other runners eating the traditional postrace beef stew—"Awful stuff, really," Flory recalls—when he overheard some other runners talking about how if you break three hours, it means you're really running. "Otherwise," Flory heard them say, "you're just a slogger."

"That was when I decided to train even harder and come back a year later and knock five minutes off my time and be a real runner," Flory says. "No way was I going to be a slogger."

Whether or not one really has to run the 26.2 miles from Hopkinton to Boston in less than three hours to be a real runner is open to considerable debate, of course (and we hasten to add that you never have to run the Boston Marathon, or any marathon, or any race even remotely similar to a marathon, to achieve optimal health through exercise).

But no matter, Flory had a new goal, and the more he ran, the better he felt. For several years after he broke three hours in Boston (in 1968) and became a real runner, Flory continued to keep a cigarette and wooden match rolled up in his shirtsleeve for a postrun smoke. In fact, Flory never made a conscious effort to give up either smoking or his devotion to beer or vodka, but over time his desire for both alcohol and tobacco dwindled, until one day, more or less unnoticed, he no longer indulged in either.

When Flory says he "felt better," he didn't necessarily mean in the sense that he felt physically healthier; certainly he did, but Flory's experience with the active life was actually much more complex than that, and thus much like the experiences of all of us who've gotten up out of our easy chairs for a brisk walk around the block.

Flory had taken up and was maintaining an active life for a variety of reasons, none of which at first glance had to do with physical health. "I slept better," Flory recalls. "I felt better physically. I felt better emotionally. And I felt better about myself. My relationships with others improved. I was simply a better person when I took up running."

But along the way, as he was beginning to look better, feel better, and feel better about himself, Flory was also slowly, steadily transforming himself physically, lowering his risk of heart disease, stroke, hypertension, diabetes, at least some types of cancer, and a host of nonfatal but nonetheless debilitating conditions such as mental decline and depression. We'll consider each of these in the chapters that follow.

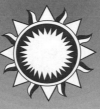

chapter 5

THE HEART OF THE MATTER

Together, Stage One and Stage Two activities will increase your heart's ability to pump blood throughout your body, improve the ability of your lungs to take in oxygen, and produce beneficial changes in your blood, all of which will reduce your risk of heart disease, heart attack, stroke, peripheral artery disease, diabetes, and probably at least some of the mental decline typically associated with aging. You'll live longer, and you'll enjoy more energy and zest for life, free of the pain, exhaustion, and disability that characterize these diseases.

Like Clyde Henry, a great many of us take up physical activity after a brush with cardiovascular disease—a heart attack, a bout of chest pain, or even a stern warning from the physician. Or maybe it's just that we're concerned. Heart disease, high blood pressure, circulatory problems, and all the other aspects of cardiovascular disease (CVD) are so pervasive in this country that they have all the markings of inevitability, especially as we grow older. Certainly no aspect of physical functioning seems to be affected more profoundly by age than the system of heart, lungs, and blood vessels that takes in oxygen and transports oxygenated blood throughout the body. But the good news is that by taking up and maintaining an active way of life, we can significantly cut our risk of cardiovascular disease and gain years of vital, engaged life.

THE HEALTHY AGING HEART

There does appear to be a decline with age in the ability of the cardiovascular system to take in oxygen and to pump oxygenated blood throughout the body and in the ability of the muscles to use that oxygen efficiently. In a practical, everyday sense, this ability to take in and use oxygen determines the body's ability to perform work, to run or walk or climb stairs, to do housework, to shop, to think, and in all ways live a vigorous, engaged, and more satisfying life. You know someone's aerobic power is on the wane when he or she huffs and puffs just climbing the half-dozen steps to the front porch.

The ability to use oxygen is commonly referred to as "oxygen uptake," or sometimes as "oxygen transport" or "aerobic power." Most often, oxygen uptake is measured as "maximal oxygen uptake" ($\dot{V}O_2max$), the maximum amount of oxygen an individual's body can use during exertion. Measures of $\dot{V}O_2max$ provide a good indication of how well the heart, lungs, blood vessels, and muscle are working together and how healthy they are. It's generally recognized that $\dot{V}O_2max$ declines by about one percent per year from a peak at about age 20 or slightly younger to half that at age 80.[1]

But is a precipitous decline inevitable, or any decline? Perhaps not. It seems, again, that what is typical of a huge population of sedentary men and women is assumed to be normal and what is normal is thus assumed to be inevitable. But much of the decline in aerobic power

---

LIFEFIT PRINCIPLES

- There is a decline with age in the ability of the cardiovascular system to supply oxygen to the body, but this decline can be slowed with regular exercise.

- Cardiovascular diseases (CVD) kill almost as many Americans each year as all other diseases combined. But the pervasiveness of CVD does not mean these diseases are inevitable. Both Stage One and Stage Two activities will *significantly* reduce your risk.

- Insulin resistance may underlie not only non-insulin-dependent diabetes mellitus (NIDDM) or adult-onset diabetes, but also two of the other biggest killers we face today: cardiovascular disease and hypertension.

- The risk of insulin resistance and NIDDM increases steadily as we age.

- Regular physical activity, primarily Stage Two activity, will significantly lower your risk of ever getting NIDDM, and if you have NIDDM, regular physical activity will reduce the severity of the disease and the risk of health- or even life-threatening complications.

---

associated with aging is not a result of aging at all, but rather of lifestyle, particularly weight gain and lack of exercise.

Although it appears that no one can entirely prevent at least some decline in oxygen transport with age, the heartening news is that men and women who remain or become active experience a much slower decline compared with sedentary individuals.[2] A study conducted by NASA and the Cooper Clinic in Dallas, for example, found that lean, active adults lost only 7 percent of their aerobic power between the ages of 30 and 70, compared with a 50 percent loss among the sedentary and overweight (see figure 5.1).[3] Better yet, you'll find that even if your aerobic power has declined more severely than it should have during years of sedentary living, once you adopt an active life at any age, you'll reverse that abnormal decline and your aerobic power will increase, along with your energy and ability to go about the tasks of daily living.

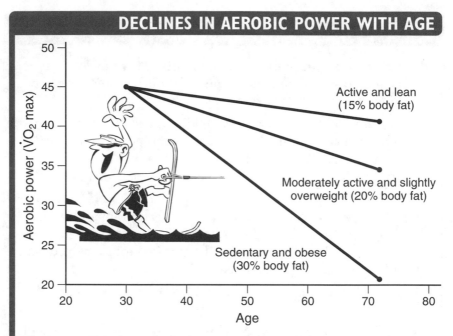

Figure 5.1   This shows the decline in aerobic power with age, the ability to take in and use oxygen. The sedentary and overweight typically lose about half their aerobic power between the ages of 35 and 70. Those who remain lean and active, however, have only a very slight decline, contradicting the common assumption that severe declines in aerobic capacity with aging are inevitable.

Adapted, by permission, from A. Jackson et al., 1995, "Changes in aerobic power of men, ages 25-70," *Medicine and Science in Sports and Exercise* 27: 113-120.

And along the way, of course, you'll also reduce your risk of cardiovascular disease.

IS CARDIOVASCULAR DISEASE INEVITABLE?

Just as the overall functioning of even a healthy cardiovascular system seems to decline slightly with age, the risk of heart disease and other diseases of the cardiovascular system increases steadily. Worse, diseases of the cardiovascular system are now so pervasive in our society, and the mortality data linking age with an increased risk are so stark and seemingly unequivocal, that cardiovascular diseases, like declines in aerobic power, have taken on all the aspects of inevitability. But are they inevitable?

The conventional thinking would have us believe that aging causes cardiovascular disease, which causes declines in functioning, reduced activity, increasing frailty, and eventually death:

aging = CVD = declines in functioning = premature death

But the chain of cause-and-effect relations between CVD and age is more properly a two-way street. Although age may increase the risk somewhat, the oncoming "lane" looks like this:

increased activity = reduced CVD = slower aging =
longer, more vigorous life

Cardiovascular diseases encompass diseases of the heart and blood vessels, and all of these related diseases are characterized by the same deleterious changes. These include changes in the blood that lead to an increased risk of blood clots in the arteries, a weakening of the heart muscle and loss of ability to pump blood efficiently, loss of elasticity in the walls of the blood vessels, and most significant, narrowing of the arteries caused by atherosclerosis—a buildup of fatty deposits called plaque.

Cardiovascular diseases—primarily coronary heart disease (chest pain and heart attack), peripheral vascular disease, and stroke—remain the number-one cause of death in the United States, together killing nearly as many Americans each year as all other diseases combined.[4] According to the American Heart Association, nearly 70 million Americans (28 percent of a population of nearly 250 million) have one or more forms of heart or blood vessel disease.[5] Coronary heart disease accounts for almost 500,000 of these deaths each year, with heart attack the leading cause of death in Americans. This year, about 1.5 million Americans will have a heart attack, and remember, for about a third of these, sudden death will be the first and only significant symptom of their disease. Overall, an estimated six million men and women alive today have a history of heart attack, angina, or both, and the vast majority of them are older adults.

RISK FACTORS YOU CAN'T CONTROL

The risk factors for cardiovascular disease are well known and fall into two basic categories: those that cannot be altered and those that can.

Age

The risk of cardiovascular disease increases steadily with age among men and women living in advanced industrial societies such as ours, and as noted above, a normal decline in cardiovascular functioning does seem to occur with age, but this is not disease, and whether or not age itself is inevitably a risk factor for CVD is open to debate. More likely, the increased risk of disease that comes with age is mostly the result of the accumulating consequences of years of bad habits; in cultures where people are generally more vigorous, atherosclerosis, hypertension, heart attack, and stroke are rare or all but nonexistent at any age.

Gender

We typically think of CVD, particularly heart attack, as almost unique to middle-aged or older men, but heart disease is also the number-one cause of death among women, claiming the lives of about 240,000 women each year. The disease is not just a man's disease that sometimes afflicts women; in fact, it's a woman's disease as well. Indeed, since 1984, more women have died each year from heart disease than have men.

Where men and women do differ is in the age at which they tend to show up in their doctors' offices with symptoms of CVD. Whereas men typically begin appearing with symptoms of CVD in their fifties, women generally don't begin showing similar symptoms until their sixties.

Women seem to be somewhat protected from CVD by estrogen, one of the hormones essential to reproduction. Estrogen acts as a vasodilator; that is, it tends to relax blood vessels, opening them up. Thus, even when decades of poor health habits have led to a build-up of plaque in a woman's coronary arteries, thanks to estrogen, the arteries are more likely to remain open, reducing the risk of blockages that shut off blood flow to the heart and cause chest pain or heart attack. Estrogen may also have some beneficial effects on blood cholesterol levels.

Until menopause, that is. Once a woman reaches menopause and her estrogen levels begin to fall, she also begins to lose the protective effects of the hormone. Very quickly, her risk of heart attack and other cardiovascular diseases rises sharply to equal that of men. Because women tend to be older than men when the first symptoms of CVD appear, the disease is also often complicated by other health problems such as diabetes, making effective treatment more difficult. Thus the mortality rate from CVD among women very quickly catches up with that for men.

Heredity

Your heredity is also a factor; if one or both of your parents had heart disease, stroke, or other diseases of the cardiovascular system, you're at increased risk as well. Thus, if you have a family history of CVD, it's imperative that you take control of those risk factors that can be changed.

RISK FACTORS YOU CAN CONTROL

Although we can't do anything about our age, gender, or genetic heritage, we can control the other risk factors that affect our hearts. The four major controllable risk factors currently recognized by the medical establishment are

- high blood pressure (higher than 140/90 millimeters of mercury);
- an unhealthful blood cholesterol profile (more than 200 milligrams per deciliter, with a high level of low-density lipoproteins, or LDLs, and low levels of more healthful high-density lipoproteins, or HDLs);
- cigarette smoking; and
- physical inactivity.

We're adding a fifth controllable risk factor, however:

- insulin resistance.

For decades, it's been known that people with hypertension (HTN) and adult-onset diabetes, otherwise known as non-insulin-dependent diabetes mellitus (NIDDM), are likely to develop cardiovascular disease. Thus the presence of the first two has long been considered a major predictor for the third, although the precise chain of cause-and-effect relations among all three has been uncertain. Recently, some investigators have begun to suspect a common cause for diabetes, hypertension, and cardiovascular disease and that these diseases are actually manifestations of the same underlying disease — insulin resistance. Insulin resistance is a controllable risk factor because it is largely the result of health habits that can be altered, including exercise and dietary habits, as we'll see shortly.

HAVE YOU BECOME HEARTSICK?

Taken together, age, gender, one's genetic predispositions, and health habits all contribute to the variety of physiological changes that increase the likelihood of disease, and these changes are manifested in several different ways, producing a variety of distinct health problems.

HEART DISEASE

The heart is a muscle roughly the size of an adult's fist. It works tirelessly throughout a lifetime to pump blood throughout the body, and when it's working properly, it never misses a beat. Never. The typical adult heart will beat about 31 million times in a year, or upward of two billion beats in a lifetime. And all it asks for all that effort is plenty of blood to keep it oxygenated and supplied with essential nutrients. Like any muscle, the heart has its own blood vessels, the coronary arteries. When healthy, these arteries keep the heart supplied with all the oxygen and nutrients it requires. And it's in these arteries that problems most often develop.

A buildup of fatty deposits inside the coronary arteries—atherosclerosis—will eventually restrict the flow of blood to the heart muscle. The buildup occurs slowly and probably begins in childhood, and it can take decades for the buildup to become severe enough to cause clinically manifest symptoms. But well before these deposits begin to affect our physical health, we're likely to experience a sense of disquiet, a subtle sense of early fatigability, a loss of zest for life, perhaps even low-grade depression.

The first clinical manifestation of atherosclerosis is often unmistakable: chest pain or angina pectoris, which occurs when the heart's need for oxygen increases beyond the ability of clogged arteries to supply it. Any demand on the heart can bring on angina; increased exertion, for example, or even a strong emotion. The pain is a dull, crushing sensation, usually, that may extend into the shoulder or arm, often on the left side. The pain is the heart's warning that it's not getting what it needs.

Heart attack occurs when the blood flow to the heart is restricted so severely that the heart muscle is damaged. Most often, a heart attack occurs when a blood clot forms in an artery, entirely cutting off the flow of blood through that vessel. Blood clots naturally in the presence of foreign substances; unfortunately, sometimes the blood reacts to plaque deposits in the arteries as if they were foreign bodies, particularly when the deposits crack and damage the vessel walls, as sometimes happens when the artery is under unaccustomed pressure due to exertion or extreme emotion. Blood clots also tend to form where the flow of blood slows; for example, where thick deposits of plaque inside the arteries have formed. Blood clots rarely form in healthy arteries.[6]

Heart attack can also occur when the coronary arteries go into spasm, often in the presence of atherosclerosis. More rarely, a piece of plaque inside the artery will break off and flow downstream to lodge where the artery narrows. And sometimes when the heart isn't getting the oxygen it needs because of narrowed coronary arteries, it will go into ventricular tachycardia, a rapid heart beat, which can lead to fibrillation, an irregular beat, loss of consciousness, and even death.

MENTAL DECLINE AND STROKE

Of all the body's organs and organ systems, the brain is the most sensitive to oxygen levels in the blood; thus anything that compromises the blood supply to the brain or the amount of oxygen available in the blood can have an impact on how the brain functions. In the worst cases, stroke occurs when the flow of blood to a portion of the brain is cut off entirely, killing or damaging brain cells.

Most strokes are caused by essentially the same processes that lead to angina or heart attack—plaque builds up in an artery in or leading to the brain, squeezing off the flow of blood. Sometimes, a clot will form in the artery, cutting off the bloodflow entirely. Other times, a clot will form somewhere else in the body, then travel to the brain to lodge in an artery there.

A stroke can also occur when a diseased artery in the brain bursts, and the risk of this happening rises sharply with hypertension. When a blood vessel bursts, cells nourished by the damaged artery are deprived of blood. At the same time, blood from the hemorrhage puts pressure on the brain, impairing function.

The brain can reroute nerve impulses around damaged areas when the damage isn't too severe, to restore at least some function, but injured brain cells can't be replaced, so prevention of stroke is vital.[7]

PERIPHERAL ARTERY DISEASE (PAD)

PAD results from the buildup of plaque in the blood vessels of the arms and legs, restricting the flow of blood to the muscles. Typically, PAD occurs in the legs, resulting in exercise-induced muscle cramping or claudication, which results in increasing difficulty simply getting up and moving about. PAD can prevent its victims from meeting the occupational, social, and personal demands of daily life, which leads to increasing sedentariness, which leads to still more of the problems that result from lack of exercise, a downward spiral to increasing disability. In the most severe cases, PAD can result in ulceration, gangrene, and ultimately amputation of the limb.

NON-INSULIN-DEPENDENT DIABETES MELLITUS (NIDDM)

Although it is not usually thought of as one of the cardiovascular diseases, we're including NIDDM here because of the underlying role of insulin resistance in both NIDDM and other CVD, and because adult-onset diabetes almost invariably accompanies one or more cardiovascular diseases.

Insulin is the essential hormone for the proper metabolism of blood sugar, regulating the way the muscles use glucose for energy. For reasons that aren't well understood, in some people, particularly the sedentary and overweight, insulin doesn't function properly; it seems that in these individuals, the cells themselves somehow become resistant to the action of insulin, so the insulin can't mediate the processes that make the glucose available to the tissues that need it. The result is that tissues starve for energy, even though ample fuel is available.

As the cells become resistant to the action of insulin and blood glucose levels rise, the body secretes more insulin in a futile effort to get energy to the cells, resulting in hyperinsulinemia. Researchers have recently found that hyperinsulinemia reduces secretion of sodium from the body, increasing blood volume and thus the risk of high blood pressure (hypertension or HTN) and the host of health problems that result, including increased risk of heart disease, kidney disease, and stroke. Hyperinsulinemia also triggers the nervous system to narrow blood vessels and causes vessel walls to thicken, making it more difficult for blood to flow through the vessels, further predisposing victims to HTN and increasing the strain on the heart. It also appears that insulin resistance is the condition underlying high levels of triglycerides and decreased levels of HDL or "good" cholesterol in the blood, both predictors of CVD, although the precise mechanism is not clear.

When insulin resistance becomes severe enough, the result is type II diabetes, also known as non-insulin-dependent diabetes mellitus, or NIDDM. The other type of diabetes, type I diabetes, or insulin-dependent diabetes mellitus (IDDM), most often occurs in men and women under the age of 20. It results from the destruction of insulin-producing beta cells in the pancreas, which investigators believe occurs when the body's own immune system attacks these cells, a malfunction that may be precipitated by a viral infection.

Because NIDDM occurs later in life, it's also called adult-onset diabetes and constitutes about 90 to 95 percent of all cases of diabetes, affecting 10 to 12 million Americans over the age of 20. The risk of NIDDM increases steadily with age, from about 20 new cases for every 10,000 adults aged 25 to 44 to about 50 new cases for every 10,000 adults over 65.

NIDDM is characterized not only by an increased resistance of the body's muscle cells to the action of insulin, but sometimes also by impaired secretion of insulin, although in some cases, those with NIDDM can actually have more insulin in their systems than normal. In his book *Staying Well*, Harvey Simon, MD, characterizes adult-onset diabetes as "starvation in the midst of plenty," a good description because in those with NIDDM, blood sugar levels can be excessively high even as the cells are starved for sugar for energy and nutrition.[8] Patients with NIDDM tend to lose weight; they drink huge volumes of liquids and are often intensely hungry. Despite voracious eating and the consumption of huge volumes of liquids, they remain hungry and thirsty because their bodies aren't able to use the energy in food. They become chronically fatigued.

Although NIDDM and IDDM are different diseases, they have similar outcomes if untreated. Together, type I and type II diabetes are the fourth leading cause of death in the United States, claiming 160,000 lives each year, with complications from the disease contributing to thousands more deaths annually.[9] All types of diabetes have the same general symptoms, including frequent urination, excessive thirst, fatigue, weakness, and weight loss. Other symptoms include tingling of the extremities, increased number of infections, blurred vision, sometimes impotence (in men) or amenorrhea (in women). The symptoms of type I diabetes can develop rapidly. Symptoms of type II come on more slowly and may not appear until months or years after the disease has begun.

As chronic diseases, both types of diabetes create enormous suffering. Diabetes is the leading cause of blindness in people aged 20 to 74 and is responsible for about one-quarter of all end-stage renal disease in the United States. Forty-five percent of those with diabetes have peripheral vascular disease, including diabetic ulcers on the feet or ankles; diabetes is the cause of an estimated 40 to 45 percent of all nontraumatic amputations in the United States.[10]

HOW TO MAKE A HEALTHY HEART

All of the risk factors contributing to CVD and NIDDM are intertwined, and when you make a favorable change in one factor, you are likely to affect them all favorably. For example, obesity raises the risk of insulin resistance, which increases the risk of high blood pressure, NIDDM, and heart disease, and lack of exercise increases the risk for both obesity and insulin resistance. High blood pressure alone increases strain on the heart, leading to heart disease and an increased risk of heart attack. Being overweight adds to the burden on the heart as well, contributing further to the risk of heart attack or chest pain. Chronic emotional stress increases blood pressure and may increase the risk of NIDDM. A high-fat diet raises cholesterol and increases the risk of atherosclerosis. Such a diet will also contribute to obesity, which again contributes to hypertension, insulin resistance, and so on.

PREVENTING CVD

The good news is that regular exercise can keep your cardiovascular system working as efficiently and as disease-free as possible throughout your life. Regular physical activity works to alter or control each of the intertwined risk factors for CVD. For example, exercise strengthens the heart muscle; exercise increases insulin sensitivity and lowers blood pressure and blood cholesterol levels; exercise appears to reduce the craving for cigarettes, making it much easier

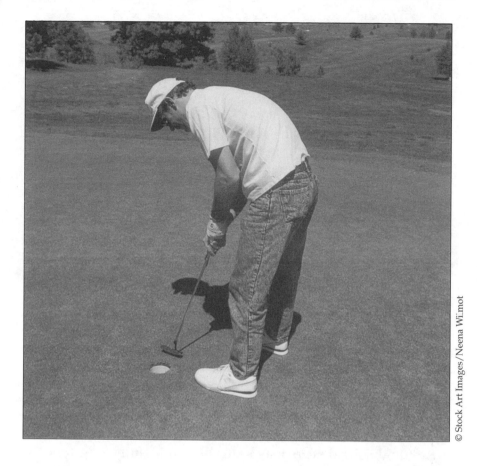

© Stock Art Images/Neena Wilmot

to quit; exercise helps us lose weight and keep it off; exercise seems to suppress the appetite and reduce the craving in some for fatty foods; and exercise even reduces stress and the likelihood of depression, which may also contribute to a risk for CVD.

Once Upon a Time

In their intriguing book, *The Paleolithic Prescription*, Eaton, Konner, and Shostak take a look at what we can learn about healthy living from the lives of our hunter-gatherer ancestors and note that, even today, in societies where everyone is more active and where diets contain much less saturated fat (fats from animal products and hydrogenated—solid—vegetable oils), cardiovascular disease is almost nonexistent.[11]

Eaton and coauthors note that the way people in traditional societies age is much more like the natural human pattern of aging than what we see in industrialized nations today. Over millions of years, they write, our bodies evolved to adapt to a hunter-gatherer or what they call a "Paleolithic lifestyle," one characterized by regular physical activity—plenty of walking, running, and, come to think of it, spear-throwing not unlike Shirley Dietderich's—and simpler diets much lower in fats and much higher in the complex carbohydrates and fiber found in fruits, vegetables, and grains.

Granted, these hunter-gatherers had a short life expectancy at birth, and many of them died in childhood from accident and infection; but according to Eaton and his colleagues, those who survived childhood and avoided death later from accident or violence could expect to live a relatively long, fit life untroubled by the diseases that plague us today.[12]

What Went Wrong?

What we like to think of as civilization is generally thought of as beginning with the development of agriculture some 10,000 years ago. With agriculture and animal husbandry came a more abundant, more regular food supply, which meant less running around chasing after dinner. Also with agriculture came villages, which meant less packing up and moving on, which hunter-gatherers were wont to do from time to time as they followed food supplies.

Although 10,000 years may seem like an awfully long time, it's practically "yesterday" compared to the millions of years humans lived as hunter-gatherers, without the benefits—or hazards—of a settled life. Ten millenia is hardly long enough for human biology to adapt effectively to our new environment. Thus our bodies and our physical needs remain those of our Paleolithic ancestors. Our flesh, at least, longs to be running through the forest, chasing or being chased. Our bodies long for a spare, healthful diet, regardless of what our civilized cravings may demand.

With the Industrial Revolution, the pace of change has accelerated even more, increasing what Eaton and coauthors call "discordance" between the conditions of our lives today and the conditions in which we evolved:

> For us, discordance between our current lifestyle and the one in which we evolved has promoted the chronic and deadly "diseases of civilization": the heart attacks, strokes,

cancer, diabetes, emphysema, hypertension, cirrhosis, and the like illnesses that cause 75 percent of all mortality in the United States and other industrialized nations.[13]

We've substituted the diseases of civilization for early death by starvation, exposure, infection, or being eaten by a predator of some sort. And although a perhaps lingering death from heart disease at 55 or 65 may seem preferable to being eaten by a bear at the age of 20 or 40, there's no reason we should be plagued by chronic disease, either. If we become more active, cut fats from our diets, eat more fiber, quit smoking, and reduce stress in our lives—that is, if we adopt a lifestyle more like that of our Paleolithic ancestors, or even more like that of traditional societies today—our risk of becoming ill or dying from the cardiovascular diseases can be significantly reduced.

College Study Findings

Among the college alumni, for instance, the most active of them experienced a reduction in their risk of death from cardiovascular diseases—primarily heart attack and stroke—of one-quarter to one-third compared with the risk among their sedentary colleagues. There was also a definite "dose-response"—the more active these alumni, the lower their risk (see figure 5.2).

The experiences of the sedentary alumni began to diverge from those of the more active men relatively early in life, so that by about age 50, sedentary alumni were already beginning to die from heart disease at a faster rate than their more active peers, and the gap widened with increasing age. The message here? Youth does protect us from many of our follies, including an unhealthful diet and lack of exercise. But by middle age, these bad habits will begin to catch up with us and take their toll.[14-19]

The Benefits of Change

Fortunately, even if you've been inactive for years, that doesn't mean it's too late to benefit from a more active way of life. Alumni who changed from sedentary to active had essentially the same experience as alumni who had always been active—or more precisely, active throughout the course of the study. Likewise, alumni who had always been sedentary or who dropped activity had almost identical experiences. Alumni who had always been active had a 37

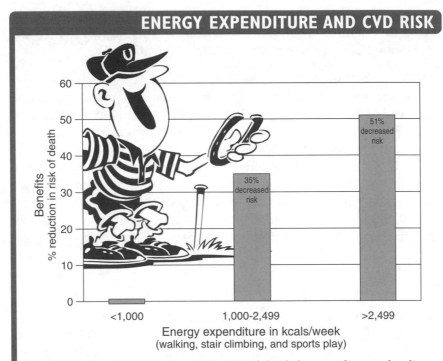

Figure 5.2   As activity increases, the risk of death from cardiovascular disease decreases.

percent reduced risk of death from CVD compared to their sedentary peers; men who took up activity had a 46 percent reduced risk (see figure 5.3).

The fact that those who took up exercise actually had a somewhat lower risk of heart disease than those who had always been active needs some explanation. First, the differences aren't statistically significant; in real-world terms, their experiences really are more or less identical. But as we discussed in part I, there is also a reasonable explanation for why those in the College Study who took up activity fared slightly better than their always-active peers. Typically, when we make one healthful change in the way we live, we tend to make other beneficial changes as well—we take up activity, we cut fats in our diets, we make changes to reduce stress, and so on—all of which contribute to a reduced risk. On the other hand, it may be that those who had always been active had a sense of their own invulnerability; they may not have been as careful about their diets or other habits as the converts.

Any physical activity—both Stage One and Stage Two—will ben-

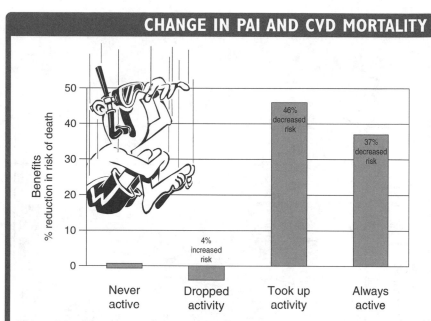

Figure 5.3 It's never too late to get cardiovascular benefits from activity. Sedentary alumni who took up activity enjoyed about the same cardiovascular benefits as the alumni who had always been active.

efit the cardiovascular system and reduce the risk of CVD. Anything that gets you up on your feet and moving about is going to help cut your risk. When it comes to preventing CVD, it appears that although intensity is important, so is consistency and duration of the activity; you need to be active regularly, without long breaks of days or weeks between exercise, and you need to strive for longer periods of activity, say 30 minutes or more in each session.

PREVENTING NIDDM

Considering the suffering that diabetes can cause, prevention and effective treatment are vital. The good news is that physical activity operates in two ways. It prevents NIDDM, and when the disease does occur, it moderates its harmful effects (see figure 5.4).

Although the causes of insulin resistance and NIDDM are not well understood, we know that the strongest predisposing factors for NIDDM are a family history of the disease and obesity (75 percent of those with NIDDM are overweight), and although you can't do anything about your genetic heritage, you can do something about your weight, as we've seen. Thus exercise has long been advocated

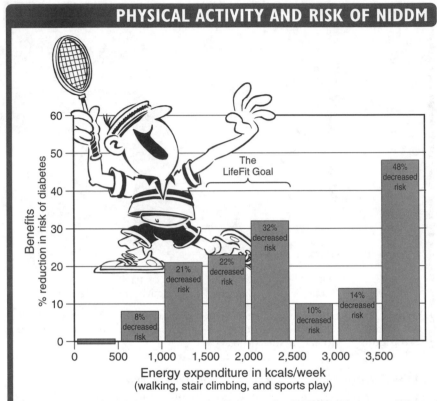

PHYSICAL ACTIVITY AND RISK OF NIDDM

Figure 5.4   As you become more active, your risk of NIDDM drops steadily and you enjoy the benefits of improved health, vigor, and reduced risk of CVD and all the ills associated with NIDDM. Those who achieved the LifeFit goal for activity (2,000 kcals/week) had the best outcomes; those who were more active appear to have a slightly higher risk than those somewhat less active, though their risk is still lower than that of the sedentary. How do we explain the very low risk of the most active? It's likely that the number of subjects active at this level was too small to yield meaningful results.

for the management of NIDDM through weight loss. More recently, exercise has also been found to directly increase insulin sensitivity, reducing the symptoms and the need for medication when the disease has already occurred.

Until quite recently, however, it wasn't entirely certain that physical activity was also effective in preventing insulin resistance and NIDDM, although the arguments in favor of exercise's protective effect are compelling:

1. Physically active societies have less NIDDM.

2. As populations become more sedentary, the incidence of NIDDM increases.

3. Physical activity increases sensitivity to insulin.

4. Greater physical activity is associated with decreased prevalence of NIDDM in a variety of studies.

Direct evidence that physical activity protects against NIDDM was demonstrated in a prospective study of college alumni aged 35 to 74. The occurrence of NIDDM in the alumni was reduced by six percent for every increase of 500 kilocalories per week in walking, stair climbing, and moderately vigorous Stage Two leisure-time activities, the amount of energy burned during an hour of jogging at 5 miles an hour, or an hour of cycling at 10 miles an hour, or swimming laps at a moderate effort.

Light Stage One activity is effective in preventing NIDDM, but it doesn't seem to be as effective as more vigorous Stage Two activities that get the heart beating and sweat flowing, a finding recently substantiated by a study of 87,253 American nurses aged 34 to 59 (see figure 5.5). During eight years of follow-up, women in that study who engaged in vigorous exercise at least once a week had only two-thirds the risk of NIDDM compared with women of the same age who did not exercise vigorously.[20,21]

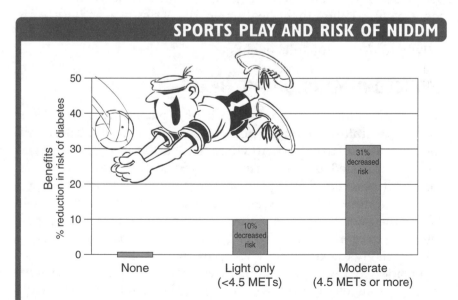

Figure 5.5 Those who participated in moderately vigorous Stage Two activity (4.5 METs or more), had only one-third the risk of NIDDM as those who were active, but who did not include Stage Two activities. The message here? The greatest benefits in terms of risk reduction come from Stage Two activity that works up a sweat and elevates the heart rate.

This inverse relation between exercise and NIDDM persisted even when other factors such as body composition, weight gain since college, history of high blood pressure, and parental history of diabetes were taken into account. In other words, exercise seems to improve insulin sensitivity and reduce the risk of NIDDM, even in the presence of high blood pressure, obesity, or a genetic predisposition to the disease. If you exercise, you'll be less likely to get NIDDM, and even if you exercise and remain overweight, even if you exercise and continue to have high blood pressure (which aren't likely), even if you have a genetic predisposition to NIDDM, if you exercise regularly, you'll still reduce your risk.

HOW ACTIVITY REDUCES RISK

Physical activity reduces the risk of CVD and NIDDM in several ways. Some of these mechanisms work to prevent "acute" disease, such as heart attacks or strokes. Other mechanisms work to reduce the risk of "chronic" disease, such as atherosclerosis, angina, and peripheral artery disease, which contribute to the occurrence of acute events. Although the health benefits of physical activity begin with step one, it will take about six months of regular physical activity to realize the full benefits.

REDUCED DEMAND ON THE HEART

Perhaps the most significant benefit of a physically active life is reduced overall strain on the heart during any activity. Chest pain and heart attacks usually occur when the heart's demand for oxygen can't be supplied because arteries going to the heart have been narrowed or even blocked by plaque, or when blood clots form where plaque occurs. Through regular activity, however, you can reduce the overall demand on the heart in any given activity; then, even if your arteries have been clogged by years of bad habits, you're still less likely to experience chest pain or heart attack.

Consider, for example, a slightly overweight middle-aged American male—an average guy we'll call Joe. He hasn't been physically active since his high school football days, and now he's on his way to Hawaii for a two-week vacation.

Joe has hypertension. He smokes. He is overly fond of hamburgers and extra mayo. If we were to examine the interiors of Joe's arteries, we would find they are badly narrowed with plaque. Joe is also under considerable stress on the job, and now he's under still more stress because he's late for his flight and will have to hurry to make it to the gate in time. But when he gets to the airport, he finds that the conveyor that moves people from one end of the terminal to the other has been shut down for repairs, and of course, as is always the case when one is late, Joe's flight leaves from the most distant gate, seemingly beyond the horizon. Joe is also a savvy traveler who knows not to check luggage if he can help it, so he has all of his clothes, toiletries, and other travel paraphernalia stuffed into a carry-on bag that seems to weigh as much as a small imported car.

Joe sets off at a slow jog through the terminal, lugging his carry-on with him. At once, he's sweating and puffing in a way he hasn't for years; his working muscles are demanding more oxygen, and his heart begins to beat faster to pump more blood to his working muscles, which means his heart is working harder and needs more oxygen as well, so his coronary arteries try to expand to allow more blood to flow through.

And there's the rub. His coronary arteries, clogged by years of imprudent eating and lack of exercise, can no longer expand effectively to supply his heart with enough blood to meet this new demand for oxygen, and quite suddenly, Joe feels a crushing pain in his chest. It's severe angina. But Joe pushes on—he has had chest pains like this before and dismissed them as indigestion. Joe ignores the pain, or tries to. Besides, the gate is just ahead. Joe figures he can rest then.

Unfortunately, as Joe's coronary arteries try to expand under the unaccustomed pressure, the plaque in one of them cracks like an old, stiffened rubber hose, damaging the wall of the artery. A blood clot quickly begins to form at the site of the crack. As Joe stops at the gate and fumbles for his ticket, the clot completely shuts off blood to a portion of his heart muscle. It suddenly feels as if someone has slugged him in the chest with a sledgehammer. Joe has just had a heart attack.

The new Joe: But let's change the scenario somewhat. Let's say for the past year before his vacation, Joe has been walking briskly for 30 minutes, three times a week. Let's also say that, now and then, feeling increasingly frisky, he's even thrown in an occasional jog. He has also increased the amount of Stage One puttering about through-out each day, including taking the stairs instead of the elevator at work and walking the dog each evening.

Now Joe gets to the airport just as late as in the previous scenario, finds the conveyor closed for repairs, and still lugging his overstuffed carry-on, breaks into a slow jog. But because Joe has been exercising regularly, the muscles in his legs are larger and stronger. Also, his muscles now can use oxygen more efficiently—an increased number of capillaries in the muscle, the result of regular exercise, allows more oxygen to be pumped to the cells that need it, which means they can work harder without fatigue. And within each muscle cell, other changes have taken place, including an increase in the size and number of mitochondria, tiny bodies that are the cell's "power-house." The mitochondria convert the energy in food into the energy currency the cells can use, a molecule called adenosine triphosphate (ATP). Having more and larger mitochondria in each cell means each cell can convert more food to more energy and thus do more work without fatigue. Thanks to regular exercise, Joe's muscles have also learned how to store more glycogen and fat, so the muscle cells have a richer supply of food to convert to energy.

Joe's arteries and lungs have also benefited from his regular exercise. His arteries have become more elastic, better able to expand to let more blood through, and his lungs have a greater "tidal volume"; that is, they can take in more air with each breath. Joe has also learned to breathe more rapidly with less fatigue, all of which means he can take in more oxygen.

Most significant, Joe's heart has also become stronger, thanks to his active life. The heart is a muscle, and like any muscle, it benefits from regular physical activity by becoming stronger. The walls of Joe's heart muscle have thickened as a result of his increased activity, which means his heart can contract more forcefully and pump more blood with each beat, which means that at any given workload, it doesn't have to beat as fast as it once did to supply blood to the rest of the body. In other words, it can supply blood with less effort, which means it needs less oxygen at any level of work, which means less risk of heart attack or angina.

Joe is still jogging just as quickly, and the carry-on bag is just as heavy—he is still performing the same amount of work—but be-cause his ability to perform work has increased due to all the changes in his heart, lungs, and muscles, the effort isn't as demanding relative to his expanded capacity. Now Joe can jog through the terminal with a significantly better chance of making it to the gate feeling grand and ready for two weeks in Hawaii.

Furthermore, as we've seen, regular exercise is the most effective means of weight loss, so it's quite likely Joe will have lost a few pounds during the year since he took up a more active way of life. Thus the new Joe will have less weight to lug through the terminal (even if his carry-on is as heavy as before), which means overall he'll have to do less work getting to the gate, and thus his risk of reaching the limits of his cardiovascular system and having a heart attack is even lower.

Even if Joe's arteries are still as clogged with plaque as they were before he took up activity a year ago, even if he still smokes, even if he still has high blood pressure, even if he's still overweight, if he has engaged in brisk walking regularly and reduced his body's demand for oxygen at any given level of effort, he'll still have reduced his risk of heart attack.[22]

Of course, after a year of walking and jogging three times a week, it's not likely that Joe would still be as overweight, still a smoker, or still hypertensive. When people begin exercising regularly, they tend to make other healthful changes in their lives; it's quite likely Joe would have quit smoking, or at least cut back, and perhaps he would have modified his diet to eliminate some of the fats, contributing to additional weight loss and perhaps a reversal of his atherosclerosis, or at least a slowing of its progression. Regular exercise will have reduced Joe's risk of CVD in a variety of other ways, and thus his risk of dying while he makes his way through the terminal.

CHANGES IN BLOOD COAGULATION

As we've noted, heart attacks and strokes most often are caused by blood clots forming in arteries that have been narrowed by plaque. By some estimates, fully 90 percent of heart attacks are brought on by clot formation at the site of arterial narrowing. But there's good evidence that after a period of regular exercise, changes occur in the blood's tendency to clot; exercise seems to reduce the "stickiness" of platelets (clot-forming components of the blood) in arteries. These platelets are less likely to stick together and form clots, thus reducing the risk of clot formation where arteries are narrowed by atherosclerosis. Exercise also seems to produce changes in what is called "fibrinolytic activity" in the blood. Fibrinogen is a protein essential to the formation of clots to stop bleeding from injury. This is important, of course, when you've cut yourself. However, the body also considers the lesions caused by plaque formations on arterial walls to be injuries, and that's not so good when a clot forms in a narrowed artery. But regular exercise increases fibrinolysis, the dissolution of fibrinogen.

Thus, even if Joe's arteries remain narrowed by atherosclerosis, if he has taken up and maintained an active life, his blood is much less likely to form clots where his arteries are narrowed and his risk of heart attack is greatly reduced.[23-26]

REDUCED BLOOD LIPIDS AND LIPOPROTEINS

Of more importance to those of us contemplating change to an active life after years of artery-clogging sedentary living and dietary indiscretions, it's also clear that atherosclerosis can be reversed through exercise, diet changes, smoking cessation, and stress reduction.[27-29]

Exercise reduces lipids (fats) and lipoproteins (cholesterol) in the blood, meaning that there are fewer fats and less cholesterol to be deposited on the walls of our arteries. Exercise also changes the nature of lipoproteins in the blood, increasing by 5 to 15 percent the level of high-density lipoproteins or HDLs, the so-called good cholesterol that is known to reduce the risk of heart disease, apparently by scouring plaque deposits off arterial walls, thus reversing atherosclerosis to increase blood flow through the arteries and further reduce the risk of heart attacks, stroke, angina pectoris, and other maladies associated with atherosclerosis.[30,31]

LOWERED BLOOD PRESSURE

Hypertension (high blood pressure) is a problem of epidemic proportions in industrialized countries. Yet in less advanced cultures where men and women consume fewer fatty foods, use less salt and less alcohol, and do more physical labor, hypertension is rare.

Blood pressure is a measure of the resistance to blood flow in the blood vessels. With each beat, the heart pumps blood throughout the body. The amount of pressure in the arteries while the heart is pumping is called the systolic blood pressure, the higher of the two numbers in a blood pressure reading. Diastolic blood pressure, the second (lower) reading, records the pressure in the arteries when the heart relaxes between beats so its chambers can refill. The higher your blood pressure, the harder your heart must work to pump blood throughout your body.

Our blood pressure is in constant flux throughout the day. During physical or mental activity, blood pressure tends to rise; during rest or sleep, it's lower. Emotional stress can elevate the blood pressure significantly. Certain drugs can as well, such as the caffeine in coffee and the nicotine in cigarettes. There's also considerable variability from person to person as to what is normal blood pressure, but it's clear that the lower your blood pressure, in general, the better your health. The most widely accepted standard for "healthful" blood pressure is less than 140/90 millimeters of mercury; "borderline" high is 140-160/90-95; and a blood pressure higher than 160/95 is considered hazardous.

Men with hypertension — blood pressures greater than 160/95 — have a threefold increase throughout their lives in their risk of developing CHD and a fourfold increase in their risk for congestive heart failure. High blood pressure also increases the risk of stroke, kidney failure, and a host of other diseases. The same trends exist for women, although their risk of disease is lower at any given level of blood pressure.

The bad news is that the risk of hypertension (HTN)—and thus of all the ills that hypertension leads to—seems to increase steadily with age, and as many as 50 to 60 percent of people over 60 probably have at least low-grade hypertension. As with so many other changes that occur with aging, however, and given the fact that in more active societies HTN is virtually nonexistent, it's not clear that this increase is inevitable.

The good news is that regular physical activity lowers both systolic and diastolic blood pressure by about 10 millimeters of mercury in men and women with mild hypertension, and it appears that for the greatest benefits, this activity should be moderately vigorous Stage Two activity.[32] Although any activity is better than none at all, among the alumni, those who engaged in some Stage Two activities each week had a significantly lower risk of developing HTN. Even the relatively inactive (500 kilocalories per week) had a much lower risk of HTN if they worked up a sweat (see figure 5.6).

Not only does exercise lower hypertension in most cases, among hypertensives who exercise, there is also a protective effect; that is, even if you are hypertensive, even if exercise doesn't lower your

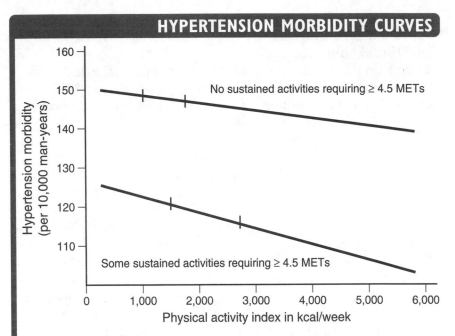

HYPERTENSION MORBIDITY CURVES

No sustained activities requiring ≥ 4.5 METs

Some sustained activities requiring ≥ 4.5 METs

Hypertension morbidity (per 10,000 man-years)

Physical activity index in kcal/week

Figure 5.6 Those who add at least one session of moderately vigorous Stage Two activities (4.5 METs or more) to their weekly routine have a significantly lower risk of hypertension than those who are active, but not as vigorously. For the most benefit in terms of hypertension, then, and particularly if you are pressed for time, the message here is that it helps to work up a sweat.

blood pressure—though it probably will—exercise still protects you from many of the ills that hypertension causes. Hypertensive men and women who are physically active have a lower all-cause mortality than their unfit but normotensive peers.[33] Among hypertensive college alumni, the most active had only a third the risk of heart disease compared with the least active, and their experiences compared rather favorably with their normotensive peers. Even those alumni whose parents had hypertension, suggesting a genetic predisposition to the disease, enjoyed significant protection through activity—the most active had about one-fourth the risk of heart disease compared with the least active.[34-38]

LARGER, MORE ELASTIC BLOOD VESSELS

Upon the death of 70-year-old Clarence DeMar, who competed in 33 Boston Marathons (his last at age 66), an autopsy reportedly re-

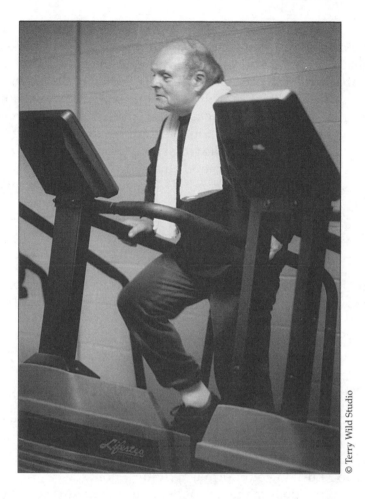

© Terry Wild Studio

vealed DeMar's coronary arteries to be two or three times larger than average.

Of course, skeptical researchers wonder if DeMar had larger than normal arteries because he ran, or was he able to run so well because he had larger than normal arteries? (And again, one has to wonder if DeMar's arteries were larger than normal, or were his arteries normal and "the norm" merely typical of the undertrained and unfit?)

Actually, it may not be the size of the arteries that is important as much as the ability of the arteries to expand during exertion, to carry more blood when needed. William Haskell at Stanford examined cross sections of the arteries of superfit, moderately fit, and sedentary older men and found there wasn't much difference in the size of their arteries, oddly enough (DeMar's huge arteries may in fact have been the products of good genes, not his training). However, Haskell did find that during exertion, the arteries in the more fit individuals were able to dilate more than those of the sedentary. What this could mean for people like Joe or the rest of us is that even if a coronary artery remains narrowed by atherosclerosis despite exercise, the artery will be able to expand more fully as needed, reducing the risk of fatigue, chest pain, or, in the worst case, a heart attack. More elastic arteries also mean a better blood supply to other areas of the body, such as the brain and extremities, preventing PAD, stroke, and perhaps even some dementias.

THE BIG PICTURE

To summarize, the many changes in the cardiovascular system that occur with regular Stage One and Stage Two activity contribute to an overall reduction in the risk of heart attack, stroke, PAD, NIDDM, and all the other ills associated with these diseases. Even if you smoke, as mentioned previously, physical activity has a protective effect. Even if you are obese or have high blood pressure, physical activity has a protective effect. A physically active life even protects against a hereditary risk of CVD; even if you have a family history of heart disease, your risk is almost completely offset by physical activity. And if you do have a heart attack—an active lifestyle is no absolute guarantee against heart attack; nothing is—it's less likely to be a fatal heart attack, and you'll recover more quickly and be more likely to return to your normal activities sooner.

These reductions in the risk of death from cardiovascular disease and diabetes account for about half of the added years of life enjoyed by active individuals. As mentioned earlier, though, all of this is merely an average of the experiences of a large number of individuals. This average obscures the experiences of men and women who, by becoming active, avoided a fatal heart attack at age 55 and gained one, two, three, or more decades of life. And these figures regarding reductions in risk and added years of life don't reflect the many years of increased quality of life. Before cardiovascular disease has advanced to the point where it increases the victim's risk of premature death, the chronic fatigue, pain, and worry associated with CVD almost certainly will have exacted a toll on vitality and enjoyment of life. Again, the reduced risk of death from CVD and added years of life that result from activity are in a sense a by-product of many more years of active, vital, enjoyable life.

Clyde Henry, for example, actually views his heart attack as a beneficial turning point in his life because it provided the motivation to get active. "It changed my life, and for the better," he says. "When I was sedentary and overweight, I was tired all the time. I didn't have energy for anything. I didn't realize until after the heart attack, and after I started walking every day, just what a toll that constant fatigue had taken on my life. My mind's much sharper now; before my heart attack, my memory was going too. In my business, that's fatal. You have to be sharp; the customer base is always changing, and you have to take a different approach with each. You can't start forgetting names or phone numbers, or what you talked about last. But the biggest single benefit is to have more energy. Now I want to live, not sleep."

chapter 6

CANCER PREVENTION AND PHYSICAL ACTIVITY

It's estimated that fully one-third of all cancers can be avoided simply by eliminating smoking and excessive drinking. Eating foods that are low in fats and high in complex carbohydrates and avoiding carcinogenic agents are also essential in reducing your risk of cancer. And now there is increasing evidence that physical activity may also be effective in reducing cancer of some specific sites.

Cancer is second only to cardiovascular disease as a cause of mortality in this country, accounting for one of every five deaths in the United States today. The American Cancer Society estimates that more than one million new cancer cases will occur in the United States this year and that a half million Americans will die of cancer.[1] According to the U.S. Department of Health and Human Service's *Healthy People 2000*, cancer is responsible for 11 percent of the total cost of disease in the United States.[2] Although some cancers ultimately are fatal, more and more are curable and many others have become chronic diseases thanks to improved detection and treatment; thus these diseases can easily consume the physical, emotional, and financial resources not just of the patient but of the patient's family.

THE CANCER BOOM

It seems that the incidence of cancer is increasing, although there is some debate over this issue. The U.S. Department of Health notes that in recent years, the incidence of all cancers has increased in the United States, and that increase has been more rapid among blacks than whites and more rapid among men than women, although the incidence of premenopausal breast cancer among women has shown a steady rise in recent years to what some now call epidemic proportions.

Of particular concern is that the huge population of men and women born between 1948 and 1957, the so-called baby boom generation, seems to have a significantly greater risk of developing cancer compared with men and women of the same age from earlier generations, according to a report in the *Journal of the American Medical Association*.[3] However, the risk of cancer among the boomer generation (the oldest are nearing 50) is still quite low, even if it is rising, so it's not certain yet what the implications are, if any. If boomers really do have an increased risk, in the years ahead, this huge generation with its increased cancer risk could place a backbreaking burden on limited health care resources as it moves into late middle and old age.

WHY THE INCREASE?

No one is certain why the incidence of cancer seems to be rising among either boomers or other populations. Environmental factors such as radiation and carcinogens in our water, food, or air are certainly implicated, as are some viruses. Smoking, of course, is the primary cause of lung cancer, and since the 1980s, the incidence of smoking-related cancers has fallen steadily among men while it has skyrocketed among women. Women born in 1950, according to the *Journal of the American Medical Association* report, have five times the risk of smoking-related cancers as their grandparents, not surprising considering how heavily the tobacco industry has marketed cigarettes to women in recent years.[4] But this study found that even among nonsmokers, the incidence of all cancers seems to be increasing.

One obvious reason a higher percentage of men and women are encountering cancer is that the risk of cancer rises steadily with age; more of us are living longer, on average, so there is more time for something to go wrong with a cell's reproduction or growth. In chapter 2, we discussed one theory that suggests aging occurs when "noise"—that is, errors in information—builds up in a cell's DNA. When this occurs, cell function declines, the cell dies, or sometimes the cell makes the transition from a normal cell to a cancer cell, characterized by uncontrolled cell division and the development of a tumor, an accumulation of "renegade" cells. In earlier generations, people tended to die younger of other causes such as tuberculosis, pneumonia, or accidents, before this "noise" had time to cause enough coding errors to result in tumors. But this doesn't explain the apparent rise in cancer incidence among the baby boom generation, none of whom at this point can be considered old.

Thus one key to cancer *prevention* is to avoid whatever can inject "noise" into the system, including known carcinogens such as cigarette smoke and other environmental toxins. Another aspect of cancer prevention is to enhance the body's defense mechanisms to eliminate cells that have begun to make errors, and as we'll see shortly, regular physical activity, particularly Stage Two activity, does just that. Regular Stage Two activity also strengthens all of the body's systems so that when cancer does occur, we're better able to withstand both the disease and the sometimes very debilitating treatments, improving the chances of survival and full recovery.

THE RESEARCH DILEMMA

Although the incidence of cancer is increasing, the death rate for some cancers is falling due to earlier detection and more effective treatments, particularly improved treatments for many childhood cancers that once were universally fatal. In truth, though, the data on cancer incidence and death rates aren't entirely clear. Thus we have alarming reports on the rising incidence of cancer among the boomers on the one hand, while an encouraging report in the *American Journal of Epidemiology* declares that we can expect a reduction in the total age-specific incidence of cancer, "and a substantial reduction in mortality, in the years to come."[5]

One reason for all the uncertainty is the nature of the disease—or more accurately the *diseases*. What we think of as cancer is really a multitude of different diseases, all characterized by uncontrolled growth of cells. Each type of cancer can be caused by quite unique factors. For example, smoking causes lung cancer but probably not

LIFEFIT PRINCIPLES

- The incidence of cancer seems to be rising, and the increase has been more rapid among blacks than whites and more rapid among men than women.

- Environmental factors such as toxins and carcinogens in our water, air, and food may be contributing to this rise. Another reason for the rise is that more of us are living longer, so we have more time to develop cancer.

- Strategies for preventing cancer include two approaches: First, avoid those external factors that contribute to the risk. Next, strengthen the body's own defense mechanism, the immune system, so that when a tumor does appear, the body can eliminate it before it impacts health or spreads.

- Stage One and especially Stage Two activities can contribute to both strategies. Among the college alumni, for example, those who were most active (expending 2,000 kilocalories or more per week in Stage One and Stage Two activities) had a third less risk of all cancers than did the least active.

- It appears that 30 minutes, three times a week, of moderately vigorous Stage Two activity is most effective in preventing all cancers.

- There is a point at which physical activity is no longer helpful in improving health. Overtraining depresses the immune system, so it's important to get adequate rest and to be aware of how your body reacts to activity.

colon cancer; diet and other factors probably increase the risk of colon cancer but probably have little to do with the risk of lung cancer. And physical activity appears to offer protection from some types of cancer but probably not others, as we'll see.

What makes the study of cancer still more complex is the disease's uncertain *induction period*; that is, the time between transition of a cell from a normal to a malignant state, its multiplication and development into a tumor, and the clinical diagnosis of cancer. Indeed, many or perhaps most of us may have small, subclinical tumors that continually develop, then are eliminated by the body's own defense systems. Perhaps only rarely does one of these tumors continue to develop, and when it does, it may develop very slowly, taking months or years before the disease has advanced enough to be diagnosed, and in the meantime the patient may have made all sorts of lifestyle changes. All of this makes it difficult to observe relations between the disease and external factors such as environmental toxins or sedentary living (the cause-and-effect link between smoking and lung cancer, of course, is well documented). Thus questions such as whether or not physical activity will prevent the transition of a normal cell to a malignancy, or delay the point at which the disease causes recognizable symptoms, remain difficult to answer. Nor are investigators certain that physical activity provides lifetime protection from the disease. Most studies of cancer follow subjects for 5 or 10 years, through the lifetime of the study itself, not the lifetimes of the subjects. What happens to physically active subjects beyond the limits of these studies? Again, no one knows.

Not that any of these uncertainties matter much when you consider the problem of cancer prevention from the perspective of the man or woman who hopes to avoid these dread diseases. What is important is that physical activity and improved physical fitness seem to play a direct role in reducing the risk of at least some cancers of specific sites.

WHAT RESEARCH SAYS ABOUT PHYSICAL ACTIVITY AND ALL CANCERS

Studies of physical activity, physical fitness, and the risk of cancer have usually either looked at all cancers or at cancers of specific sites.

Generally, studies that looked at all cancers have produced somewhat equivocal findings.[6] But this makes sense if you remember that cancer is actually a number of different diseases with different causes; physical activity might be expected to impact some types of cancer but not others.

Despite that, the findings from some studies of all cancers are compelling. The College Study found a clear gradient of decreasing cancer risk with increasing activity levels (figure 6.1).[7] Alumni were divided into three categories, from least active to most active, and their cancer mortality rates were, respectively, 28.9 (relative risk, or RR, of 1.00), 20.0 (RR of 0.69), and 19.6 (RR of 0.68) per 10,000 person-years of observation. Similar associations between occupational activity and decreasing risk of all cancers have also been observed by other investigators.

Steven N. Blair and colleagues at the Cooper Institute for Aerobic Research in Dallas conducted a study of 13,000 men and women, measuring their fitness and following them over the course of eight

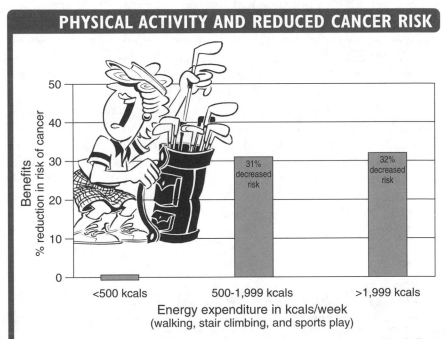

Figure 6.1   In analysis of data on phyiscal activity and all cancers, the College Study found that as activity increases, the risk of all cancers clearly decreases.

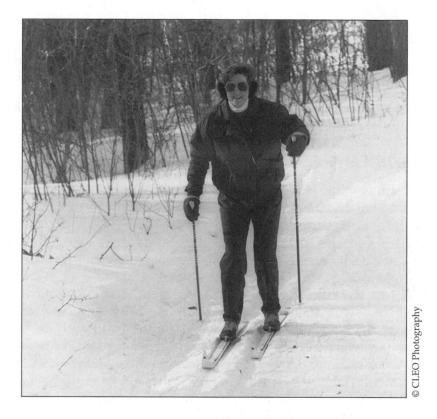

© CLEO Photography

years for their experience with cancer. The study found that the least fit men and women had twice the deaths from all cancers compared with the next-to-least fit group.[8] Because improved physical fitness is at least in part a result of increased physical activity, it's probably safe to conclude from Blair's findings that increasing physical activity is beneficial.

However, it's not clear from that study whether the cause of the reduced cancer deaths among the most fit was their fitness—we think it is—or whether they pursued other health habits such as eating a low-fat, high-fiber diet, not smoking, and so on, all of which may have reduced their risk. Most likely, the most fit were the most physically active, and the most physically active would probably tend not to smoke, significantly reducing their risk of lung cancer. The most fit might also be more likely to eat foods low in fat and high in fiber, dietary habits that might reduce their risk of colon and some other cancers.

THE RELATIONSHIP OF EXERCISE TO CANCERS OF SPECIFIC SITES

Most likely, the reduced risk of all cancers found in many studies results from significant reductions in cancers of specific sites.

COLON CANCER

According to the National Cancer Institute, colon cancer will strike about 34 of every 100,000 Americans this year, and only about half of those afflicted will survive five years or longer. Data from a variety of studies, including the College Study, demonstrate that the risk of developing this particular type of cancer can be reduced through exercise.[9-15] The most active college alumni, for example, had half the risk of colon cancer during 12 years of follow-up compared with their sedentary peers, perhaps because exercise speeds "transit time," or the movement of feces through the large intestine, which may decrease the time the walls of the colon are in contact with potentially carcinogenic substances.[16] Diet may play a role in this reduced risk as well; physically active people generally follow more healthful diets that are lower in animal fats and higher in fiber, a type of diet known to reduce the risk of colon cancer. There may also be other factors at work here. Moderate physical activity seems to strengthen the immune system, which may help reduce the risk. Physically active people may also engage in other healthy habits that play an as yet undetermined role.

BREAST CANCER

According to the National Cancer Institute, the U.S. incidence of breast cancer increased 32 percent between 1982 and 1987. Cancer is the leading cause of death for women age 35 to 50 (among older women, the leading cause is CVD), and breast cancer is the most common malignancy, although lung cancer is rapidly moving up to first place. One woman in nine will get breast cancer in her lifetime.

And again, the risk seems to be rising, at least in part because we are an aging society. More than half of women who die of breast cancer are age 65 or older, and because more women are living longer, it's not surprising that more women are at risk. But there are other factors at work here as well.

KNOWN RISK FACTORS FOR BREAST CANCER

- A "primary" relative (mother or sister) with the disease
- Advancing age
- Early onset of first menstruation (menarche)
- Late onset of menopause
- Late age at first pregnancy
- Early age at last pregnancy
- Premenopausal leanness
- Postmenopausal obesity
- No pregnancies
- Alcohol consumption
- Perhaps prolonged estrogen use
- Perhaps a high-fat diet in childhood or adolescence
- Lack of exercise

Family History

For example, a family history of the disease is a significant and unfortunately unmodifiable risk factor. Thus a woman is at a much higher risk if her mother or a sister has had breast cancer, and she'll want to be very careful to change other risk factors that can be modified.

Alcohol and Diet

Alcohol consumption may also increase the risk, and a high-fat diet is thought to be a factor.[17] Women in countries such as Japan, where they consume much less dietary fat, have a significantly lower risk of breast cancer than American women. Japanese women who move to this country and who, over time, adopt more American-style eating and other habits eventually come to have the same risk as other American women.

Obesity

As noted in chapter 4, being overweight is also associated with an increased risk of breast cancer, particularly in the menopausal years. Because obesity can be a result of both diet and activity patterns, dietary changes to reduce fats will also likely reduce calories consumed, and as we've seen, increasing activity to expend more calories will further contribute to weight loss, thus reducing the risk.

The Hormone Connection

The female hormone estrogen is thought to play a role in the risk of breast cancer and perhaps some other cancers of the reproductive system; tumors grow rapidly in the presence of the hormone, thus the risk of breast cancer probably fluctuates with changes in estrogen levels throughout a woman's life. The risk of breast cancer appears to increase with early onset of menstruation (before the age of 12), late age of first pregnancy or early age of last pregnancy (30 or older), late menopause (45 or older), or no pregnancies. The risk of breast cancer may also increase with prolonged use of estrogen in hormone replacement therapy (HRT), although this is still a matter of debate. Many women take estrogen around the time of menopause to help alleviate symptoms such as hot flashes, and the use of estrogen for a limited time around menopause seems to carry little or no risk. But long-term hormone replacement therapy may increase the risk of breast cancer. The Nurses' Health Study of over 120,000 registered nurses around the nation found that those over 60 who had undergone HRT for five years or more had a slight increase in risk of breast cancer.[18] Long-term hormone replacement therapy is sometimes used in reducing CVD in older women with heart disease or those who are at high risk (if they have hypertension, NIDDM, unhealthful blood cholesterol levels, are overweight, have a family history of CVD, or don't exercise). Long-term hormone replacement therapy is also useful in treating osteoporosis, because estrogen slows or prevents bone mineral loss.

The message here? If you're a woman around the age of menopause and are contemplating estrogen replacement, you'll need to weigh the benefits of estrogen replacement against the risks. On the one hand, estrogen replacement will help cut your risk of CVD and osteoporosis. On the other, it may slightly increase your risk of breast cancer. Depending on your risk factors for CVD, osteoporosis, and breast cancer, the benefits of reduced risk of CVD or osteoporosis from estrogen replacement may far outweigh any increase in your breast cancer risk; heart disease kills many more women than breast cancer. If you have a family history of breast cancer, though, you'll want to weigh this risk carefully against other possible benefits and discuss your situation with your physician.

The Exercise Connection

In any case, the effect of physical activity on estrogen levels is what makes the protective effect of exercise so plausible. Physical activity and leanness tend to decrease estrogen levels, thus a lower lifetime exposure to estrogen that might result from a physically active life would likely lower the risk of breast cancer and perhaps also cancer of the uterus and ovaries.

Regular exercise, control of body weight, reduced consumption of dietary fats, and moderate or no alcohol consumption all appear to reduce the risk of breast cancer. Even if you have other risks over which you have no control—a genetic risk revealed in a family history of the disease, for example—your risk will still be lower if you avoid the precursors mentioned above.[19] Indeed, if your mother or sister has had breast cancer, it's absolutely imperative that you reduce those risk factors over which you do have control.

One study of former college students found that former college athletes had an 86 percent lower risk of breast cancer later in life, an apparent benefit of athleticism that was independent of family history, age, body fat, and so on.[20] What this implies for women who weren't college athletes but who later take up physical activity such as walking, jogging, swimming, and the like remains to be seen. However, because leanness is associated with a reduced risk of breast cancer, and because women who exercise regularly usually become and remain lean, it's likely that exercise would have a protective effect.[21] This notion is supported by a later study that looked at the incidence of breast cancer by occupation and found that women in more physically demanding occupations had a lower risk, suggesting a protective effect from *contemporary* physical activity.[22]

PROSTATE CANCER

The prostate is a walnut-sized gland that is part of the male genital and urinary system; the gland secretes a fluid that is part of semen. Prostate cancer is the second most common type of cancer among men, behind lung cancer, with about 80 percent of prostate cancers appearing in men over age 65 (on autopsy, incidentally, fully 80 percent of men over the age of 80 have subclinical, usually nonmetastasized prostate cancer). Since the early 1970s, the incidence of prostate cancer has increased about 2.2 percent per year, according to the U.S. Public Health Service, again most likely because more men are living long enough for subclinical prostate cancer to advance to the point where it causes identifiable symptoms.[23]

But there's some good news. Very high levels of physical activity, at least in older men, may reduce the risk of prostate cancer.[24] Preliminary observations in the College Study suggest that men who expended 4,000 or more kilocalories a week in physical activity may have a lower risk of prostate cancer compared with men who expended less than 1,000 kilocalories a week.[25] We know there's a link between high levels of the male hormone testosterone and an increased risk of prostate cancer. Likewise, we know that especially heavy exercise decreases testosterone, suggesting a link between high levels of exercise and a reduced risk of prostate cancer.

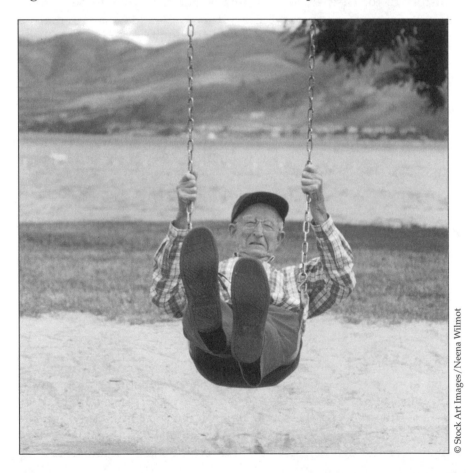

© Stock Art Images/Neena Wilmot

Obesity and high-fat diets are also associated with an increased risk of prostate cancer, and again, because men who exercise regularly tend to cut their intake of dietary fats, and because they tend to be leaner than average, it makes sense that physical activity might be associated with a reduced risk, although it may not be a cause-and-effect relation.

Not all studies find such a relation between activity and reduced risk, however; thus men should weigh the uncertain reduction in risk of prostate cancer from high levels of activity against the risks posed by the activity itself.[26] Very high levels of activity lead to overtraining, perhaps an increased risk of infection, an increased risk of injury, and even a reduced libido, all of which raise questions about quality of life.

LUNG CANCER

In the College Study findings and those of a handful of other studies, there was a clear link between an increased level of physical activity and a decreased risk of lung cancer.[27-29] In the College Study, for instance, moderately active alumni had a 21 percent reduction in the risk of lung cancer compared with inactive alumni. The highly active alumni enjoyed a 61 percent reduction in risk. Also, men over 60 achieved the same benefits from exercise in terms of reduced risk of lung cancer as younger men.[30]

Findings such as these are plausible. If you exercise, you're much less likely to smoke, and again, smoking is *the* primary cause of lung cancer. But more significantly, among the alumni, active nonsmokers also had a lower risk of lung cancer compared with inactive nonsmokers; likewise, physical activity also was found to provide some protection from lung cancer, even for those who indulged in the noxious habit. Thus physical activity may offer protection from lung cancer through some mechanism other than control of the nicotine habit. Just what that mechanism might be is open to considerable debate, but one possibility is increased ventilation of the lungs. When you exercise, you breathe more deeply and rapidly. This may help flush the lungs of carcinogens, even those found in cigarette smoke.

Physical activity also may work to reduce the risk of lung cancer as well as all other cancers through other mechanisms, and one of the most promising avenues of investigation concerns the effect of physical activity on the immune system.

CANCERS AT OTHER SITES

Physical activity may provide some protection from other cancers as well. There's some evidence that more active women have a lower risk of cancers of the uterus, cervix, vagina, and ovaries, and of endometrial cancer. Among men, investigators in Great Britain found that active men had a lower risk of testicular cancer than the sedentary, who had twice the risk compared with the most active men.[31-33]

HOW EXERCISE CAN PROTECT YOU FROM CANCER

What type of exercise is best for reducing your risk of all cancers or cancers of specific sites? The definitive answer to this question isn't in yet, but it appears that moderately vigorous Stage Two activities might offer the most protection.

As just discussed, regular exercise may offer protection from specific cancers in a variety of ways, but the most important preventive mechanism may be the impact of activity on immune system function. Regular exercise of moderate intensity—Stage Two activity—appears to reinforce the immune system, helping to fight off infectious diseases and perhaps some types of cancer.[34-37] Light exercise, although certainly helpful, probably isn't going to be as beneficial as moderately vigorous Stage Two activities. On the other hand, too much exercise will suppress the immune system.

The body's immune system is a surveillance system that helps it recognize "self" from "notself," attacking and destroying whatever it perceives to be notself, whether that happens to be an invading virus or one of the body's own cells that has begun dividing uncontrollably as a cancer. The system has several lines of defense, including T-lymphocytes (or T-cells) and B-lymphocytes (B-cells), which protect against a number of viral, bacterial, and parasitic infections. An additional line of defense is provided by cells called natural killer (NK) cells, which are capable of killing a wide variety of targets, including tumor cells.

How exercise works to enhance the immune system is not fully understood, although studies have shown that moderately vigorous aerobic training such as brisk walking is associated with an increase in the number of T-cells circulating in the blood.[38] Exercise raises body temperature, which may also help kill some types of temperature-sensitive viruses or bacteria. And exercise is generally associated with habits that promote overall good health, including good nutrition and a tendency to get adequate sleep, which may aid in the body's fight against infection.

However, high-intensity exercise of long duration leading to overtraining or "staleness" may actually lower T-cell count and slow the rate of antibody synthesis, suppressing the immune system and leading to an increased risk of infection. This explains the well-known phenomenon of athletes who become prone to colds one to two weeks following a period of intense training and competition.[39]

What constitutes overtraining varies widely from individual to individual, however. Thus, as you take up and stick with an active way of life, you will want to be aware of your own limits and how your body responds to exercise. It's important to allow adequate recovery time between hard workouts and not to increase the intensity, duration, or frequency of training beyond your body's ability to adapt and recover.[40,41] We'll discuss overtraining and how to prevent it in more detail in part III.

TIPS FOR A CANCER-PREVENTION LIFESTYLE

Is there a "cancer-prevention lifestyle"? Clearly there is, and it includes the following:

- Don't smoke.
- Eat a diet high in complex carbohydrates (grains, vegetables, and fruits) and low in fats (see chapter 4).
- Supplement with antioxidants—vitamins A, C, and E, folic acid, and beta carotene (see chapter 4).
- Use alcohol sensibly, if at all.
- Engage in moderately vigorous Stage Two activities, but not to the point of overtraining.
- Avoid obesity.
- Avoid contact with known carcinogens.
- Try to control stress in your life (see chapter 7).

A LOOK BACK, A LOOK AHEAD

As we've seen here and in the previous chapters, when you take up and maintain an active way of life, you will reduce your risk of cardiovascular diseases, NIDDM, osteoporosis, obesity, frailty, and perhaps some cancers. You will add years to your life and enjoy the many physical benefits of activity, including more physical vigor, independence, and zest for life. And there are other benefits of activity that are harder to measure but no less important. We'll discuss some of these benefits in the next two chapters.

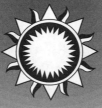

chapter 7

AGING, SOCIAL CONNECTIONS, AND STRESS

We live in rapidly changing, often difficult times in which social connections tend to fray and stress and anxiety levels are on the rise. It makes sense to try to avoid stress, but that's not always possible. A key to a long, healthy life is to use stress to your advantage. The body's physical responses to stress clear the vision and sharpen the mind, for example, which can be very useful when the job demands quick or creative thinking. But chronic, unrelieved stress can be harmful, even deadly. A physically active way of life helps us develop coping strategies and social connections that minimize stress, as well as a strong, fit body that can more effectively withstand the impact of stress and recover quickly when it does occur.

Gail Gustafson was working as a research biochemist at the University of California in San Francisco in 1969 when she gave up smoking and gained a few pounds on a subsequent trip to Europe. So she started taking an exercise class at lunchtime. She'd wear tennis shoes and shorts and do lots of sit-ups, then jog around the basketball courts while the medical students shot hoops.

"At night," she recalls, "I'd sneak out and run around in the dirt at the polo field in Golden Gate Park, when there was no one around who could see me. I thought I looked ridiculous; this was back in the dark ages when women weren't supposed to sweat. But there was something about it all that I really liked—the sweat, being outside, the sense I was taking control of my body."

The fellow who ran the lunch-hour exercise class was thrilled with Gail's enthusiasm; the more Gail kept at it, the faster and thinner she became. "He took me to my first race," she recalls, "and to buy my first real running shoes, heavy leather things, but I thought they were wonderful. And I was starting to meet people, others who liked to run, and they were wonderful people."

Among those she met was the new and improved Flory Rodd.

"There was a race around Lake Merced," Flory recalls. "Then everyone got together after. I remember walking into the room where everyone was and seeing a really pretty young woman across the room. I asked the hostess, 'Who's that?' She told me, 'Gail Gustafson.' 'How about introducing me?' I asked. She said, 'Why not introduce yourself?' So I did. I asked her if she was by any chance going to run the Port Costa 10K the next weekend, and she said she was, so I made what I call my 'airline barroom move'—I was still an airline navigator at the time. I asked her if she liked Ramos Fizzes, and she said she loved them. Then I told her I knew a bar in Port Costa that made the best Ramos Fizzes in the world, suggesting we meet at the end of the race and go there."

"I figured, why not," Gail recalls.

Flory and Gail had both just discovered something that an increasing number of runners and other athletes were discovering at the beginning of the so-called fitness boom 20-odd years ago: Sport is good not only for one's physiology, but for one's social life. Sport offers an entree to conversation and a safe place to meet and become acquainted with others who share your interests in health and self-development; and the shared effort of working up a sweat during a road race, at the gym, on the tennis courts, or wherever helps break

GAIL RODD'S TRAINING

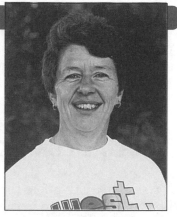

Gail Rodd (formerly Gustafson), 54, retired biochemist

Training

Every morning, Gail runs for an hour to an hour and a half at about a nine-minute-mile pace (5.4 miles per hour), for a total of about 40 miles a week. In addition, she spends an hour or so each day landscaping and working in her garden. (Total kilocalories per week in physical activity: approximately 4,000 from running; perhaps 300 or so for every hour she spends landscaping and gardening.)

Impetus to change

"I'd quit smoking and gained a lot of weight on a trip to Europe. I knew I had to do something, so I joined this lunchtime exercise class at the hospital where I worked. We did sit-ups and ran around the gym while the medical students played basketball."

What she likes most about an active life

"I like the way it makes me feel, that I can do anything I want to do. I look at my neighbors, and they can't walk up a hill. I don't want to be like that."

Advice

"I'd say do a little bit every day; never miss a day. It doesn't have to be walking or running, but walking is the easiest; anyone can walk, so there's no excuse not to. You can walk fast and get into great shape."

down the natural reticence that prevents many of us from making friends easily.

"On a long run, there's plenty of time to talk," Gail notes, "so I think you get to know people faster than you would normally. And you meet people from different walks of life. Working at the lab, I met only other scientists. As a runner, though, I meet all kinds of people and get to know them well as runners before I ever find out what they do. I think this makes for a richer social life and a broader perspective on life and society. Now my entire social life is built around running; most of my friendships and my marriage—Flory and I married—have come through people I met through running."

SOCIAL CONNECTIONS AND LONGEVITY

Physical activity offers the social benefits and emotional consolations of meeting and getting to know others within a safe, healthy environment, all of which is good for one's psyche and soul, certainly. But increased social connections may also promote longevity and increased vitality by reducing the risk of heart disease, hypertension, perhaps some cancers, and even infectious diseases. Indeed, social connectedness appears to be one of the more important factors in heart disease prevention. A Swedish study, for example, found that a person's social contacts—with a spouse, relatives, friends, church and other community involvements, and so on— were a better predictor of the risk of heart attack than any of the accepted biomedical risk factors such as hypertension and an adverse blood cholesterol profile, although this study didn't measure exercise or diet.[1]

A study of newly unemployed workers found that those who had the support of spouses had lower cholesterol levels than those who lacked such support. A 1970 study of married and unmarried individuals found that those who are not married experience a higher mortality rate than those who are; a study of pregnant U.S. Army wives found that women with rich social resources had only one-third the complications of those without social connectedness. In a recent study of on-the-job stress, investigators found that men and women with good social support networks had lower heart rates and lower blood pressures than those who lacked such social support.[2-6]

THE "CONNECTIONS" CONNECTION

What's the link between one's sociability and health and longevity? And where does an active way of life fit in? It's a complicated matter. As with any research looking at relations between presumed causes

LIFEFIT PRINCIPLES

- Social connections—involvement with others, including friends, relatives, family members, or church and fraternal organizations—preserve mental functioning and reduce the risk of heart disease, infection, and perhaps even some types of cancer, NIDDM, and osteoporosis.

- To increase your connections with others, get involved in volunteer or church activities, community involvements, continuing education, or use physical activity. Involvement in sports such as walking or swimming creates a nonthreatening milieu in which connections with others can be formed and maintained.

- One of the hazards of social isolation is increasing stress, but there are plenty of other causes of stress in these changeable, fast-paced times, and regular Stage One or Stage Two activity will help relieve stress and help protect your body and health from the ravages of stress.

- Any activity is better than none, but moderately vigorous Stage Two activity sustained for at least 30 minutes seems to provide the most stress-busting benefits.

- Use physical activity to develop coping strategies to reduce stress when it does occur. For example, exercise provides a time-out during which to think through stress-causing problems; exercise also produces many of the same relaxation responses provided by meditation.

- Don't let exercise itself become a source of stress. Make sure you don't try to do too much; get adequate rest, and be aware of the warning signs of overtraining (see part III).

and observed effects, the question of selection bias continues to nag researchers. In the case of longevity and social connectedness, for example, it's not unlikely that individuals who have a rich social life and who are also observed by epidemiologists to be healthier, more active, and longer-lived than their less sociable peers may have more social contacts *because* they're healthier, not necessarily the other way around. People who are healthy and fit may be more likely to interact with others. Someone who feels good and functions adequately and is free of debilitating illness—diabetes, arthritic knees, a bad heart—will simply be more likely to get out of the house and interact pleasurably with others. On the other hand, the observation that those with poor social connectedness tend to be less active and have a higher risk of heart disease, cancer, and other diseases may reflect the fact that when we feel lousy, we're less likely or able to get out and socialize.

Which, of course, begs the important question: If we feel bad because we're sedentary and out of shape, then take up an active life and begin to feel better and have more energy, will we be more likely to get out of the house and engage in life and enjoy the many benefits? We think so.

Whether or not you become more active, anything you can do to increase your connections with others is going to benefit your health and sense of well-being. And taking up and sticking with an active life will help. Moreover, there is growing evidence that social connections themselves act directly to improve our health, that there is a direct, biologically plausible cause-and-effect relation.

WE'RE SOCIAL ANIMALS

It's hardly a revelation that we humans are social animals. We naturally tend to seek out connections with others, and to have these connections denied for whatever reason is one of the cruelest fates. Indeed, in ancient cultures, one of the gravest punishments that could befall someone was to be ostracized—driven out of the community and denied the fellowship and protection the community could afford. (The term *ostracism* comes from the Greek word *ostrakon*, a broken piece of pottery used as a ballot when voting to ostracize someone. It was a grim business.) In ancient times, at least, ostracism could have an immediate impact on health and longevity; beyond the protective walls of the community, the ostracized person was much more likely to be eaten by wild animals or murdered by roving barbarians, if he didn't starve to death first.

This may at least hint at an explanation for why today's versions of ostracism—loneliness, lack of social contacts, the anomie of today's highly mobile society in which families, neighborhoods, and other traditional social structures are at best temporary and easily fragmented—can have nearly as direct an impact on health and longevity as being driven out of the village into the jungle. Social isolation, even in these more "civilized" times, can be as direct a threat to physical well-being as ostracism was in more ancient times. On a practical level, we all need social and community ties to fulfill some basic, tangible needs, particularly as we grow older: help when ill, help locating and acquiring goods and services, transportation, and so on.[7] People without a network of supportive friends or relatives are more likely to suffer the consequences of not having their needs fulfilled. The problem is particularly acute for older adults.

In ancient cultures, older men and women were fully integrated into their society and, in fact, were revered as sources of wisdom and experience. In our own, presumably more civilized contemporary culture, older adults are often segregated into retirement villages, planned living complexes, and nursing homes. Of course, these establishments often provide ample opportunities for socializing, but of necessity, this takes place disconnected from the larger community.

As we've charted it by age group in figure 7.1, women with the most connections enjoyed, respectively, a 78 percent, 52 percent, and 67 percent reduced death rate during the period of observation, compared with those with the least social contact. Among the men, the reduction was 61 percent, 69 percent, and 45 percent. Considering these data in terms of risk of death, we see that women with the least connections had between 2.1 and 4.5 times the risk, compared with those who had the most connections. Among the men, the relative risks were 4.6, 2.1, and 3.0. (The 33-percent increase in deaths among a small group of women, those with slightly more connections, compared with those with the fewest connections, is likely the result of small numbers, not a meaningful increase in risk.)

One way that social connectedness gives us a greater feeling of control over stressful situations could be the sense that "we're not in this alone," or that however bad things become, there will be friends, family, and others to help us out. Certainly it helps to talk to others when we're troubled, grieving, confused, or otherwise under stress; thus, when troubled, we seek out the confessional, 12-step meetings, a neighborhood bar, or the therapist's couch. Or, for that matter, the local tennis court, gym, track, or lap pool. And beyond the fact that simply talking things out can help us feel better, the perspectives of others can offer practical suggestions for dealing with a difficult situation, further adding to our sense of control and thus diminishing the harmful effects of stress.

Of course, it's not at all certain that someone who has been shy or even antisocial all his or her life can somehow suddenly develop a

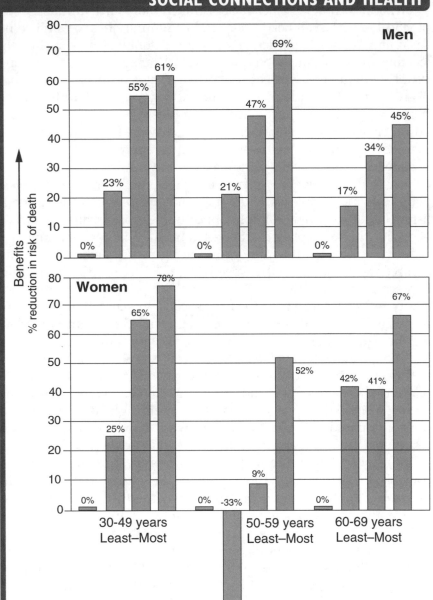

Figure 7.1 In each age group, men and women with more social connections—friends, family, religious, or community involvements—enjoyed reductions in their risk of death compared with those with fewer connections. The trends are clear: The more social connections you have with others, the more likely you are to enjoy a delay in mortality, at least to age 69, the oldest age-group studied. Data from the Alameda County Study by Lisa Berkman and Lester Breslow (1983).

richer social network. But as Gail and Flory and millions of others have found, sport creates situations in which it's easier to meet and get to know others.

A STRATEGY FOR CONNECTIONS

We can develop and maintain social connections in many ways. Involvements in church, volunteer activities, social clubs, continuing education, and other community service all help us connect with others. But if one is debilitated by being overweight, by the sort of chronic fatigue that plagues the habitually sedentary, or by outright disease, it's hard to stay involved. Thus an active way of life can contribute to social connections by promoting the vigor and self-confidence it takes to get out and meet folks and get involved.

Better yet, activity itself can become a means of staying connected. Physical activity of any kind, particularly in the context of a club, team, or other group situation, can be an effective strategy for connecting with others, and as we get older, sports can become increasingly important as a means of preserving social connectedness.

Although the notion of the "loneliness of the long distance runner" has become firmly fixed in our cultural mythology, you don't have to be alone when you run—or walk, swim, cycle, or whatever—unless you want to. Take advantage of running or walking clubs, masters swim teams, aerobics classes, the tennis courts, or Sunday morning cycling tours to make and preserve contacts with others. Take activity classes at the local Y or rec center. Or simply call a few friends and ask them to join you on the walking trails.

Next, get involved in volunteer efforts around your chosen activities. Volunteer to pass out water at local fun runs, for example, or to help organize weekend bike rides. Such involvements bring you in contact with men and women of all ages, backgrounds, and occupations, who are nonetheless united in their healthy-mindedness. This unity of spirit creates for many a safe place, a community in which to meet and talk with others, conversation from which friendships and social networks grow.[8,9]

But the connections linking social interaction, physical activity, and physical health and longevity appear to go much deeper than simple community; they seem to be "hardwired" into our basic

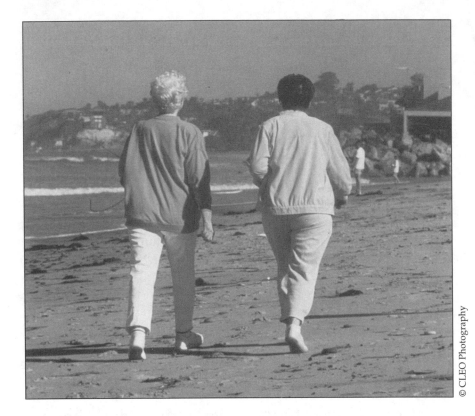

© CLEO Photography

biology and have to do with the ways in which we react to stress. We may face no more stressful a situation in life than a break in our connections with others—a divorce, for example, or the death of a loved one or friend. And there are plenty of other sources of stress in our lives as well. While helping to promote connectedness with others, physical activity also works to directly counter the harmful impact of stress.

THE HIGH COST OF STRESS

By some estimates, perhaps as many as 80 percent of all diseases are at least partially related to the effects of chronic, unrelieved stress, that stomach-knotting, teeth-gritting sense that things are closing in on us, an increasingly inescapable feature of our fast-paced, rapidly changing, and socially fragmented modern world.

Stress raises the blood pressure and increases the risk of strokes, heart disease, diabetes, and a host of other serious health problems such as kidney disease. Stress appears to weaken the immune system, increasing the risk of infection and perhaps some types of cancer. Stress also has been linked to an increased risk of asthma, arthritis, sleep disorders, eating disorders, migraines, chronic anxiety, difficulty concentrating, alcohol and drug abuse, and depression. Stress may even increase the risk of accidental death or injury.[10]

And stress can also make you age more quickly. Solid evidence is accumulating showing that hormones released by the brain during times of chronic, unrelieved stress accelerate the aging process.[11-13] In particular, glucocorticoids, hormones that help us think more quickly and clearly during brief periods of acute stress, will damage brain cells over longer periods as a result of chronic, unrelieved stress. And the result, of course, is memory loss, declining mental sharpness, and, at its worst, dementia.

Stress-related health problems cost society an estimated $300 billion annually in lost productivity, absenteeism, and medical costs, not to mention the impact of stress on quality of life. Unfortunately, these are increasingly stressful times by any measure, with an accelerating pace of change and uncertainty, the essential ingredients of stress.

EXACTLY WHAT IS STRESS?

The term *stress* is a grab-bag word that encompasses the stressor— the cause or source of stress—as well as all of the mind's and body's responses to that stressor. Anything can be a source of stress: social isolation, as we've seen, any life change, any need to adapt. All of these can put demands on an individual's physical, emotional, or intellectual resources, whether that change is positive or negative. The morning rush-hour commute, hitting your finger with a hammer, the evening news, a tax audit, and the death of a loved one are all obvious sources of stress. But so are winning the lottery, a major promotion, getting married, or a positive pregnancy test. These are all "life changes" in the vernacular of stress.

Lack of Control

Although the mythology of stress would have us believe that the hard-driving, pencil-chewing Type A male executive is the classic example of the stressed-out modern person, in fact, it's more likely that his secretary is under much more stress. It has to do with our sense of control, and quite often it's the man or woman holding a low-level job, one with plenty of responsibilities but no real authority, who is likely to suffer most from the health consequences of chronic stress—someone who worries about money, who has a family to care for, bills to pay, dinner to cook that night.

The curious thing about stress is that although the stressors may differ widely, and our individual perceptions of those stressors may differ just as widely, our physical reactions to stress from any source are remarkably similar.

The General Adaptation Syndrome

The late Hans Selye, MD, of Montreal, best described this peculiar aspect of our reactions to stress over 40 years ago in his book *The Stress of Life*. He called the phenomenon the General Adaptation Syndrome (GAS), better known as the "flight-or-fight" response. His theory is based on the belief that, biologically, we are animals, and that our biology is based on another, quite distant time. Whenever animals—rats, elephants, cats, dogs, or even humans—encounter situations that place demands on their ability to adapt, a chain of identifiable, predictable physical and mental responses take place, all of them regulated by the hypothalamus, a part of the brain that evolved to cope specifically with the rigors of a rough-and-tumble life in the jungle or on the savannah.

The hypothalamus wants to keep on being a hypothalamus, and as far as the hypothalamus is concerned, the only realistic response to any source of stress is physical action, usually accompanied by quick thinking, perhaps to run (to catch dinner or to keep from becoming dinner), to fight, to walk long and fast to find shelter or warmth, or to search for a new mate. So the hypothalamus responds at once to any stressor by preparing the body for rigorous physical activity. It directs the pituitary and adrenal glands to secrete a veritable Mulligan's stew of hormones and neurotransmitters—adrenocorticotrophic hormone (ACTH), catecholamines such as dopamine, norepinephrine, and epinephrine, and various corticosteroids.

The most immediate and measurable result of all of these surging chemicals is that your blood pressure shoots up, your heart rate increases, your breathing quickens and deepens, and the small, peripheral blood vessels in your skin constrict, diverting more blood to your working muscles while your face goes pale and your hands grow clammy. Still more blood is diverted to the muscles from various internal organs, particularly the stomach, putting digestion on hold (when this happens frequently enough, by the way, the result may be increasing inflammation of an existing ulcer).

Your pupils dilate so you can see better. More glycogen stores in your body are broken down to augment blood sugar levels for immediate energy. Your blood chemistry changes subtly to shorten clotting time in case you're injured, while blood flow to the brain increases and the brain's chemistry changes so you can think more quickly. Even the body's processes of cell repair and growth are put on hold temporarily during stress; your hypothalamus, after all, sees no point in expending energy on cell repair if you're being chased by something that wants you for dinner.

All of these changes—the GAS, as Selye called it—result in a state of physical and mental arousal for "flight or fight." All of these changes evolved to help us cope with usually short-term threats to well-being, threats that could be resolved with action, usually by either confrontation or running away, and in either case, the stress would be over quickly enough. It's this response to immediate threats that seems to be the key to understanding what chronic stress does to us today.

THE RESULTS OF CHRONIC STRESS

The problem is that although modern life has provided us with plenty of new aggravations, our bodies haven't evolved new ways to deal with them; we still confront stressors by preparing for physical action, usually vigorous. But we can't run from rush-hour traffic jams, income taxes, or obtuse politicians. We can't fight them either. They're a grim fact of life. Civilization has short-circuited the entire fight-or-flight process, and all too often our systems flood with all the chemicals of the stress response, and then we sit there in our automobiles, our offices, in waiting rooms, hour after hour, "stewing" in our own juices. Even just the thought or anticipation of a stressful event can trigger the body's stress response; the hypothalamus has a difficult time distinguishing between a real threat and an imagined one.

The results of the drawn-out, unresolved stress we face today are all the diseases of civilization.

Cardiovascular Disease

The increased cardiovascular tone (increased heart rate, breathing, and blood supply to the working muscles and brain) that prepares us to run or fight is a highly adaptive and beneficial response to immediate threats. But when sustained over long periods of time, this same adaptation may result in the disease of hypertension and all the ailments associated with it. Stress also may increase platelet stickiness, and as we saw earlier, the risk of heart attack increases when platelets accumulate at the site of atherosclerotic plaque in the arteries.

Digestive Ailments

The diversion of blood from the digestive system to the working muscles during acute stress may, after enough persistently stressful days at the office, activate the symptoms of peptic ulcers, colitis, irritable bowel syndrome, or other digestive system ailments.

Diabetes

By releasing glycogen stores into the blood, our stress-response system enables us to fight or run more effectively, but we may overdraw our energy savings account when exposed to prolonged, unrelieved stress. The result could be exhaustion and chronic fatigue. This stress-related process may also in some way contribute to insulin resistance, which, as we've seen, appears to be an underlying factor in heart disease as well, although this is still a hypothesis.

Osteoporosis

The cessation of the body's anabolic (growth) processes that takes place during acute episodes of stress may result in an increased risk of osteoporosis when the stress is prolonged, although this is also only a hypothesis at this point.

Infection and Cancer

Likewise, the body's immune system shuts down during times of acute stress to save energy for action. But the result of chronic stress and an immune system that is suppressed too long may be an increased risk of infection and even cancer.

Mood Disorders

The flight-or-fight response, as we've seen, leads to a state of arousal, which of course is beneficial in the right circumstances, whether you're a hunter-gatherer being chased by a lion or a midlevel manager who has to be at her best in a meeting with the board. But over time, when the stress isn't relieved, this arousal can become anxiety, and at its worst, panic attacks. Indeed, in these high-stress times, anxiety is a pervasive social problem, and panic attack is now the most frequent type of psychopathology.[14]

Anxiety is characterized by worry, self-doubt, apprehension, and outright fear. Of course, at low levels, a bit of fear or self-doubt can be helpful spurs to action in the proper contexts. At their worst, though, these feelings can intensify to the degree that the victim is virtually paralyzed and unable to function. The body and mind can maintain an aroused state for only a limited time before becoming exhausted. Then the individual may slip slowly from an aroused, anxious state to its functional opposite, depression.

Brain Disorders

Perhaps what is most disturbing of all is the toll chronic, unrelieved stress takes on intelligence and cognitive functioning. During times of acute stress, glucocorticoids (hydrocortisone) are released in the brain. These hormones help us think more quickly and clearly for brief periods, just what you'd want before an important business meeting, for example; you want to be aroused—alert and quick on your feet.

But these hormones that are so helpful during brief episodes of acute stress may wreak havoc on the brain over a longer period; they damage, perhaps even kill, neurons, essentially accelerating the aging of the brain.

More alarming still, glucocorticoids released during chronic stress take a particularly heavy toll on the hippocampus, a part of the brain that regulates the stress response itself. It's the hippocampus that turns off the stress response, shutting off the glucocorticoids, among other things. But when the hippocampus can't perform this function, the result is what neurologist Robert Sapolsky of Stanford calls a "degenerative cascade," resulting in further aging of the brain, accelerated memory loss, and declining mental acuity; we become less able to think quickly and respond to novel situations.[15]

WALK (OR RUN, SWIM, OR CYCLE) FROM STRESS

All of this sounds dire. Fortunately there are a number of ways to shut off the stress response, even in this revved-up, high-stress age of ours. You *can* control stress in your life and reduce its harmful effects. Both Stage One and Stage Two activities will help, but for the most stress-busting benefit, 30 minutes of Stage Two activity at least three days a week—or certainly whenever you feel the effects of stress getting to you—is best. Anything that gets the heart beating and brings a bit of sweat to the brow—brisk walking, jogging, swimming, or any other aerobic activity—is ideal. But weight training, chopping wood, heavy housework, gardening, golf, or anything else that gets you up on your feet and moving about will be effective.

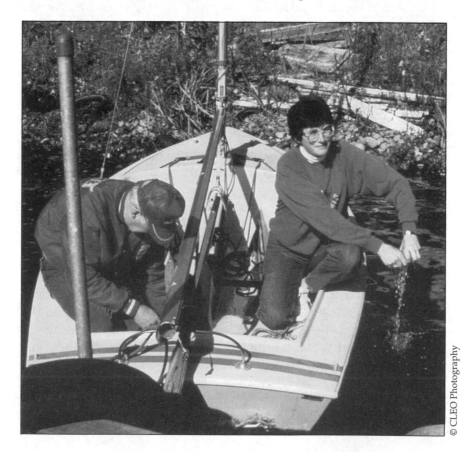

SWEAT FOR YOUR LIFE

Although exercise may not keep you from lying awake at night brooding about the job or the mortgage or taxes, it can give you the opportunity to do what the hormones released under stress prepare us to do, thus effectively "resolving" the stress response. Exercise supplies the one ingredient in the whole stress-response system that has too long been missing from our high-pressure but sedentary lives, a burst of physical activity.

These days, much research on the link between stress and health is focusing on catecholamines, the hormones of stress that arouse the body and prepare it for fight or flight and may also mediate at least some of the relation between social connectedness and health. For example, one study found that subjects with poor social networks had high urinary catecholamine excretion. This suggests that some subjects weren't reacting to stress as healthfully as those who had more social contacts and lower catecholamine levels.[16]

Catecholamines depend on oxygen for their metabolism, and by revving up the metabolism through exercise and increasing oxygen supplies throughout the body, exercise literally burns off all of the chemicals released in response to stress. In a study conducted at the Cooper Institute for Aerobics Research in Dallas, a group of men and women with diastolic blood pressures of 90 to 104 millimeters of mercury (anything higher than 90 is considered a threat to health) were put on a 16-week program of regular exercise involving walking, jogging, or running three or four times a week. After training, the subjects showed significantly lower catecholamine levels—and blood pressures—than a sedentary control group.[17]

Of course, it's not as if you can always get up and go hang out with friends, or run around the block, or go for a swim when your boss dumps a weekend's worth of work on you on Friday afternoon. But the sooner you can get out and talk to others or work up a sweat, or better yet, do both, the better off you'll be.

Over time, the improved physical fitness that comes with regular exercise also works to directly counter the health impact of chronic stress. Aside from reducing platelet stickiness and thus the acute risk of heart attack resulting from stress, exercise strengthens the heart so it's less susceptible to the damage caused by stress. And as we've already seen, exercise lowers blood pressure, strengthens the immune system to fight infection and perhaps some types of cancer, and increases insulin sensitivity and reduces the risk of diabetes, all benefits of a physically active way of life that will help you stay healthy in these stressful times.

PRACTICE RELAXATION TECHNIQUES

Exercise also works to protect us from stress in another way. Herbert Bensen, MD, of Harvard, popularized the importance of relaxation to general health and well-being in his book *The Relaxation Response*. Relaxation techniques such as yoga, tai chi chuan, meditation, breathing exercises, and prayer counteract the harmful effects of stress.[18] All of these practices lower blood pressure, produce alpha waves in the brain—the mental state of relaxation—and slow the heart rate and breathing. Studies at the University of California School of Medicine in San Francisco found that relaxation techniques even enhance the immune system's ability to fight infection, and that T-lymphocytes (the body's natural "killer" cells that attack invading viruses and bacteria) increase in number after meditation or other relaxation practices.[19]

Rhythmic large-muscle exercise such as swimming, walking, or jogging can also be a form of relaxation for many of us. The rhythmic motion of the legs and arms while walking or running can have an almost hypnotic effect, and running long distances at a comfortable pace appears to produce exactly the same changes in brain-wave activity as deep meditation.

Prolonged, large-muscle exercise also apparently stimulates the release of endorphins, the body's own natural painkillers, which have a soothing, calming effect and may account for the state of euphoria that some experience, typically after 30 minutes or so of exercise. Although this phenomenon is widely known as the "runner's high," you don't have to run to experience it. The essential prerequisite is sustained, moderately vigorous (Stage Two) activity of about 30 minutes' duration, and duration is important here; it takes about 30 minutes for metabolic changes to result in increased endorphin levels. This activity can be anything—brisk walking, swimming, cycling, aerobic dance. Whether or not resistance training also offers similar benefits hasn't been studied extensively, but we suspect that for the appropriate personality, it's just as effective and beneficial.

And at a more basic level, a fatigued muscle is a relaxed muscle; even if exercise doesn't remove the source of stress, or even if exercise doesn't result in a "runner's high," the physical fatigue following

Stage Two activity provides an important refuge from the physical tension and resulting high blood pressure that accompany stress.

DEVELOP COPING STRATEGIES

Our physiological response to a stressful situation, and the resulting impact on our physical, emotional, and mental health, also depend to no small degree on whether or not we perceive the situation as stressful. And our perceptions depend very much on our sense of control over the events in question, the predictability of the events, or a host of other factors such as our ability to vent our frustrations. Thus the same situation may be merely an interesting challenge for one person and a health-threatening source of unrelieved anxiety for another. It depends on how you look at it, but regular exercise can help change your perspective.

How does a physically active way of life contribute to a sense of control over stressful situations? Simply understanding that, through exercise, you can mitigate some of the harmful effects of stress can give you that sense of control. Exercise also teaches strategies that further strengthen your sense of control. For example, psychologists note that much of what constitutes stress in our lives results when we don't examine our own thinking patterns around an issue that may be causing problems. An activity such as running or walking becomes a time-out, a chance to think about things you might not have seen at the time of stress, things that might help you cope more effectively with the situation.

Exercise also builds self-esteem, an important weapon against stress. When your self-esteem or your confidence are low, even minor, distasteful situations can become sources of stress. As you exercise and begin to feel better about yourself, your ability to cope with stress may improve. And as you exercise and become leaner, faster, stronger, and fitter, you gain a profound sense of control over your body that may translate into an improved sense of control over all aspects of life; and again, a sense of control is your most powerful weapon against stress. Even if you can't escape from the stress of rush-hour traffic, income taxes, or the prime-time news, simply knowing that later you can take time out for yourself, and take control of one aspect of your life by doing something that is good for you, might in itself help mitigate the stress response.

The key to coping with stress and living successfully and healthfully in our stress-filled world is not to avoid stress—as if anyone can—

but to use stress to your advantage, harnessing all the energy released by the general adaptation response without letting it harm your health. To do that, you need a strong, fit body that can recover quickly from that stress before it does permanent harm, and you need to develop strategies such as exercise that minimize the effects of stress when it does occur, providing a variety of stress-release opportunities.

DON'T MAKE EXERCISE A STRESSOR

Paradoxically, exercise itself is a source of stress. Indeed, the physiological changes that take place during a walk or run, for example, appear to be similar to all those changes that take place during other times of stress, with raised levels of catecholamines and adrenaline, elevated blood pressure, and so on.

How exercise can both cause and reduce stress is something stress researchers don't fully understand. Clearly, though, there are qualitative differences between the stress of exercise and the stress of a bad day at the office. Brisk walking, for example, is for most a pleasurable stress. We have complete control over our walking—we can quit when we're tired, not when the boss is done with us. And there may be significant but as yet unidentified differences between the chemistry of exercise-induced stress and stress caused by other demands on our ability to adapt to change. For example, the release of some types of endorphins during a walk does not appear to take place during other types of stress. And walking is a "self-contained" stress, short-lived and self-limited, whereas a hectic day at the office can go on and on and on. And for most of us, a brisk walk is followed by a deep sense of peace and relaxation; again, a fatigued muscle is a relaxed muscle.

But exercise can be just as harmful as stress from other sources. There can come a point at which we're overtraining—putting a load on our bodies that they can't repair. How much exercise is too much depends on the individual, of course, but there are clear signs of overtraining, and these are probably good indicators that you're doing more harm than good. In fact, these objective signs of overtraining—elevated blood pressure, reduced resistance to disease, sleep problems, depression, loss of appetite, trouble concentrating, and so on—are indistinguishable from the symptoms associated with chronic stress.

Commonsense training is the best way to keep exercise from becoming yet another source of stress in our lives, and we'll get into that in detail in part III.

chapter 8

EXERCISE AND THE MIND

Perhaps no aspect of aging is more misunderstood—or anticipated with more uncertainty or dread—than the effects of aging on the mind, particularly on memory, general intelligence, and mood. Conventional thinking holds that as we get older, declines in mental functioning are inevitable. But the conventional wisdom is probably wrong; new research is showing that an active way of life that includes physical activity can preserve full mental function well into old age.

Conventional thinking holds that as we get older, what we think of as "senility"—a general slowing of the central nervous system, a tendency to depression, memory loss, confusion, slowed reaction time, and difficulty thinking clearly and functioning normally—is an inescapable fact of life. This way of thinking insists that as we age, we inevitably and steadily lose neurons in our brains. By the time we're 60 or so, it is assumed, we've lost enough brain cells that measurable changes have taken place in our cognitive functioning.

What has long been assumed to be an inevitable decline in mental function with age, in the absence of organic factors such as stroke, real dementia, chronic depression, or the side effects of some medica-

LIFEFIT PRINCIPLES

- The supposed inevitable decline in intelligence and memory and the increasing risk of depression and other mood disorders we expect with age are at least in part the result of unhealthful habits—habits that can be changed.

- The good news is that regular physical activity seems to work in several ways to enhance cognitive function by increasing blood flow to the brain, by promoting beneficial changes in neurotransmitters and increasing neural connectivity, and by contributing to increased social interactions and reduced stress and depression.

- Compared with their less active peers, physically active men and women at any age are generally sharper mentally and have better memories; they enjoy a lowered risk of depression and possibly even less risk of Parkinson's disease, Alzheimer's disease, and other dementias.

- The ideal exercise program for peak physical and mental performance and improved mood is a total-body routine that includes sustained Stage Two activities—aerobic training and resistance training—and some complex activity that requires continual learning or refinement of motor skills.

- Better yet, do at least some activity in a social context for the benefits of staying connected with others. Add continuing education, community involvement, and the like for additional benefits.

tions, is at least in part the result of unhealthful habits—*habits that can be changed*. The important thing to remember as society bombards you with messages about what you can expect with aging is that lifestyle habits are directly within your control, and so are what have until now been viewed as the inevitable effects of aging on the brain. Is it possible to maintain a healthy brain into old age, or to achieve a healthy brain with changes in our health habits? Absolutely.

A LOOK AT MOOD

Depression may be nearly as common as the common cold, affecting as many as 90 percent of Americans at least once in their lives; it is the "headache" of mental illness, as some have labeled it. Clinical depression—depression that has been diagnosed by a physician—ranks second only to advanced coronary heart disease in the number of days patients spend in the hospital or disabled at home. Severe depression is more disabling than many other serious medical disorders, including lung disease, arthritis, and diabetes.[1] And as we grow older, the risk of depression increases.[2]

WHAT IS DEPRESSION?

A variety of mood disorders are lumped under the heading of depression. Chronic depression is a low-level sense of pessimism

---

RISK FACTORS FOR DEPRESSION

- Being a woman (women are at twice the risk of depression compared with men)
- A family history of depression or alcoholism
- A negative home environment
- Recent negative life events, particularly those involving a loss
- A lack of confiding relationships
- Giving birth in the past six months

From Weissman, M.M., et. al. 1984. The epidemiology of affective disorders. In *Neurobiology of Mood Disorders*, edited by R.M. Post and Ballenger, 60-75. Baltimore: Williams and Wilkins.

that may not interfere significantly with how one makes it through life, and that appears to others as simply a glum personality. Manic-depressive illness is characterized by wide mood swings from depression to euphoria. Major depression is the blackest despair; it's accompanied by physical symptoms, gets diagnosed by clinicians, is treated by medications and therapy, and sometimes results in hospitalization and too often in suicide. The causes of depressive diseases are not well understood and can be highly individual.

"Normal" Depression

At the most basic level, many—perhaps most—of us become depressed at times because we find ourselves in "depressing" circumstances. Certainly everyone feels a bit "blue" or down in the dumps now and then, when nothing seems to go right, when the bills pile up, when the car needs a major overhaul, or when our legislators have just done something else that's clearly counterproductive. Depression can be a normal and understandable response to the strains of our confusing, frenetic, and unnerving postindustrial society, a signal that it's time to take a breather, slow down, take stock of the situation, and maybe go to Hawaii for a week or so.

There seems to be a genetic component to depression; if there's a history of depression in your family, you may be at greater risk yourself. Those who were raised in dysfunctional families also seem to be at increased risk. And then the "external" or "environmental" factors, the depressing, stressful times in which we find ourselves, interact with whatever genetic predispositions to melancholy may exist and we end up down in the dumps. Avoid the depressing circumstances, however, and a genetic predisposition may be irrelevant.

Not-So-Normal Depression

But sometimes this quite legitimate funk we might feel while watching the evening news turns into something more profound and troubling. We lose interest in the outside world, withdraw into our own bleak inner world, lose the ability to love, and lose our sense of self-esteem until, paralyzed by self-loathing, we simply cease to function. The depressed individual becomes paralyzed by the horror of his or her own existence, like a deer caught in the headlights of an oncoming truck. For purposes of diagnosis, a *major depressive episode* is defined as a "change of mood that has been present at least two weeks and is marked by symptoms of depressed mood or loss

SYMPTOMS OF DEPRESSION

- Difficulty making decisions
- Decreased productivity
- Irritability and hostility
- Withdrawal from or extreme dependence on others
- Feelings of hopelessness or despair
- Slow speech and chronic fatigue
- Flat or blank expression (flattened "affect")
- Inability to concentrate
- Decline in dependability
- Unusual increase in errors
- Prone to accidents
- Tardiness and absenteeism
- Lack of enthusiasm for work tasks

From Goleman, D. 1993, Dec. 3. Depression Costs U.S. Billions. *West County Times.*

of pleasure or interest."[3] Mental changes with major depression include apathy, poor concentration, and memory deficits. These are accompanied by physical symptoms that include fatigue, loss of appetite or perhaps overeating, sexual dysfunction, digestive problems, and abnormal sleep patterns.[4]

What makes depression so frightening is that often the depressed person doesn't clearly understand why he or she feels this way, leading to increased anxiety, more depression, and a downward spiral that ends in suicide in 10 to 15 percent of severe, clinically diagnosed cases of depression.[5]

FREUDIANS VERSUS BIOLOGISTS

No two people respond to the loss of a loved one, or financial problems, or even the evening news in quite the same way. And why some respond with a justifiable but limited depression while others sink into suicidal paralysis of the spirit is the subject of much learned but politely heated discussion among psychiatrists, psychologists, biologists, and other mental health professionals.

The Freudians, on the one hand, believe depression is strictly a psychological ailment, a kind of grief that has gone out of control for some reason and turned inward to become rage and guilt and utter despair. But the Freudians are outnumbered these days by the "organic directed" psychiatrists, who take a more mechanical and chemical view of the mind and body; they see depression as the result of a complex and poorly understood series of biochemical misadventures in the brain. Most likely, both factors play a role in how any given individual responds to what life throws his or her way. Genetic factors—affecting both biochemistry and psychology—may play the major role.

Despite the complexity of depression and the murkiness of its causes, one thing is known for certain: Most depressed people recover eventually. Depression often lifts as mysteriously as it comes. By some estimates as many as 85 percent of the depressed patients seen by mental health professionals would improve on their own without intervention

Many who are depressed lack the patience and equanimity to await the remission of their disease, of course. And because one of the central qualities of depression is hopelessness, the severely depressed may not ever believe that by waiting, they'll recover, which further contributes to their hopelessness. Those who have the ready cash to pay for professional help can find a variety of treatments for this dark night of the soul, ranging from simple talk and analysis to drugs and even electroshock therapy.

SWEATING THE BLUES AWAY

In recent years, however, another therapy has been gaining widespread attention—exercise. The effectiveness of exercise as a treatment—some might even say a cure—for depression is gaining increasing acceptance. A variety of studies of exercise and mood over the years have looked at the therapeutic effects of exercise on depressed patients and concluded that

- exercise is a better antidepressant than relaxation or other enjoyable activities are;
- exercise is as effective in decreasing depression as psychotherapy is;

- anaerobic exercise (for example, weight training, sprinting) is as potent an antidepressant as aerobic exercise (walking, jogging, and so on) is; and

- exercise and psychotherapy together are more effective than exercise alone is.[6-9]

Considering how pervasive a problem depression has become in this country, a cheap and effective therapy could have an enormous impact on the nation's health. And exercise is, above all, cheap. Even with the most expensive jogging togs, a personal trainer, and a basement full of treadmills, weight machines, and exercise bikes, exercise is still cheaper than hospitalization, regular doses of antidepressants, or a course of weekly sessions with a therapist. Although not every depressed patient can afford a $150-an-hour Freudian, everyone can afford a brisk walk around the block. Not everyone has time to spend stretched out on a therapist's couch, but just about anyone can squeeze in a few laps around the neighborhood or a few laps in the local pool. With exercise therapy, the depressed can treat themselves with a minimum of preparation and information. And

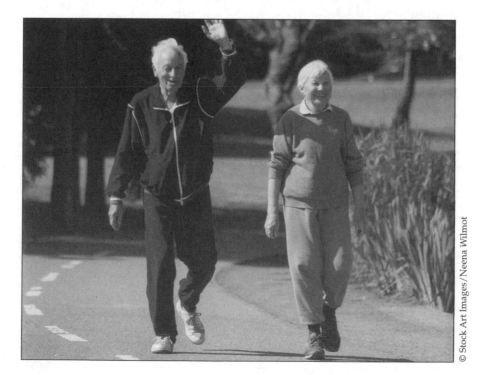

finally, unlike many antidepressant medications, exercise has positive side effects, not harmful ones.

Fewer studies have looked at the preventive benefits of exercise for "normal" men and women. Among investigators who've considered both, William Morgan at the University of Wisconsin-Madison, one of the pioneers, has concluded after much study that regular physical activity not only improves the mood of depressed patients, it also reduces the risk that normal men and women will become depressed.[10]

Professor Morgan's conclusions, and similar conclusions of other researchers, are supported by findings from the College Study.[11-13] Among the college alumni, for example, there was a direct associa-

---

PHYSICAL ACTIVITY AND SUICIDE

Interestingly, among the college alumni, there was no significant relation between level of total energy expenditure and rates of suicide, although there were trends suggesting such a relation. However, alumni who involved themselves in regular sports play had only half the risk of suicide compared with alumni who didn't.[a]

What do we make of this? Were alumni who participated in sports less likely to become depressed and take their own lives because they played sports, or did they play sports because they weren't depressed? Someone who's feeling blue is probably going to have a hard time getting out for a jog or a game of softball with the office league. Perhaps those alumni who enjoyed life more, were more engaged with life and by nature less likely to become depressed and commit suicide, were also more likely to get involved with sports. On the other hand, findings from other studies that found a preventive effect from exercise in terms of depression suggest some cause-and-effect link.

But the relation seems plausible in light of what we know about the links between social engagement and stress, stress and depression, and so on. Sports play that involves some engagement with others would seem to provide both the preventive benefits of the physical activity and the benefits of social contact.

Note. [a]Paffenbarger, R.S., Jr.; Lee, I.M.; & Leung, R. 1994. Chronic disease in former college students: LIII. Physical activity and personal characteristics associated with depression and suicide in American college men. In J. Lonnqvist & T. Sahi, eds., *Acta Psychiatrica Scandinavia 89* (Suppl. 377): 16-22.

tion between physical activity and a reduced risk of becoming depressed. The more active the alumni, the less likely they were to become depressed (see figure 8.1). Those who expended 1,000 to 2,499 kilocalories a week in walking, stair climbing, and sports had a 17 percent lower risk of becoming depressed than less active alumni. Those who expended 2,500 kilocalories or more a week were at 28 percent less risk. In particular, alumni who participated in three or more hours of moderately vigorous sports each week experienced a 27 percent lower risk of depression than those who participated one hour or less.

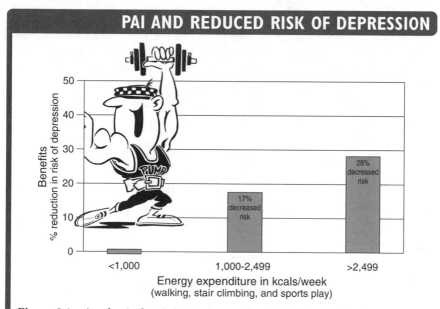

Figure 8.1 As physical activity increases, the risk of depression decreases.

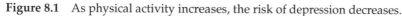

AGING, MEMORY, AND AN ACTIVE LIFE

Changes in our ability to remember things as we grow older can be particularly troubling. As we grow older, any lapse of memory sounds a tiny alarm. We forget where we left the car keys and immediately think that we have Alzheimer's disease. But, most memory loss is not a sign of impending dementia, and it's debatable whether or not memory loss associated with aging is even an indicator of physiological changes in the brain, something we'll discuss shortly.

Indeed, forgetfulness at all ages is probably more common than we realize. But most of the time, there's a balance between what we expect to be able to remember and what our memories actually can accomplish. As we grow older, however, our expectations change as we become sensitized to the issue of memory loss and aging.

The reason for the apparent poor memories of many older adults may be that the older we get, the more life experiences we've had, so we simply have more to remember. It's easy enough to find a single file in an otherwise empty file cabinet, but try to find the same file in a cabinet that's stuffed full of other files—you'll probably still find it, but it might take longer. The fact that older adults may take a bit longer to recall some things, or may have more memory lapses, could be a sign of something positive; would you rather have a mind nearly empty of memories or one that's stuffed full of material?

There are four general types of memory: immediate memory (information learned and immediately repeated); recent memory (information recalled a few days later); remote memory (facts learned in grade school, for example); and learned skills.

Each of these types of memory represents a different memory system involving different mental functions. Of the four systems, only the second type of memory—recent memory—seems to be affected by age: you're introduced to someone at a party and a week later can't recall his or her name. It can be aggravating and even embarrassing, but it's not a sign of impending disease or mental decline.

Studies looking at whether or not most of us can indeed expect to become more forgetful in this particular area have found that as we age we tend to use fewer spontaneous strategies to help us remember, such as rehearsal (repeating information) and categorization (grouping related items). Studies of both young and old subjects show that if both groups are given something to remember, and then are introduced to such memory strategies, there's little difference between them. In a sense, as we get older, we may be more prone to "forgetting to remember." We make a grocery list in the morning and then forget to take it with us when we go shopping. We meet a person at a party and "forget" to employ strategies to remember that person's name.

The question that arises, then, is why do we tend not to use these strategies to remember as we grow older? Why are we less likely to "remember to remember"? Again, it may be that as we get older, we simply have more things to remember, so we're less likely to "remember to remember" the things we want to remember. Disease, anxiety, or depression can distract us or sap the energy we might employ to "remember to remember." When we're ill, certainly, we have other things on our minds, which can impair memory. At a less acute level, it may be that as some of us grow older and become more sedentary and less fit, our energy decreases, and we have fewer energy reserves to put out the effort it takes to "remember to remember." This suggests, at the very least, that regular exercise, to the degree it "energizes" us, may have a beneficial impact on memory.

But there appears to be much more to the ways in which physical activity helps us maintain sharp minds throughout our lives, and this gets us into the inner workings of the brain itself and the complex issues of intelligence.

THE "PUMPED UP" BRAIN

At least some of the apparent declines in intelligence observed among some older adults result from lack of practice, not an inevitable biological outcome of advancing years. Much research is available demonstrating that documented declines in intelligence with age, as measured by IQ and similar tests, are quite reversible and prove to be nonexistent when subjects of all ages are coached in test-taking procedures and given opportunities to practice.[14,15]

In this country, where older adults are too often expected and sometimes are required to retire, when they're expected to separate themselves from daily discourse and are relegated to retirement villages or rest homes to sit in front of TVs for hours watching shows that often cannot be conceived of as mentally stimulating under any circumstances, apparently inevitable declines in intelligence are more likely simply cultural artifacts.

Many older adults are troubled by depression and this can have a negative impact on mental function. Likewise, anxiety, perhaps over health or money, can also impact intelligence as well as memory, often simply by making it difficult to concentrate. Lack of social interaction may also cause apparent declines in intelligence. The older man or woman whose spouse has died, whose friends have moved away, who is alone much of the day may seem to grow "duller" simply because he or she isn't putting the mind to use.

For example, take Alzheimer's disease, a progressive loss of memory and other mental functions caused by the death of neurons and loss of connections between neurons in the brain. No one understands what causes Alzheimer's, and a cure seems very far off. But most experts agree that an active, healthy life with good nutrition, plenty of social interaction, and activities to keep the mind busy, are the best hope we have so far for preventing the disease. One intriguing study of Boston residents, for example, suggests that the more years of education you've had, the lower your risk of Alzheimer's.[16,17] Of course, Alzheimer's is a disease, not an aspect of normal aging. But what's true for Alzheimer's may be true for other mental changes. Any brain thrives on novelty and stimulation.

Neuroscientist Marian Diamond of the University of California in Berkeley suggests that a healthy brain does not lose neurons or function at any age.[18] But of course that's the rub: how many of us have *healthy* brains? The key to preventing disease and keeping the brian healthy, or preventing the supposedly "normal" decline of thinking horsepower that some feel comes with age, says Diamond, is not only to preserve neurons in the brain—neurons can't be replaced once they die—but to preserve, and better yet, to build new connections between them. Diamond put old rats into new cages with new toys and their brains fairly blossomed with new neural connections and increased blood flow, and what's true of old rats is probably true of old humans (or young ones, for that matter). Mental stimulation increases or preserves neural connections. And thinking power comes both from the number of healthy, functioning neurons, and the numbers of connections between them.

Thus the link between education and a reduced risk of Alzheimer's, or any age-related mental decline, begins to make sense. The more education you have when young, and the more education you continue throughout your life, the more neural connections you have, and the more you have available to lose before any noticeable symptoms develop, producing a protective effect.[19]

And even if some loss of neurons with aging is normal, as some believe, it's possible that through various lifestyle changes, including taking up physical activity, we can increase the efficiency of the remaining neurons through exercise and thus delay or prevent the mental changes we associate with aging.

The brain is acutely sensitive to any condition that limits its supply of blood, oxygen, and nutrients. Plaque buildups in arteries to the brain can limit the amount of blood flow to the brain, which may adversely impact mental functioning. Likewise, lung disease can reduce the amount of oxygen available, and declines in heart functioning due to disease or simple inactivity may also reduce the flow of blood and oxygen to the brain.

The good news here is that activity seems to work in several ways to enhance cognitive function by increasing blood flow to the brain, promoting beneficial changes in neurotransmitters and increasing neural connectivity, and perhaps also by contributing to increased social interactions, reduced stress, and depression.

PHYSICAL ACTIVITY AND COGNITIVE EFFICIENCY

At the University of Maryland, a research team led by Brad Hatfield, PhD, has been looking at how high levels of physical endurance correlate with high levels of mental functioning, specifically in terms of mental efficiency as measured by the amount of "fast-frequency" brain-wave activity during specific mental tasks, including math problems.

Hatfield's theory—only a hypothesis as yet, but a good one—is that the fitter subjects can think better, and that aspects of this improved intellectual functioning can be measured objectively in the laboratory. This notion is based on the work of others who find that those with high IQs show less fast-frequency or "beta" activity in the brain during mental challenge. Those with higher IQs, in other words, seem to have more efficient brains; it takes them less brainpower to perform any given mental task.

To test his hypothesis, Hatfield set out to measure the beta-wave activity of highly fit and less fit individuals of a variety of ages to see how they compared. In one study, his fit subjects were very active older men (average age of 66 years) who trained by running about six miles a day. The less fit group of men the same age weren't total couch spuds, however; these men burned about 300 kilocalories a day in less strenuous physical activities such as golf or walking. Hatfield was careful to choose all of his subjects so they came from the same socioeconomic background, with roughly the same education and income levels. He hooked up his subjects to EEGs to measure beta-wave activity and then gave them a battery of tests intended to challenge their thought processes.

Hatfield's findings are enlightening: The more physically fit subjects showed roughly half the beta-wave activity of their less fit peers.[20] Hatfield notes that those in both groups had equal ability to solve problems, but the less fit were using more gray matter to do so; they were thinking more intensely to solve the same problems, and what this may mean in a real-world context is that the fitter individuals would be less mentally fatigued at the end of a tough day at the office. Fitter individuals would probably recover from mentally stressful situations more quickly as well, which has important health benefits, as we've seen earlier. Also, fitter individuals may be able to concentrate more effectively and probably have improved memories.

Even more heartening, in a companion study, Hatfield and colleagues compared fit older men with unfit older and unfit younger men in a similar battery of mental tests given while the subjects were connected to EEGs. In this study, Hatfield considered "Tau" scores for all three groups: "old trained" (OT), "old untrained," (OU), and "young untrained" (YU). Tau scores, like measures of beta-wave activity, measure cognitive efficiency (the lower the Tau score, the better, because it means you're using more specific areas of the brain to think). Hatfield found that Tau scores for the older trained subjects were .192 and .199 for the left and right hemispheres of the brain, respectively. For the older untrained subjects, the scores were .354 and .290, a significant difference. And for the young untrained, he found that their Tau scores were a dismal .386 and .355. In other words, the fit older men in Hatfield's study could think more efficiently than both the younger and older untrained men. This suggests that even if the conventional wisdom is correct, even if we do lose brain cells as we age, if we can make more efficient use of the cells we have left as we grow older, we can prevent or at least slow the apparent effects of aging on the mind.

Hatfield's research, of course, raises the ever-troubling issue of cause and effect; were the fitter men in his study more cognitively efficient because they trained regularly, or did they happen to train regularly because they were perhaps more intelligent (and perhaps understood better than others the value of regular exercise)?

To approach this question, Robert Dustman, PhD, of the Veterans Affairs Medical Center in Salt Lake City, looked at 50- and 60-something couch-spuds-turned-athletes, putting his subjects on a four-month program of walking and jogging. Before the training began, Dustman had his subjects take an extensive battery of both physical tests to measure fitness and mental tests to measure cognitive functioning, during which he also measured brain-wave activity. At the end of the four-month training program, he put them through the same battery of physical and mental tests and found that the subjects who changed from a sedentary to an active way of life had improved their physical endurance by 27 percent and their performance on a battery of mental exams by nearly 10 percent (see figure 8.2). Better still, the mental functioning of the newly fit older men compared quite well with that of much younger controls.[21-24]

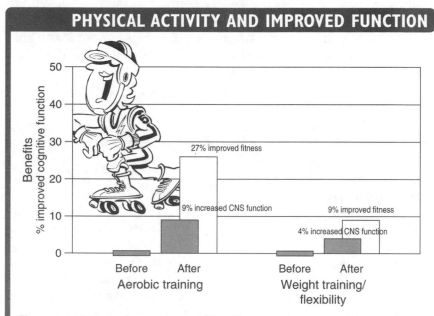

PHYSICAL ACTIVITY AND IMPROVED FUNCTION

27% improved fitness

9% increased CNS function

9% improved fitness

4% increased CNS function

Benefits
% improved cognitive function

Before After
Aerobic training

Before After
Weight training/
flexibility

Figure 8.2 Men and women aged 55 to 70 years were given a battery of tests to measure both fitness and cognitive function before and after four-month training programs. Training included either brisk walking or jogging for the "aerobic" group, and weight training and flexibility for the other exercise group.

Adapted, by permission, from R. Dustman, 1984, "Aerobic exercise training and improved neuropsychological function of older individuals," *Neurobiology of Aging* 5: 35-42.

THE "MUSCULAR" BRAIN

Think of the brain as a type of muscle; when you train a muscle sufficiently, it requires fewer muscle fibers to perform a given task. There's less strain on the trained muscle when it's taxed. It becomes more efficient so it can work better for longer. It doesn't tire as quickly. And now we're seeing that the same may be true of the brain. Even if the brain does lose functioning neurons as we age—and, remember, neuroscientist Marian Diamond says a healthy brain doesn't—if we remain physically fit and mentally active, our brains become more efficient, requiring fewer brain cells to perform any given task; any loss of neurons that may occur with age is counteracted by improved use of the cells that are left.

This may have important implications in terms of our ability to adapt to change as we grow older. You may recall from earlier chapters that one definition of aging is decreasing ability to adapt to change and cope with sudden threats to well-being. If, due to inefficiency, the brain is being taxed just to get through the day, there will be no reserves left when something novel challenges us. The healthy brain is like a well-run firehouse; when a fire occurs, only enough trucks and men as are needed are sent to deal with a particular fire; if all the trucks and men were sent out to extinguish someone's overcooked turkey, for example, there would be no reserves left to fight a second, perhaps more serious, fire, and the result could be disastrous. Likewise, the brain of the woman or man who exercises may be more efficient and thus has more reserves for use when those reserves are needed.

IS OXYGEN THE KEY?

What's the link between more efficient muscles and improved cognitive efficiency, between sweat and brains? Oxygen, perhaps.

To work at its best, the brain needs a constant supply of oxygen and glucose, which is carried to the brain by the blood. Because a constant supply of blood is so essential, the arteries supplying blood to the brain have the ability to narrow and widen as needed to ensure adequate oxygen and nourishment. Likewise, blood vessels within the brain widen and narrow to regulate the flow of blood to those areas of the brain working hardest. For example, as you read this, some parts of your brain are receiving more blood than others. But certainly there are limits to how much the vessels supplying blood to the brain can accomplish, as we'll discuss shortly.

How the Brain Works

The average human brain accounts for only about 2 percent of body weight, yet it receives 15 percent of the body's total blood flow, takes 25 percent of its oxygen, and uses a whopping 70 percent of available glucose.[25] The brain is made up of billions of nerve cells (packed 100 million to the cubic inch), and each neuron can be connected to tens of thousands of other neurons with which it is in constant communication, with messages passing from cell to cell at the synapses, millionth-of-an-inch gaps between neurons. In these synapses, all the enormously complex, fascinating, and mysterious bioelectrical activities take place to transmit messages from one neuron to another, enabling us to think, move, feel, laugh, love, hate, brood, read, and watch the news. Several chemicals called neurotransmitters are activated in the synapses to aid in the transmission of these messages between cells, and it's also here where the all-important interactions between neurotransmitters can go wrong, bringing on all the varied and sometimes spectacular inspirations, neuroses, psychoses, profound or frivolous ideas, depressions, visions, and artistic creations that have cursed and blessed us for all of civilization. Some 40 or more neurotransmitters have been identified in the past 30 years, including dopamine, serotonin, and norepinephrine, all key players in our moods, and researchers believe many more neurotransmitters will be discovered in the future.

When a neurotransmitter is released from one neuron and travels across the synapse to another neuron, it can have either an inhibitory or an excitatory effect. Because each neuron is receiving chemical messages via neurotransmitters from thousands of others in its immediate vicinity, the net effect of all these chemical inputs determines whether the neuron "fires" and passes on the stimulus to the next cell. Imagine billions of neurons, each linked to thousands of others in a network of unimaginable complexity, made more so by the fact that there are different types of synapses as well as the known and still-undiscovered neurotransmitters, all interacting with each other in ways we only vaguely understand.

What is known, though, is that the entire system is both enormously durable and frighteningly delicate. Stroke, accident, or disease can destroy large portions of the brain, yet the brain can, to an extent, form new functional pathways and networks through existing neurons around damaged areas or "reprogram" existing neurons to restore at least some of the original function and memory.

Brain Chemistry

Although the brain is enormously adaptable and durable, its ability to function at peak levels is highly sensitive to anything that can upset the balance of neurotransmitters. Even subtle changes can have a profound effect on the ability to think clearly and rapidly, and imbalances of neurotransmitters probably play a major role in schizophrenia, depression, and various other mental disorders. Lack of dopamine, which has an inhibitory function, results in the uncontrollable shaking of Parkinson's disease, and it may be that insufficiencies or excesses of other, perhaps as yet unknown, neurotransmitters produce the slowing of the central nervous system, slowing of reflexes, and memory changes we associate with aging, as well as the more severe symptoms we call dementia or Alzheimer's disease.

Serotonin, dopamine, and norepinephrine are all amines, a specific class of nitrogen-based chemicals. It is known that depressed individuals have abnormally low levels of serotonin in their brains, and that exercise of at least 30 minutes stimulates the production of serotonin. Indeed, theory has it that when we exercise for about 30 minutes, the serotonin rises to a level at which its effects can be felt, a "lightening" of the step, an energized feeling.[26]

Another class of chemicals receiving much attention these days is endorphin, a morphine-like substance produced by the body. A natural and apparently quite effective painkiller that increases with the stimulus of physical activity, endorphin perhaps also contributes to the improved mood many experience during exercise and may provide some of the relief depressed individuals experience when they exercise.

Much of this is speculative, of course. But adding weight to the idea that exercise affects brain chemistry is the quite observable fact that patients receiving antidepressant medications who take up exercise become increasingly sensitive to the drugs, as if their own "internal pharmacopoeia" has kicked in along with their sweat; typically, patients begin to decrease their medications as their exercise increases, often discontinuing them entirely.

The Oxygen Connection

In any case, all of these neurotransmitters depend on oxygen for metabolism, and although the brain's own blood vessels do a marvelous job of keeping the flow of blood to and within the brain at optimal levels, there may be limits. If you're sedentary and out of shape, your cardiovascular system won't work as well; it won't be able to pump as efficiently; your arteries will be clogged with plaque, and eventually this puts limits on the amount of oxygen available in the blood. In theory, when that happens, your brain won't get as much oxygen- and glucose-rich blood as it needs, even after the vessels supplying blood have opened as widely as possible; you can turn the kitchen faucet on all the way, but if the well's gone dry, you won't get any water. There's much debate on this particular point; some theorize that the brain always takes all the oxygen it needs, no matter how compromised the cardiovascular system may be, even at the expense of other organ systems. But there's some question about just what we mean by the brain's "needs." When the cardiovascular system has been compromised by sedentary living, smoking, and so on, and less oxygen is available throughout the body, the brain may ratchet down its needs, making do with less oxygen and operating, not at peak, but at a somewhat lower level, although still operating, more or less. But we shouldn't settle for "more or less." Our goal should be to continue functioning at peak levels throughout our lives.

Lack of oxygen may cause brain cells to die off or cause connections between neurons to break down. And lack of oxygen may also interfere with the metabolism of neurotransmitters. In research done on the dutiful white lab rat, for example, it was found that, compared with sedentary rats, aerobically trained rats produce higher levels of the neurotransmitter dopamine. Of course, it's always risky to generalize from the experience of the ever-accommodating rat and try to draw conclusions about how humans should conduct their lives, but such findings fit nicely with data from the College Study, for example. These findings suggest that physical activity offers at least a slight protection from Parkinson's disease, suggesting that what's true of the rat really is true for us humans. Moderately active men in the study had about a 17 percent reduced risk of Parkinson's compared to men who were more sedentary. More active men had a slightly increased risk compared with the moderately active, although their risk was still less than that of the sedentary group.[27] These findings could mean that alumni who subsequently suffered Parkinson's had a prolonged subclinical phase before the onset of obvious symptoms, a time during which they may have been able to function quite normally in daily activities but were impaired when required to do more demanding activities, and thus selected themselves out as more sedentary. But research with rats at least suggests protection, not merely selection.

All of this supports findings such as those of Hatfield and Dustman and others: As we exercise and become more physically fit, our cardiovascular systems are able to pump more blood throughout the body, including the brain, and this improved oxygenation facilitates the metabolism of a variety of neurotransmitters—not just dopamine, but perhaps also acetylcholine for good memory, norepinephrine for mood regulation, and other neurotransmitters we don't even know about yet.[28-30]

All of this is still highly speculative, but it's not excessively wild conjecture. And all of this may have important implications for those who are concerned about reducing the risk of Alzheimer's disease (and who isn't?). Like Parkinson's disease, Alzheimer's results from cell death in the brain.[31] If physical activity can help maintain blood flow to the brain into old age and thus prevent the death of brain cells, and if this increased blood flow can enhance the metabolism of neurotransmitters in the case of dopamine and Parkinson's, wouldn't the same sort of mechanism be at work in the case of Alzheimer's? Maybe. On the other hand, the mechanisms leading to Alzheimer's could ultimately prove to be quite different than those of Parkinson's; much more research is needed is this area.

STRUCTURAL CHANGES IN THE BRAIN

Not only does the chemistry of the brain change with increased physical activity and improved cardiovascular performance, but physical changes appear to take place in the brain that correspond to physical changes in the rest of the body. Just as blood vessels in the working muscles increase in size, and just as there's a proliferation of new vessels to carry more blood, likewise there's an increase in the size and number of blood vessels that serve the brain. William Greenough, PhD, of the University of Illinois in Urbana, and James Black, MD, of the University of Utah, found a 20 percent increase in the number of blood vessels nourishing the cerebellum of rats that were aerobically trained for four weeks.

More intriguing still, whereas Greenough and Black found that aerobically trained rats had an increased blood flow to their brains, rats trained in what they called "acrobatic" activities—that is, complex physical tasks that require a period of learning to master—showed a surprising increase in synaptic connections between brain cells.[32] Thus it may be that an additional benefit of exercise—or at least the appropriate type of exercise—is the preservation and perhaps even growth of neural connectivity as we age.

EXERCISE AS MEDITATION

Physical activity can contribute to peak mental functioning and particularly to improved mood in many other ways.

Physical exercise that involves the rhythmic movement of large muscle groups—swimming, cycling, running, walking, rowing, and so on—seems to be most effective in relieving stress or preventing depression, both of which impair cognitive functioning. The routine rhythmic motion of running or walking, in particular, requires little thought or attention. Anyone who has run or walked regularly for even a few minutes knows how the mind seems to open to a flood of thoughts and emotions; solutions to nagging problems suddenly appear like flashing 100-watt bulbs. Fantasies arise. You find your-self thinking of all the smart things you should have said to the cop who gave you that speeding ticket. In fantasy, there's no limit to your power and ability, and during that magical time, with the blood flowing and the legs pumping steadily, many people find the key to

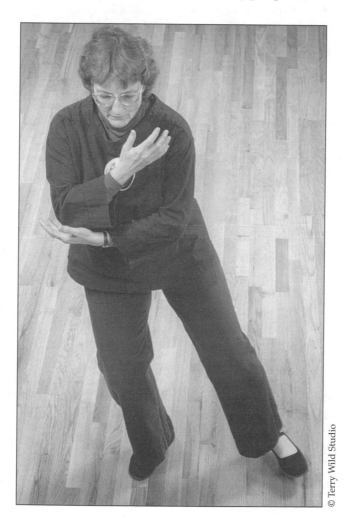

solving whatever problems plague them. It's a creative, mentally stimulating time for many.

And for those who are troubled by depression, in particular, exercise may unlock the chains of their despair, or at least offer a break from it. Think of an exercise period as a sort of vacation from all the negative thinking and nagging sense of guilt or "what's the use" that characterize depression. The benefits of this time-out reverberate long after the run or walk is over. It's like a weekend in the mountains, and some researchers such as William Morgan believe that this "vacation" or time-out may be exercise's primary benefit when used as a therapy or prevention, providing a chance to break away from the routines of daily life.[33]

EXERCISE PRESCRIPTION FOR A HEALTHY BRAIN

All of this has important implications for the older man or woman who wants to stay mentally sharp. The ideal mind/body program for optimal mental functioning includes sustained Stage Two aerobic activities as well as activities involving complex motor skills.

30 MINUTES

On an acute level, as noted, 30 minutes of sustained, moderately vigorous exercise seems to have the most immediate impact on brain chemistry and cognitive functioning. Intensity does seem to matter; the more intense the activity, to a point, the more pronounced the influence on brain chemistry, so as much as possible, strive for sustained Stage Two activities. Whether activities such as resistance training are as effective remains to be seen; most likely, any type of exercise—brisk walking, jogging, or pumping iron—will be beneficial if it raises the heart rate, keeps it elevated, and brings a bit of sweat to the brow.

OVER TIME

"Chronic" effects of regular activity could lead to an increase in blood vessels in the brain as well as beneficial effects on the cardiovascular system, ensuring a richer supply of oxygen and nutrients for the brain. Aerobic activities such as brisk walking and jogging are particularly popular because they're simple and don't require a lot of equipment or special facilities.

ADD SOME COMPLEXITY, TOO

Although aerobic activities and strength training develop the cardiovascular system and thus improve the flow of blood to the brain, they may not provide all the benefit we would hope for in terms of neural connectivity. For younger adults, these activities may be sufficient, because neural connectivity may be preserved or developed through social interactions and the demands of the job. But for the retired man or woman whose opportunity for social involvements and intellectual challenge may be more limited, involvement

---

KEEPING THE MIND HEALTHY

Here are some simple things you can do to keep your mind in good working order:

- Engage in regular Stage One and Stage Two exercise.
- Eat a healthful diet that is low in fats and high in complex carbohydrates.
- Drink alcohol in moderation, if at all.
- Don't smoke.
- Read; participate in continuing education programs.
- Avoid rigid adherence to routine; seek variety.
- Practice stress reduction.
- Maintain as many friendships as possible.
- Keep engaged in community activities—volunteering, continuing education.
- Develop intellectually stimulating hobbies, but these should be things you like: Learn a new language, take up painting, learn an instrument, and so on.
- Learn, learn, learn.

in a complex physical activity such as tai chi chuan, yoga, aerobic dance, tennis, or squash becomes increasingly important, about which more in part III.

The ideal exercise plan for peak physical and mental performance thus would be a total-body routine that includes aerobic training such as brisk walking, weight training for strength, and some complex activity that requires continual learning or refinement of skills. Even better, do at least some of this in a social context for the benefits of staying connected with others. Add continuing education, community involvement, and the like for additional benefits. Learn a new language, take up an instrument, join a book discussion group, or enroll in extension classes at the local college.

In the next three chapters, we'll discuss how to get started in an active way of life, how to stick with it for a lifetime of good health and vitality, and how to train sensibly.

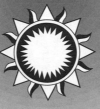

part III

A PROGRAM FOR CHANGE

Not less than two hours a day should be devoted to exercise, and the weather shall be little regarded. I speak this from experience, having made this arrangement of my life. If the body is feeble, the mind will not be strong.

—Thomas Jefferson
Letter to Thomas M. Randolph, Jr.
August 27, 1786

chapter 9
<hr>

FIGURING IT OUT

If you're just starting out in an active life, or if you've been only haphazardly active because you've had a hard time sticking with it, you'll have the best chance of changing successfully if you know what you want and what works best for you.

We hope you're convinced by now that taking up and sticking with physical activity will add years to your life and life to your years. Now you'll want to know exactly what to do and how to do it.

In chapter 1, we sketched out the basics of the two-stage LifeFit program for optimal health and longevity. To review: Stage One includes a total of at least an hour a day simply being up on your feet using the large muscles of your legs, puttering about in activities of daily living. Any activity—other than sitting quietly—can be a Stage One activity. Stage Two activities include at least three 30-minute sessions each week of sustained, moderate physical activity that elevates your heart rate and brings sweat to your brow—brisk walking, jogging, swimming, and so on.

Together, Stage One and Stage Two activities will amount to a weekly energy expenditure of about 1,500 to 2,000 kilocalories if you weigh about 155 pounds, or about 10 percent more or less for every 10 pounds above or below 155 pounds. This is the least amount of physical activity that will provide you with the most health benefits at the least risk of injury, burnout, or discouragement. Stage One and Stage Two together will be your long-term LifeFit goal.

Although we should all strive for the LifeFit goal, there is no single right way to go about it. This chapter suggests a number of ways to learn more about yourself, your likes and dislikes, your abilities and inclinations, and thus how to find those activities that will best suit your needs and work best for you in your own program for optimal health.

Chances are you're already well on your way to this goal, but if you're like most adults, you may need to employ a few simple strategies to bring you closer. Reaching Stage Two will likely take a bit more determination and planning, but as you'll see, this needn't be difficult. In fact, in this chapter and the next, we'll specifically show you how.

After you've gone through this chapter, you'll have the basic information you'll need to get started by creating an individualized beginning program that is best for you and thus easiest for you to stick with. Chapter 10 helps you use the information you've discovered about yourself to develop and fine-tune your progression toward your LifeFit goal. Chapter 11 offers some useful strategies for sticking with activity for the long haul.

LIFEFIT PRINCIPLES

- Although we should all strive for the LifeFit goal, there is no single right way to go about it.

- One of the best ways to become more active, and then to stick with an active life while reducing your risk of discouragement or injury, is to engage in activities that best suit your body and your temperament.

- Acknowledge such nuts-and-bolts issues as potential barriers due to conflicting commitments, lack of time, or lack of facilities.

- You'll have the best chance of sticking with an active life if you approach activity in the spirit of a child, open to the possibility that whatever you're doing, whether puttering or walking briskly, running, cycling, swimming, or playing tennis, can also be fun.

- One of the best ways to stick with exercise, and reduce your risk of discouragement or injury, is to engage in activities that best suit your body. Consider physiological impediments such as old injuries or health concerns.

- Try to anticipate the difficulties you'll face becoming and staying active, then choose activities that best help you work around those barriers. This will reduce the number of excuses too many of us manage to find for not being active.

- Be aware of the specific results you want.

- Set clear goals; having goals will help you stay motivated, particularly when you think you are too tired to exercise after a tough day at work, or you think you don't have time, or it's too chilly out.

- Keep a record so you know if you are progressing toward your goals.

- Reward yourself when you achieve specific goals.

WHO ARE YOU?

One of the surest ways to become more active, and then to stick with an active life while reducing your risk of discouragement or injury, is to engage in activities that best suit your body and your temperament; not everyone is built to be a runner or even a walker; and not everyone likes—or knows how—to swim. If walking makes your feet ache or chlorinated swimming pools make your eyes burn, you'll be unlikely to stick with these activities. Some find cycling in city traffic an exercise in sheer terror. Others may be uncomfortable in an aerobics class where the walls are covered with mirrors. To give yourself the best chance of reaching your LifeFit goal, the program you create for yourself will have to be one that's realistic and acknowledges such nuts-and-bolts issues as potential barriers due to conflicting commitments, lack of time, or lack of facilities. You'll also want to consider physiological impediments such as old injuries or health concerns. Your LifeFit program should bring you the specific results *you* want. And your program should, above all else, involve activities that you like to do.

There is an endless variety of activities from which to choose. But which ones are right for you? You won't know for sure until you've tried a variety of things. The answers to the following four questions will help you narrow the possibilities.

QUESTION 1—WHAT DO YOU LIKE?

Ultimately, what is right for you will be something you *like* to do; in other words, something that's fun. The idea that exercise might be fun and that we should have fun may seem something of a stretch in this frenetic, competitive, no-nonsense world of ours. What sensible, responsible adult has time for fun, after all? And at the outset, making the transition from a sedentary to an active life may not seem much like fun; all change can be stressful, as we've seen. And getting out and walking, jogging, or aerobicizing can make your muscles ache, at least at first. Besides, fun's really for kids, isn't it?

Indeed, but then we have much to learn from our children. For one thing, once kids have been pried away from the TV and video games, they spend most of their waking hours in action—playing. And notice *how* they play, and thus how it is they can keep at it hour after hour. It's not just their youth that gives them such stamina, but also the fact that they're having fun while they play, and children are very good at keeping things fun.

First, they do things they like; if it's not fun, they won't do it, unless, of course, Mom or Dad makes them. And kids continually change their activities for variety. Once something becomes a bore, or if it hurts, then it's not fun, and kids won't do it, a very important lesson for us adults as we grow older and perhaps less durable. True, kids at play will get banged up, but when left to themselves, they'll rarely "play" themselves into the sorts of overuse injuries that plague adults and too often result in a return to sedentariness. Of course, we adults need to learn the difference between the "good" pain of getting in shape and the "bad" pain of incipient injury, and we'll cover that in chapter 11.

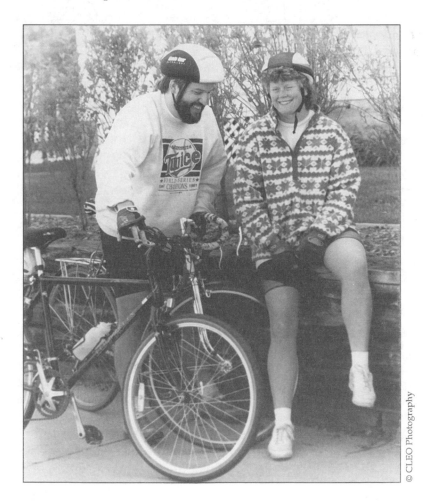

© CLEO Photography

You'll have the best chance of sticking with an active life if you approach activity in the spirit of a child, open to the possibility that whatever you're doing, whether puttering or walking briskly, running, cycling, swimming, or playing tennis, can also be fun.

Here are some things to think about when deciding what might be fun for you.

Alone or With Others?

Think back to your high school physical education days. Did you enjoy playing baseball? Or did you prefer more solitary activities such as swimming or running?

Training with others is unquestionably a matter of personal taste. Some prefer to train alone; for some, a long, solitary walk is a special time to think, to work through problems on the job, to come up with new ideas for family solidarity, or just to have some peace and quiet away from ringing telephones and other intrusions.

And yet, if you've made a commitment to others to meet at a certain time and place for a walk or jog together, it becomes much more difficult to sit at home. The prospect of coffee or lunch with friends after exercise provides an additional powerful inducement to keep at it. Most communities of any size have jogging or walking clubs, health clubs, and aerobics classes that provide many opportunities to meet others of like mind. Forming friendships around exercise provides not only additional motivation, but also the benefits of social connectedness discussed earlier in chapter 7.

Likewise, building family outings around physical activity—weekend hikes, camping trips that include walks, backpacking, evening bike rides with the kids, family excursions to the local health club—will help ease some of the tensions in our busy lives that arise when we try to balance commitment to our families and careers with commitment to an active life.

Of course, not all activities lend themselves readily to sociability; although the "loneliness of the long-distance runner" has made its way into popular lore, there is probably nothing more solitary than swimming laps—how do you strike up a conversation with your neighbor in the next lane, after all? (But joining a masters swim team is a great way to make friends before and after workouts.)

Training with partners is not without hazards; you need to find training partners who are simpatico, who train at your pace if you're having a bad day (likewise, you need to be sensitive to your partner's needs, and be willing to back off a bit if your partner is dragging). And there may be times when your body needs rest, no matter how badly you would like to join your friends on the hiking or jogging trails; at times like these, arrange to meet your training comrades for snacks or drinks after they've completed their workouts and you've had a rest.

Some activities such as walking lend themselves to either group or individual effort. Lap swimming, as noted, is inevitably a solitary pursuit. Other activities such as basketball demand group effort and require sociability on your part.

Indoors or Out?

If you prefer the great outdoors, activities such as walking or cycling are definitely for you. If snow and wind discourage your outdoor exercise, or if you're not certain you want to be seen by your neighbors in shorts and a T-shirt, there are plenty of indoor activities from which to choose; for example, aerobics classes set to music, lap swimming, or weight or circuit training.

Structure or Freedom?

Some of us thrive on rules and structure, some of us lean more toward anarchism; you'll want to examine your own preferences in this regard. Walking is arguably the ultimate "anarchist's sport." It has no rules or structure. You simply lace on your shoes, walk out the door, and do it. Team activities such as volleyball and basketball are more structured; they come with all the official rules of the game as well as less official but no less strict conventions governing one's behavior or deportment. For some, this is all part of the fun; for others, it's a nuisance. Think back to your youth—did you enjoy arguing endlessly about rules during sandlot ball games? Or were you more anxious to get back to the game?

Some activities are structured by nature. For safety's sake, weight training requires close attention to how you practice, a type of structure some find to be either a distraction or a source of added interest. Lap swimming and aerobics classes might be structured around the schedules of the club or instructors. Tennis is structured around rules, court availability, the bounds of the court, and whether or not you and your partner can keep the ball in bounds with any regularity.

To Compete, or Not to Compete?

This question is relevant only in terms of Stage Two activities—it's difficult to turn housecleaning, gardening, or walking the dog into a competitive activity—and almost any recreational sport activity can be competitive if you want it to be. But some sports are inherently competitive, such as tennis, racquetball, handball, or basketball, which involve an opponent or teams. When choosing the activities that will be right for you, you'll want to examine your own attitudes about competition. If you reach that point in your active life when you decide to enter the realm of competition, you need to be aware of both the benefits and the hazards.

Masters competition in various sports such as road running, track and field, swimming, cycling, and the triathlon provide not just incentive to become and remain physically active, but impetus to make other beneficial changes in diet, sleep habits, and so on for the sake of top performance. Masters competition also creates a social network that provides the many significant benefits of connections to others we've already discussed. And winning, of course, is always a pleasure. Competition can also teach us such lessons as how to seek and find the positive in defeat, such as what will help "next time," or the personal victory of improved performance despite defeat, a thought process that might be applied in all areas of life.

But one of the joys of walking, running, or cycling is that they provide a respite from the day-to-day "competitions" that permeate our culture—negotiating rush-hour traffic every morning, competing for a table at lunch, the sometimes petty competitions of office politics, the more serious competition to provide a stable, secure environment in which to raise a family when so much around us—an uncertain economy, rising crime, drugs, violence on TV—makes that difficult. A long walk or bike ride provides a period of solitude during which to "think one's thoughts."

Keep in mind, though, that competition need not be with a single opponent, as in tennis, or with others in your age group in a local bike race; competition could just as well be between you and your own past best performance, and when the desire to beat your own best begins to bump against the fact that maybe your best already is your *best*, the competitive spirit can become yet another source of stress and anxiety, leading to discouragement, frustration, illness or injury, and ultimately a return to a sedentary life and all that implies.

The activity characteristics chart on pp. 240-243 shows at a glance how several different activities stack up in terms of the issues you've just read about.

QUESTION 2—WHAT *CAN* YOU DO?

One of the best ways to stick with exercise and reduce your risk of discouragement or injury is to engage in activities that best suit your body. If you're very overweight, even walking may be out of the question, at least at the outset, although cycling may be ideal. An old knee injury might make cycling unrealistic, but perhaps you can swim. A low-impact aerobics class can provide a balanced, total-body workout that might be perfect for someone with tender joints. Tennis might be out for someone with problem shoulders, but walking might be the perfect activity. If you're physically frail from years of sedentary living, weight training, water aerobics, or yoga or tai chi are good starting points to build your strength and balance for other activities. There's really no end of possibilities (refer to chapter 10 for more detail on each of these activities).

Consider your physical and medical condition. Conventional medical wisdom regarding change from a sedentary to an active life holds that anyone over 40—especially any typically overweight, overstressed, hypertensive American male—probably should have a medical exam beforehand to make sure working up a sweat isn't going to result in a sudden heart attack or worse. In truth, there's less risk in activity than in continuous inactivity. It's probably more advisable to pass a careful medical examination if you intend to be sedentary to establish whether your health is good enough to stand the inactivity![1] Certainly, if you've been sedentary for years, it wouldn't hurt to have a checkup to see what harm that inactivity may have caused. At which point your physician will probably advise you to "get a little more exercise."

Age and CVD Risk Factors

If you have concerns about your health, or if you are overweight, have hypertension, diabetes, or a family history of heart disease, you probably should check with your physician, and again, he or she will likely advise you to "get a little more exercise."

Certainly, if you've had a previous heart attack, or any symptoms that could indicate heart disease such as chest discomfort, shoulder or arm pains, shortness of breath, palpitations, or undue fatigue, a

Activity Characteristics Chart   Stage One Activities

Activity	METs[a]	Kcals/hr at 155 lb	Group or Individual[b]	Low or High Impact[b]	Outdoor or Indoor[b]	Structured or Unstructured	Competitive?	Special equipment required?	Builds Endurance, Strength, Flexibility, or Balance[b]
Carpentry	6.0	420	(G)I	L(H)	(O,I)	U	No	Yes	(E)S,F,B
Child care	3.0	210	G	L	(O,I)	U	No	No	(E,S)F,B
Cleaning (heavy)	4.5	315	I	L	I	U	No	Yes	(E,S,F,B)
Cleaning (light)	2.5	175	I	L	I	U	No	No	(S,F,B)
Cooking	2.5	175	(G)I	L	I	U	No	Yes	(S,B)
Gardening (general)	5.0	350	(G)I	L(H)	O	U	No	Yes	(E)S,F,B
Golf (with cart)	3.5	245	(G)I	L	O	S	Yes	Yes	(S)B
Ironing	2.3	161	I	L	I	U	No	Yes	(S)B
Lying quietly	0.9	63	I	L	I	U	No	No	
Mowing lawn (push)	6.0	420	I	L	O	U	No	Yes	E,S,B
Playing cello	2.0	140	(G)I	L	I	U	No	Yes	
Playing piano	2.5	175	(G)I	L	I	U	No	Yes	
Playing violin	2.5	175	(G)I	L	I	U	No	Yes	
Playing with kids	4.0	280	G	L(H)	(O,I)	U	No	No	(E,S)

Notes. [a]MET values taken from Ainsworth et al. 1993.
[b]Letter in parenthesis means activity has some of the characteristic.

Stage One Activities

Activity	METs	Kcals/hr at 155 lb	Group or Individual	Low or High Impact	Outdoor or Indoor	Structured or Unstructured	Competitive?	Special equipment required?	Builds Endurance, Strength, Flexibility, or Balance
Raking leaves	4.0	280	I	L	O	U	No	Yes	(E)S,B
Scrubbing floors	5.5	385	I	L	I	U	No	No	(E)S(F,B)
Shopping (no cart)	2.3	161	I	L	I	U	No	No	(S)B
Shopping (w/cart)	3.5	245	I	L	I	U	No	No	(E,S)B
Shoveling snow	6.0	420	I	L	O	U	No	Yes	E,S(F)B
Sitting	1.0	70	I	L	I	U	No	No	
Standing quietly	1.2	84	I	L	I	U	No	No	
Standing teaching	2.5	175	G	L	I	U	No	No	(B)
Sitting reading	1.3	91	I	L	I	U	No	No	(B)
Sweeping	2.5	175	I	L	I	U	No	Yes	(S,B)
Walking (slowly)	3.0	210	(G)I	L	O,I	U	No	No	E(S,F)B
Washing dishes	2.3	161	I	L	I	U	No	No	(B)
Watering lawn	1.5	105	I	L	O	U	No	No	B
Writing at desk	1.8	126	I	L	I	U	No	No	

Activity Characteristics Chart   Stage Two Activities

Activity	METs[a]	Kcals/hr at 155 lb	Group or Individual[b]	Low or High Impact[b]	Outdoor or Indoor[b]	Structured or Unstructured	Competitive?	Special equipment required?	Builds Endurance, Strength, Flexibility, or Balance[b]
Aerobics (low impact)	5.0	350	G(I)	L	I	S	No	No	E,S,F,B
Aerobics (high impact)	7.0	490	G(I)	H	I	S	No	No	E,S,F,B
Badminton	4.5	315	G	L(H)	O,I	S	Yes	Yes	(E,S,F)B
Basketball	8.0	560	G	H	O,I	S	Yes	Yes	E,S(F)B
Cycling (leisure)	6.0	420	(G)I	L	O	U	(Yes)	Yes	E(S)B
Cycling (vigorous)	10.0	700	(G)I	L	O	U	(Yes)	Yes	E(S)B
Golf (without cart)	5.5	385	(G)I	L	O	S	Yes	Yes	(E,S,F)B
Handball	12.0	840	G	H	I	S	Yes	Yes	E,S,F,B
Judo	10.0	700	G	H	I	S	Yes	Yes	(E)S,F,B
Racquetball	7.0	490	G	H	I	S	Yes	Yes	E(S)F,B
Rowing machine	9.5-12.0	665-840	I	L	I	U	(Yes)	Yes	E,S(F)
Running (6 mph)	10.0	700	(G,I)	H	O,I	U	(Yes)	No	E(S,F)B
Running (8 mph)	13.5	945	(G,I)	H	O,I	U	(Yes)	No	E(S,F)B

Notes. [a]MET values taken from Ainsworth et al. 1993.
[b]Letter in parenthesis means activity has some of the characteristic.

Stage Two Activities

Activity	METs	Kcals/hr at 155 lb	Group or Individual	Low or High Impact	Outdoor or Indoor	Structured or Unstructured	Competitive?	Special equipment required?	Builds Endurance, Strength, Flexibility, or Balance
Softball	5.0	350	G	L(H)	O	S	Yes	Yes	(S,F)B
Stationary cycling	5.0-10.0	350-700	I	L	I	U	(Yes)	Yes	E(S,F)
Ski machine	9.5	665	I	L	I	U	(Yes)	Yes	E(S,F)
Ski (downhill)	5.0-8.0	350-560	I	(L,H)	O	U	(Yes)	Yes	(E)S,F,B
Ski (light cross-country)	7.0	490	(G)I	L	O	U	(Yes)	Yes	E,S,F,B
Ski (vigorous cross-country)	9.0	630	(G)I	L	O	U	(Yes)	Yes	E,S,F,B
Swimming (general)	6.0	420	I	L	O,I	U	(Yes)	No	E,S,F(B)
Swimming (vigorous laps)	10.0	700	I	L	O,I	U	(Yes)	No	E,S,F(B)
Tai chi chuan	4.0	280	G,I	L	O,I	S(U)	No	No	(E)S,F,B
Tennis	8.0	560	G	H	O,I	S	Yes	Yes	(E,S,F,)B
Walking (brisk, 4 mph)	4.5	315	(G)I	L	O,I	U	No	No	E(S,F)B
Weight training	6.0	420	I	L	(O)I	U	(Yes)	Yes	(E)S(F)
Yoga	4.0	280	(G)I	L	(O)I	S(U)	No	No	S,F,B

talk with your physician is in order before you embark on an exercise program, and your physician's recommendation will probably be that you "really ought to get some exercise."

Your physician might have you take an exercise stress test that can reveal some types of heart disease, or he or she may order a battery of more sophisticated tests intended to reveal the precise extent and location of blockages in your coronary arteries, if any; at which point your physician will probably advise you to "get some exercise."

Indeed, only in the instance of the most severe disease is your physician likely to advise you *not* to get more exercise, and in these cases, more invasive treatments such as angioplasty or bypass surgery might be used to help improve blood flow to the heart muscle, and *then* your physician will probably advise you to exercise to prevent future problems.

Hypertension

If you have high blood pressure, you may want to lean toward lower intensity aerobic activities such as walking, jogging, cycling, and swimming and away from activities such as weight or circuit training, at least until your hypertension is under control.

Prescription Medication

If you're taking any prescription drugs, you might want to tell your physician you're about to embark on an exercise program; regular physical activity over time can change the body's reactions to certain medications. For example, the body's sensitivity to insulin increases with activity, so if you're taking medication for NIDDM, you may find your need for it will decrease. Exercise may increase your sensitivity to some psychoactive medications—antidepressants or tranquilizers. And if you're taking medication for high blood pressure, you may find that with regular exercise, your need for the drug will decline over time.

Bone and Joint Problems

Some preexisting health problems may preclude specific activities from your range of choices. If you have osteoarthritis or old joint injuries, activities such as basketball, court sports, and the like might not be a good choice because the abrupt stops and starts during play could inflame tender joints. Running might also aggravate knee problems, and tennis can irritate shoulders and elbows (walking, swimming, and cycling are all relatively safe for the joints). This doesn't mean you should automatically exclude any of these activities from your list of possibilities; if you think you might like tennis despite a tender shoulder, give it a try and see how your body reacts (and refer to chapter 11 for more on the subject of injury prevention).

Women with osteoporosis will want to be especially careful in choosing activities that won't overstress weakened bones. Low-impact aerobics, exercise classes in water, and walking are ideal. Light weight training is very effective in preserving bone mineral density, and there is good evidence that such training can even reverse the course of the disease. However, weight training should be approached with extreme caution if severe osteoporosis has already developed, and you'll want to check with your physician before taking it up. You may also want to be cautious about undertaking any activities that increase the risk of falls.

Diabetes

People with diabetes will want to be very active, as exercise is one of the most effective means of controlling the condition, but they should be very careful of their feet and evaluate activities with the health of their feet in mind. Swimming is an ideal activity for most, but those who have diabetes should be wary of barefoot journeys through locker rooms and the increased risk of infection from unsanitary floors. Running or walking are excellent, but beware of blisters from ill-fitting shoes.

QUESTION 3—WHAT'S AVAILABLE TO YOU?

Try to anticipate the difficulties you'll face becoming and staying active, then choose activities that best help you work around those barriers. This will reduce the number of excuses too many of us manage to find for *not* being active. Depending on your schedule, location, and so on, some activities will be more convenient—and thus you'll be more likely to keep at them. Start by listing all the barriers you might face along the path to a more active life, along with proposed strategies for overcoming each.

How Much Time Do You Have?

Lack of time is perhaps the most common barrier—or excuse—many of us encounter when starting out or trying to stick with exercise, and although some activities sound great "on paper," they aren't necessarily ideal for busy men and women. You can do yourself a favor by choosing activities that fit well into your schedule of work, family, and other commitments.

Write out your schedule for a typical week looking for gaps here and there where a few minutes of brisk walking, for example, can be worked in. Can you get up 30 minutes earlier for a before-work walk or bike ride? Does that mean going to bed 30 minutes earlier? If so, can you adjust your evening activities accordingly? What about at lunchtime? Are there recreation facilities or a pool or park near your work? Can you take a few minutes during lunch for a swim or walk? How important to you is a leisurely lunch? In your mind, do the benefits of that free time outweigh the benefits of exercise? Are there opportunities for exercise in the evening? Can dinner be delayed for the sake of a sweat? Can you exercise after dinner? And what about weekends? Can you schedule some time for catch-up activities?

Swimming, for instance, is an excellent overall exercise, but unless you have your own pool, you're limited to the hours the community or health club pool is open for laps, and it takes time to get to and from the pool. If your own schedule of meetings and travel doesn't coincide with the pool schedule, it's sometimes easier simply *not* to exercise at all. Walking, on the other hand, is something you can do almost anytime, anywhere, weather permitting, thus it fits more readily into full schedules. But if you live where the winter weather gets really wet or cold, walking may not be the solution either, so be sure to give some thought to prevailing weather patterns throughout the year and the appropriateness of potential activities.

Where Are You?

Another consideration is the availability of exercise facilities. This is particularly important if you have to fit activity into a busy day. Swimming becomes a more realistic option if there happens to be a pool around the corner from your work, for instance. Explore exercise facilities near your job or home. Bike or jogging trails, aerobics studios, or gyms nearby all make these activities viable options. On the other hand, if such facilities aren't handy, you may want to develop activity options that require little in the way of facilities, equipment, or scheduling.

Give some thought to weather patterns where you live. If you live in Minnesota, you'll probably want to develop a variety of exercise options for the sometimes brutal winters—indoor activities or cross-country skiing. If you live in Florida, you'll want to develop options that offer safety in heat and humidity—swimming or various indoor activities such as mall walking or aerobics (assuming the facilities are air conditioned).

How Much Money Are You Willing to Spend?

Some activities cost money, which can be either good or bad, depending on a variety of factors, not the least of which is the depth of your wallet. Certainly, you'll want to weigh the benefits against the costs of involving yourself in sports that require special—often expensive—equipment. Cycling is great exercise, but you need a bike, which these days can easily cost a thousand dollars or more. An annual membership in a decent health club can cost you nearly as much, and annual fees for some golf clubs can cost more than a small car. On the other hand, walking and jogging are probably the best deals in town when you weigh their costs against their benefits. A decent pair of walking or jogging shoes will likely cost less than $50 (of course, you can easily spend two or three times that if you want) and will last for months.

One of your goals is to eliminate as many reasons as possible for *not* being active, such as bad weather or darkness. Another goal is to exercise in safety. Walking is cheap, but if your schedule means walking at night, or if the weather where you live can get ugly, you'll want other convenient options if conditions threaten to interrupt your chosen activities.

For some, a well-equipped home gym is an excellent solution, assuming you have the space for it and the money to buy the equipment. And the equipment doesn't come cheap. A stationary bike or rowing machine, a stair-climbing simulator, a ski machine, or a set of weights can each easily cost $500 or more. But a home gym can make a workout more efficient, more convenient, safer, and more fun. If you're self-conscious about your appearance in shorts, even hidden under baggy sweats, you may like the privacy a home gym can offer. Plus, there's nothing like the thought of what you paid for the gym to motivate you to use it. Of course, you don't need a lot of equipment for a home gym. A cheap set of barbells and weights used along with sit-ups, pull-ups, and jogging in place will provide numerous activity options at negligible expense.

QUESTION 4—WHAT RESULTS DO YOU WANT?

After considering what sorts of activities you might like, what might best suit you physically and psychologically, and finally, what's most convenient or available, next give some thought to the specific results you want.

The LifeFit program emphasizes moderate aerobic activities for improved endurance and cardiovascular health. These are sustained physical activities that engage large muscles groups—primarily the legs and arms—and elevate the heart rate and get the sweat flowing. With these activities as a foundation and your LifeFit goal in mind, you can develop your own program to produce the specific results you want. Although any activity will be good for your health and will count toward your LifeFit goal, different activities provide other, more specific results. The activity characteristics chart (pp. 240-243) shows you what activities bring certain results. Here are some things to consider.

Reduced Risk of Disease

As discussed in part II, physical activity confers a variety of benefits in terms of reduced risk of the so-called diseases of civilization. Any activity will be beneficial, but sustained aerobic activities vigorous enough to elevate the heart rate will most directly produce the results you want.

The term *aerobic* refers to activities performed at a level of effort at which your cardiopulmonary system—that network of heart, lungs, and blood vessels—is capable of supplying the working muscles with sufficient oxygen to continue working. These activities strengthen the working muscles, and of most importance, they also strengthen the cardiovascular system. Aerobic activities include walking, jogging, cycling, swimming, cross-country skiing, and racquet sports (as long as you don't spend a lot of time wandering around looking for lost balls), among others.

Lower Blood Pressure

Sustained aerobic activities work best. Again, if you have very high blood pressure, be especially cautious about resistance training or other intense activities. Over time, high-intensity exercise will contribute to reductions in blood pressure, but *during* such exercise, your blood pressure can shoot way up. Start with gentle aerobic exercise; as your blood pressure comes under control, only then should you consider activities such as resistance training.

Increased Strength

Any activity will improve strength, but resistance training works directly toward this result. Aerobic dance and calisthenics such as push-ups, sit-ups (always with the knees bent), and pull-ups directly produce this result as well. Increasing the intensity of any aerobic activity—sprinting, walking, running, or cycling uphill, swimming fast laps, and so on—will also help. These more intense activities are performed at a level of exertion near or beyond the body's ability to supply oxygen to the working muscles, thus they're called "anaerobic" activities. Although you might be able to walk or jog comfortably for hours, anaerobic effort can only be sustained for a brief period, perhaps a few seconds or minutes, and there's no mistaking that moment when your level of effort has taken you across the line separating aerobic from anaerobic effort. At that point, the wastes of the anaerobic metabolism—lactic acid—begin to build up in the muscles; it feels as if someone is digging hot pokers into your flesh. Very quickly, the exhaustion of the working muscles and increasing discomfort bring the activity to a halt.

There are fewer data showing that anaerobic training provides the same health benefits as aerobic activities, most likely not because anaerobic training doesn't, but simply because this area hasn't been studied extensively. Anaerobic activities do clearly provide significant health benefits, and as noted previously, strength training, in particular, becomes more important as we grow older.

Although aerobic activities in themselves will help maintain strength, incorporating resistance exercises into your LifeFit program as a supplement to aerobic exercise is a good idea. This will help prevent injuries resulting from muscle-strength imbalances. A steady diet of running, for example, tends to create imbalances between the muscles of the front and back of the legs, which sometimes can lead to injury; if you're hurt and can't exercise, you're not getting the benefits of exercise. Also, aerobic training tends to develop strength only in those muscles used—the legs in walking or running or the upper body in swimming, for example.

Total-body strength training provides a more balanced, total-body fitness.

Weight Loss

As noted in chapter 4, weight loss is a national obsession; most of us, it seems, are trying to lose weight, or thinking about trying, or have tried and failed, or have tried and succeeded and then gained it all back, and then some. Any activity will help contribute to weight loss; the bottom line, as we've seen, is to expend more calories than are consumed. A weight-loss program that combines exercise with prudent eating is the most effective means of shedding pounds.

For the very overweight, Stage One activities will be the best place to start. As weight decreases and fitness improves, gradually add gentle Stage Two aerobic activities. As noted earlier, however, resistance training may be the most effective means of weight loss and weight control; not only does resistance training expend calories *during* exercise, like any other activity, it also results in a greater energy expenditure *after* a workout is over. And the added muscle developed through weight training expends many more calories than fat tissue, even at rest.

Keep in mind that this desired result will—and should—come slowly. Don't weigh yourself after every workout expecting big changes; if it seems as if "it's taking forever" to lose that spare tire, that's probably a good thing. Crash diets and too-rapid weight loss are not only bad for the health, they almost invariably result in "rebound" and discouragement.[2] If weight loss is a desired result for you, consider it a very long-term goal.

Improved Functioning for Daily Activities

Any activity will contribute to the goal of staying independent and fully functioning, but some activities are more helpful than others. Activities such as swimming, rowing, stationary cycling, and weight training will contribute much to improving cardiovascular function and improving or preserving strength. Resistance training, in particular, addresses the needs of the very old to remain strong. Strength training helps keep bones strong and reduces the risk of injuries from falls, as we've seen.

Another important aspect of staying independent is balance. As we grow older, our sense of balance becomes less acute, and the risk of falls increases. But like other declines we associate with aging, this decline is more often the result of lack of use, not an inescapable result of aging. Too many older adults become inactive and simply never do enough to keep their sense of balance in good tune. Yoga and the gentle Asian martial art of tai chi chuan are particularly helpful. Walking, jogging, and cycling also help keep the sense of balance sharp. Weight training and activities such as swimming, rowing, or stationary cycling probably aren't as helpful in this regard. A well-rounded program that includes aerobic activity, resistance training, and activities that sharpen the sense of balance is the best approach.

Stretching is also important. Most exercise prescriptions recommend stretching before or after exercise to help prevent injuries, but truly devoted stretchers seem to be rare. As we grow older, stretching, like strength training, becomes increasingly important to help prevent or delay the stiffening that contributes to increased frailty and risk of falls. Stretching also helps prevent injury, as a flexible muscle or tendon is less prone to pulls or tears than a tight one; thus,

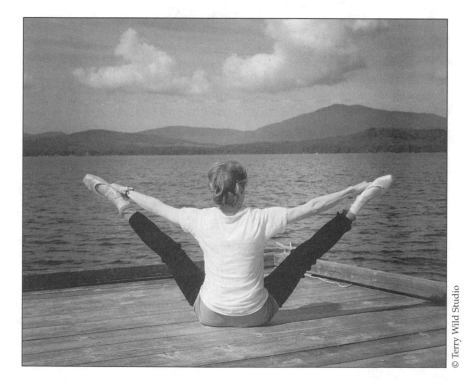

although stretching is not a substitute for either aerobic or anaerobic activities, it is an important supplement to any effective program of physical activity. (*Note:* Stretching, yoga, and tai chi contribute to your Stage One goal; they shouldn't be counted toward Stage Two, as they don't elevate the heart rate sufficiently.)

Feeling Better

Feeling better may seem a somewhat amorphous or abstract result, but it's also one of the most important results of an active life, and one you can achieve every time you go for a walk or take a few laps in the pool at the local Y. When you set out to achieve the simple result of feeling more energetic, more alive, and more positive about yourself and your prospects, you automatically become aware of how good physical activity will make you feel, and once you've become aware of this, sticking with it becomes much easier. Feeling better is a powerful positive reinforcement for adherence to an activity, even when the weather's inclement, you're pressed for time, and you feel "too tired." Any activity will help toward achieving this important result.

Looking Better

Of course, one reason so many of us want to lose weight is so we'll look better, and looking better is for most perhaps the *number one* motivation for taking up and sticking with activity. But weight loss is only part of improved body image; increased muscle tone and definition, improvements in posture and carriage, and changes in one's attitude don't necessarily result from weight loss alone, but rather are the result of regular physical activity, particularly resistance training. If looking better is something you want, you'll certainly want to include some regular weight training in your activity plans.

However, be aware that changes in body image come slowly and require much effort—which doesn't for a moment prevent countless hucksters on late-night TV from promising you an improbably svelte body in just six weeks, or even two weeks, if you call now to order this or that tummy-tightening, thigh-sculpting exercise gizmo or this or that bottle of diet pills, thigh creams, or food supplements.

If a general improvement in body image is one of the results you want, recognize that it won't happen overnight. Be patient and forget the hucksters.

WHERE DO YOU START?

Now that you have some insights into what activities you like, what's realistic for you, and what specific results you're after, the next step is to write out a list of options based on these insights.

CONSIDER YOUR OPTIONS

Suppose you're a woman in your late fifties, a retired teacher living in Illinois. You're busy with volunteer work and your grandchildren—toddlers—so you don't have a lot of time. Your weight is within acceptable limits and you have no significant health problems except for a twinge of what is probably arthritis in your left knee. But you have never done much in the way of exercise, and now you want to change that. You understand the value of exercise, particularly for women of your age. You know that the risks of heart disease and osteoporosis rise steadily in women as they grow older. You also want to feel better and have more energy to keep up with your grandkids, and you want to feel better about yourself and, of course, wouldn't mind looking better as well.

You've thought back to your youth and recall that in high school, you particularly liked running, but you were never much inclined toward team sports. You like the outdoors, and you relish rare moments of solitude in which to think your own thoughts, uninterrupted by ringing telephones. On the other hand, you have an active social life and enjoy being with friends. You like to walk, but even better, you like to swim, although the nearest pool is across town and you're not sure how to fit swimming into your full schedule; nor are you sure how swimming would fit into an Illinois winter. You have no interest in cycling, however. You might like to try slow jogging, and you're intrigued by the idea of firming up and getting stronger through weight training. Considering your daily living activities, you suspect you're not really on your feet enough, so you decide to give some attention to this as well.

Taking all of these factors into consideration, write out a list of options for both Stage One and Stage Two activities—and here you might want to check the activity characteristics chart again (pp. 240-243), and also refer to chapter 10 for a discussion of how you can tell how active you are in Stage One activities and how you can build in more.

Under Stage One, you write:

  Expand garden? Plant earlier, grow more?

  Skip the elevators and use the stairs.

  Whenever safe, park in a far corner of the lot and walk to the store.

  Weekend hikes with friends or family

Under Stage Two:

  Brisk walking (enlist some friends to go with me; start a walking club)

  Swimming (get lap-swim schedule)

  Aquatic exercise (get schedule of classes)

  Jogging???

  Weight training

Or suppose you're a 40-something manager in a large corporation. You're routinely putting in 10-hour days at the office, with plenty of weekends thrown in for good measure. You're a bit overweight with slightly elevated blood pressure, not surprising considering all the pressure you've been under at work. Otherwise, you're in pretty good health. You play softball with some of the guys from the office now and then, plus a little obligatory golf with clients, and you go for weekend bike rides with the kids. But that's about it. On occasion, your wife has suggested, gently and circumspectly, that you ought to get a little exercise. Which is exactly what your physician told you at your last checkup. And that's fine—you'd like to get a little more exercise as well. But how?

Realistically, increasing your Stage One puttering about is probably impractical. You can take the stairs more often at work, and during breaks maybe take walks around the office complex rather than sit in the lunchroom trying not to have one of the jelly donuts someone brings in on a regular basis. But given the little free time you have, you'll probably want to concentrate on Stage Two activities instead, as these give you the most health benefits for the time you spend at them.

What are the possibilities? You like softball, but it's not practical as a regular opportunity for exercise, and in truth, it's not that much exercise; you spend most of your time in right field, with bursts now and then when you get a hit or someone hits a ball your way. You're not sure you're up for jogging just yet, and besides, you still recall with distaste how your old high school gym teachers used to make you run laps as punishment whenever you were late to class. You still tend to view jogging as punishment. You don't live near a gym, so that's not practical, and because you travel a great deal on the job, it's a good idea to choose activities that you can do on the road as well as at home.

Your feet are in good shape, and you have no preexisting joint problems, so it looks like brisk walking is it. You can go for walks wherever you are, whenever you can fit them in.

Your list of possibilities might look something like this:

Stage One:

Take more stairs at work.

Walk around during breaks.

Stand and shuffle while on the phone.

Do whatever I can, when I can.

Stage Two:

Take *brisk* walks (buy some good shoes; carry shoes and walking shorts in car or when traveling).

With a list of possibilities in hand, your next step is to put the pieces together into a workable plan.

SET CLEAR GOALS

The LifeFit program is based on the long-term goal of a combination of Stage One and Stage Two activities for optimal health and a longer, healthier, more vital and engaged life. But that's not the only goal you can or should have.

For some, Stage One puttering about may be the final goal. For others, however, it will be only the first step toward Stage Two and beyond. Whatever your long-term goals, you'll want to set intermediate and short-term goals toward which to strive along the way.

Having precise goals will help you stay motivated, particularly when you think you're too tired to exercise after a tough day at work, or you think you don't have time, or it's too chilly out. Psychologist Mihaly Csikszentmihalyi writes that "a goal is necessary so that a person may get feedback to his or her actions, so that at any given moment they know whether the responses were appropriate to the challenges. Without a goal there can be no meaningful feedback, and without knowing whether one is doing well or not it is very difficult to maintain involvement."[3]

And if you've set some goals for yourself, then you'll have the distinct pleasure of achieving those goals, another powerful motivation to stick with an active life; if you haven't set any goals, of course, you'll never meet them. Here are some things to consider about goals, especially if you're just starting out in an active life, or if you've been somewhat haphazard about activity in the past.

Goal 1—Adherence

Adherence is the key at this point and should be your first goal. Everything that follows is intended to help you achieve the goal of adherence. Considering that so many men and women abandon an active life, the simple goal of adherence may be the most important one of all, the foundation on which all else rests. Especially if you've been sedentary for years, or at best inconsistent in your exercise habits, you shouldn't just start out trying to exercise at a high level during your first week, or even the first month. Therein lies discouragement and possibly injury. Your first objective along the way to your LifeFit goal should be adherence, the development of activity as a habit.

Habits are behaviors you do naturally, without having to think much about them, or certainly without having to make yourself do them. You will know activity has become a habit for you on the day you feel frustrated or a bit edgy, with the nagging sense of important things left undone, when circumstances prevent you from being active.

Forming the habit of activity typically takes about six weeks of conscious effort and involves three distinct steps: (1) the decision to take up an active life; (2) activity along with behavior changes such as juggling schedules so there's time for activity; and (3) long-term maintenance.[4]

Step 1—Make the Decision

If you've read this far in *LifeFit*, we hope you've already made the decision to become more active. And perhaps you've actually begun being more active as well.

Step 2—The First Week

Choose light activities that you might like. You've already given some thought to this, so pick one or two simple activities from your list of possibilities. At this point, you shouldn't be concerned about how much or how intensely you exercise. Your exercise should be well within your comfort zone, and it might be anything from gardening to walks around the block to taking the stairs at work.

Your primary effort right now is devoted to learning how you can adjust your life so that physical activity becomes as natural a part of your day as brushing your teeth or eating dinner. This will probably mean rearranging your schedule and changing other habits such as when you eat dinner, when you go to bed, when you get up in the morning, or how much time you spend on Sunday mornings perusing the papers or watching "Meet the Press."

You've already given some thought to your daily schedule, looking for gaps where you can fit more activity. Now literally schedule activity into your day: Write a time for activity into your daily schedule, just as you'd write in an important appointment. Think of that physical activity as simply another part of doing business; the immediate benefits of exercise—more vitality, relaxation, a chance to think without interruption, improved mood, a quicker mind—will all contribute to your performance on the job.

For example, schedule 10 minutes of walking every weekday at noon, before lunch. Or schedule 15 minutes of cycling each evening after work, or even just five minutes of walking each morning before leaving for the job. It all counts. Another way to approach this is to make a resolution that every time you drive to the market, you will park at the far end of the lot and walk. Or resolve to park at a lot several blocks from work and walk to your office, then take the stairs rather than the elevator.

Having established a schedule or routine, stick with it for one week. The adherence goal chart on page 258 shows how you might record these goals.

Step 3—Week Two and Beyond
As you begin the second week, evaluate how the first week went. Consider how well your schedule worked and whether or not it needs to be adjusted. Perhaps too many competing involvements in the evening make that 15-minute evening walk impractical, so it's time to consider a morning walk or some other activity. At this point, you're still experimenting and finding out what works for you, and the important thing to keep in mind is that you're trying to develop the habit of activity, nothing more.

Suppose you resolved that for the first week, at least, you would

Adherence Goal Chart

Goal: Walk 10 minutes, 3 days, before dinner							
Reward: Buy a magazine, read in hot bath							
Week 1	Mon ✓	Tue	Wed ✓	Th	Fri ✓	Sat	Sun
Week 2	Mon ✓	Tue ✓	Wed	Th	Fri ✓	Sat	Sun
Goal: Climb stairs daily to office							
Reward: Buy 1 pound gourmet coffee							
Week 1	Mon	Tue ✓	Wed ✓	Th ✓	Fri ✓	Sat	Sun
Week 2	Mon ✓	Tue *Try again!*	Wed ✓	Th ✓	Fri ✓	Sat	Sun

simply walk for 15 minutes every evening before dinner, and that worked fine for the first three days. Then on day four it was raining, and you didn't feel like slogging through puddles. On the fifth and sixth days, though, the weather was better and you walked again. On the seventh day, a Sunday, you took an hour walk with friends around the city park.

At the end of the first week, you have perhaps realized two things. First, you should find alternative activities in case of bad weather, something that becomes increasingly important once winter sets in. Second, you've done pretty well despite the one missed day. Maybe it's time to call the local Y for a schedule of when the pool is available for lap swimming and the gym for weight training or use of the treadmill. Perhaps a new goal is that one morning a week—rain or shine—you'll go to the Y for some laps in the pool or an 8 A.M. aqua aerobics class. While there, maybe you'll want to stick your head into the weight room as well, just to see what it looks like.

The important thing at this point is not what you do, how much of it you do, or how intensely. What is important is that you *do something*, and do it regularly, and that you experiment to find what you can do consistently, in such a way that it's convenient, practical, and fun.

You'll want to establish short-term goals along the way. First a week of consistent activity, then perhaps set a new goal of two weeks of consistent activity, then perhaps four weeks, by which time activity should be taking on all the aspects of a cherished habit.

Along the way toward the goal of adherence, begin to give some thought to another important goal—performance.

Goal 2—Performance

After three or four weeks, once the idea and practice of physical activity have become more habitual, once you've begun to establish a pattern of activity and a schedule that works for you, begin to think about the goal of performance, which will take you from Stage One to more vigorous Stage Two activities (see the performance goal chart at the bottom of the page.)

Some Performance Goals

Start by considering what sorts of physical activity you do that can add to your Stage One activities and that can contribute to Stage Two. Performance goals can come in a variety of forms:

- Increase intensity: If your activity involves covering a specific distance, such as in walking or cycling, increase the intensity by

Performance Goal Chart

Goal: Walk 1 mile in 20 minutes							
Reward: New pair of walking shoes							
Week 1	Mon	Tue	Wed	Th	Fri	Sat	Sun
	29 min		$27\frac{1}{2}$		27		24
Week 2	Mon	Tue	Wed	Th	Fri	Sat	Sun
	$24\frac{1}{2}$	22		$22\frac{1}{2}$	24		$19\frac{3}{4}$
Goal: Walk 1 mile without stopping							
Reward: Weekend at health spa							
Week 1	Mon	Tue	Wed	Th	Fri	Sat	Sun
	$\frac{1}{4}$ (10 min)		$\frac{1}{4}$	$\frac{1}{4}$	$\frac{1}{2}$ (slow)		$\frac{1}{2}$
Week 2	Mon	Tue	Wed	Th	Fri	Sat	Sun
	$\frac{1}{2}$ rest $\frac{1}{4}$	$\frac{1}{2}$	$\frac{1}{2}$ rest $\frac{1}{2}$		$\frac{3}{4}$		1 mile!

covering that same distance in less time. In the case of lap swimming, you might want to see if you can swim the same number of laps in less time.

- Increase the quantity: You might want to add to the time you engage in some activity—increase the distance you cover, the number of laps you swim, or whatever.

- Or increase both the intensity and the quantity.

You can also build your performance goals around the specific results you've already decided are important for you.

- Weight loss: For example, if weight loss is one result you want from an active life, you might want to set specific weight-loss goals, say a half pound or a pound a week for a specific number of weeks. (Remember, too-rapid weight loss is bad for the health and almost always results in weight rebound—don't become obsessed with the scale.)

- Improved strength: If improved strength is important, establish specific goals in terms of weight lifted or number of repetitions.

- Improved health: It's more difficult to measure results such as reduced risk of heart disease or cancer, but there are some signs you're headed in the right direction.

Measuring Performance Goals
Your resting pulse can serve as a general measure of improved cardiovascular health, so a reasonable goal might be a steady decline in your resting pulse over a period of weeks. Start by taking your pulse at rest at the beginning of your exercise program, then check your resting pulse once a week at the same time each day, for instance, in the morning on rising. Chart the decline. If you don't see a decline, you may want to adjust your program until you see the desired results (also see chapter 11; a *rise* in resting pulse can be a sign of excessive fatigue and overtraining).

If you have hypertension, you may want to set the goal of a lower or normal blood pressure; this will mean either taking your blood pressure yourself or having someone do it for you, but it can be a reasonable measure of favorable changes in your health. You should take your blood pressure three or four times over a period of a week or two, preferrably at the same time each day, to get an accurate picture.

If you have the time, resources, and inclination, you can even establish goals such as beneficial changes in your serum cholesterol, if you don't mind the needle prick and the expense. If you have NIDDM, of course, control of that condition is an important goal, and self-monitoring will be a useful indication of progress. If you have the money and time for periodic treadmill tests to measure oxygen consumption at given workloads, this is a very accurate way of measuring your aerobic fitness; thus improved aerobic fitness can become a goal as well.

If feeling better and looking better are your goals, they'll be a bit harder to measure, but certainly you'll become more aware of changes in how you feel and how you look—narrowing waist, firming buttocks, larger biceps—so you can decide for yourself if you're progressing satisfactorily in the direction you want.

KEEP A RECORD

Keep a record so you can see how well you are progressing toward your specific goals. This might include time spent puttering about or time spent walking briskly, miles walked or jogged, or laps swum. You might also keep a record of declining waist measurements, expanding biceps measurements, or decreasing weight (or increasing weight, if muscle gain is your goal).

Record keeping has motivational benefits as well. If you start keeping a chart of miles walked or time sweating, after a few weeks you begin to realize how much time and energy you've invested in the activity, and this makes it hard to stop. It's like building two-thirds of a house; once you're that far, you'd be crazy to quit.

Charting other factors such as increased strength or endurance, slowed resting pulse, improved recovery time from exertion, or weight loss will also be valuable motivational tools, particularly when put in the form of graphs; when you feel your enthusiasm flagging, take a look at the chart to remind yourself how far you've come and how much you've already benefited.

Record keeping is not entirely without hazards, however, if you become too determined to keep the graph of miles walked or jogged always sloping upward, for instance, or the chart of decreasing weight always sloping downward. This can lead to injury if you ignore the body's warnings to take a break (refer to chapter 11), or to boredom if you persist in an activity that's no longer interesting. If you keep a record, also bear in mind that you will reach plateaus where no amount of effort seems to provide the improvements you want, or times when illness or fatigue produce dips in the graph. At times like these, it might be wise to close the record book and do what feels right to you at the time, not what past accomplishments or present goals demand. Don't become obsessive.

REWARD YOURSELF

If you've established some specific goals and you're keeping a record, you have the opportunity to reward yourself for reaching those goals. Added years of life, reduced risk of disease, weight loss, improved appearance, a better self-image, and improved vitality are all "rewards," of course, but they usually come only after several weeks or months of consistent activity. To keep yourself motivated in the meantime, offer yourself more immediate gratification.

Set up a "token economy." For example, if you like beer—or an alcohol-free substitute—allow yourself one can for, say, every five

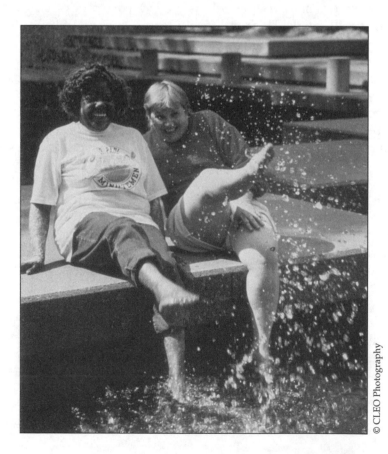

© CLEO Photography

miles of walking or jogging. Or reward yourself with a weekend at your favorite bed-and-breakfast once you've logged 100 miles of walking, or the equivalent in laps in the pool (roughly speaking, a quarter mile of swimming is equivalent in energy expended to one mile of walking or running). If you'd like a new dress that costs $100, set up a token economy around that dress: For every 100 kilocalories burned in exercise (or 10 kilocalories if you can't wait), drop a dollar in a jar. Soon enough you'll have enough money for the dress. You may even fit into a size smaller than you would have without the token-economy approach to exercise.

Each of us must decide which rewards are attractive and powerful enough to keep us motivated, of course; for some, it might be a vacation in the Bahamas; for others, merely a blueberry Danish.

TIPS FOR SUCCESSFUL GOAL SETTING

Setting goals can be a tricky business, particularly goals for physical activity. If you set inappropriate goals, or goals that are too ambitious, or if you try to achieve your goals in an inappropriate way (say too quickly), you could be setting yourself up for discouragement or even injury and a return to sedentary living. For example, if you decide to lose five pounds a week for a month, you've probably set an inappropriate goal. If you've decided that after a year of steady activity, you'll compete in the Boston Marathon, you may be setting yourself up for disappointment, if not injury; it would probably take well more than a year of steady training, and for many of us, training for and competing in a marathon is simply out of the question (and certainly not necessary for optimal health).

On the other hand, if you set goals that aren't ambitious enough, you could become bored by the endeavor and lose your motivation, or miss out on the many physical, emotional, and mental benefits of an appropriately active life.

Be flexible when approaching your goals, and be willing to modify them if circumstances require. A too-rigid adherence to goals can lead to injury, or at least discouragement. Ironically, sometimes it is those individuals who are most motivated—those we view as the most goal-oriented—who have the most difficulty sticking with exercise; this is because when such people decide, say, to jog two miles *today* at noon, and something prevents them, they may not run at all. A more flexible approach to goals, however, might leave room for other options: *Okay, a two-mile run at noon today isn't possible, but perhaps a 10-minute walk is.* And a 10-minute walk is definitely preferable to nothing at all.

You'll probably find that one of the best ways to achieve your intermediate and long-term goals is to take them a day at a time. Keep your long-term LifeFit and other goals in mind, but don't dwell on them at first, or they could seem dauntingly far away and difficult to achieve. Rather, start slowly and take it a day at a time: *Today*, tell yourself, *I will be a little more active. Just for today, I will take the stairs rather than the elevator. Today I'll go for a short walk at lunch or a walk before dinner.* Don't worry about what you'll do tomorrow. Don't worry about what you'll be doing a month from now, or how long— and steep—the road ahead appears to be. Just worry about today.

And when tomorrow becomes today, start again: *Today maybe I'll be just a bit more active than I was yesterday. Today I'll go for that walk before dinner, but this time maybe I'll walk just a little farther than I did yesterday.* Or *today I'll walk a bit more briskly.*

And if, for whatever reason, today isn't the best day, then tell yourself: *Okay, today I'll walk just a bit less. Just today, though, and then tomorrow, we'll see.* It's like investing in high-quality conservative stocks for the long haul; maybe *today* your stocks dip in value, but you don't worry about it, because you have confidence that with time their value will increase. Likewise, with an active life, all the "todays" add up, and looking back, you'll see how very far you've come and how much you've benefited.

Ultimately, the LifeFit program is one of self-exploration. It will take time to learn how your body responds to exercise, how long it takes to progress from goal to goal, how prone you are to particular injuries, or how necessary it is to vary your routine and adjust your goals to keep yourself interested and motivated. Think of goals as a means toward self-exploration, not as absolutes that must be achieved at all costs. Goals are "mirrors" in which to consider your own reflection and thus learn more about yourself, your skills, talents, and inner resources. As you set goals and work toward them, you will want to be attentive to what you see in these mirrors and what you learn about yourself, and as you learn, you'll need to be willing to adjust your goals accordingly.

Such mindfulness becomes increasingly important as we grow older. The resilience of youth protects us from all sorts of foolishness, but as we've seen, as we grow older, our bodies become less adaptable and less able to cope effectively with demands to adapt; the risk of injury and discouragement increases, and with it comes an increased risk of return to a sedentary way of life.

Think of yourself as an athlete, and adopt the athlete's mindfulness. The best athletes have clear goals, but they know that if they are physically worn out, mentally exhausted, or injured, they will never achieve those goals. So the best athletes are always watchful of how their bodies and minds cope with their training, and they are always willing to adjust their goals and how they work toward them as they learn more about their capabilities and limitations.

Of course, thinking of ourselves as athletes may seem like a bit of a stretch, particularly as we get older, and especially if we've been sedentary for years and find ourselves huffing and puffing just to get around the block. But we are talking here about the concept of *athlete* in the original sense of the word. In the original Greek, an athlete is anyone who contends for a prize. In the original Olympics, athletes included dancers, dramatists, and even poets along with boxers, runners, and wrestlers, all of whom competed for the victor's olive wreath. As a society, we typically tend to restrict the definition, inappropriately, to include mostly *young* men and women (Nolan Ryan, Martina Navratilova, and George Foreman notwithstanding) who compete at high levels for gold medals, or for huge salaries and even richer endorsement contracts for this or that athletic shoe or candy bar.

But there is no greater prize than life itself, and that's our goal. "We're all athletes in the game of life, and an athlete in this game," writes George Leonard, "plays voluntarily and wholeheartedly, even while realizing that this Game is not all that is; knows the rules and limitations of play, and sees beauty in the order thus imposed; seeks to expand any frontier available and yet is not unmindful of ethical imperatives and the needs of others. This athlete contends in a game for a prize, and the prize is play itself, a life fully experienced and examined."[5]

WHAT'S NEXT?

You have explored your preferences, your circumstances, and your schedule, and now you have a good idea what's best for you. And you have begun a program of increasing activity designed around the specific goals of adherence and performance. In doing so, you have also developed clearer insights into what works and what doesn't. Stick with it for about six weeks to firmly establish the *habit* of being more active and to further refine your program of adherence and improving performance. In the next chapter, we'll show you how to build an individualized LifeFit program based on the information you have discovered about yourself so far.

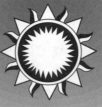

chapter 10
_____

PUTTING IT TOGETHER

To give yourself the best chance at achieving your LifeFit goals and sticking with an active life, find out where you are now, then set goals for getting to where you want to be. The LifeFit program for optimal health, a combination of Stage One and Stage Two activities, provides general guidelines. You can customize these guidelines to develop a program that works best for you.

Now it's time to stretch yourself a bit toward your long-term LifeFit goal by writing a specific activity program for optimal health, longevity, and vitality. This program will include both Stage One and Stage Two activities.

PLANNING STAGE ONE ACTIVITIES

Every day, as we've seen, you should be on your feet for at least an hour moving around, using the large muscles of your legs while

LIFEFIT PRINCIPLES

- It's likely most of us will have to make a *conscious* effort to add a few minutes of Stage One puttering around periodically throughout the day to achieve an hour a day for optimal health.

- Most American women in all likelihood already come very close to an hour a day of what we call puttering around, especially if they're homemakers.

- Be creative; life offers endless opportunities to be active; we simply have to be open to them.

- Moderate activities are activities that are intense enough to elevate the heart rate, increase your rate of breathing, and bring sweat to your brow.

- You'll get the most health benefits for time spent in moderate activities.

- The benefits of physical activity, whether Stage One or Stage Two, increase most rapidly at the lowest levels of effort as we move from sedentary to even moderately active; anything you can do to be up on your feet is going to help.

- When just getting started in an exercise program, keep in mind that even very light Stage One activity may seem extremely intense because your body isn't used to the effort.

- There are many ways to achieve your LifeFit goals; you can create your own balance of Stage One and Stage Two activities that best suits your needs and provides the results *you* want.

walking, climbing stairs, working in the garden, shuttling about the kitchen, playing with the children, or anything but sitting quietly in front of a TV. This need not be continuous activity, remember, nor is it necessary to work up a sweat. Stage One activities are primarily activities of daily living.

HOW MUCH IS AN HOUR OF PUTTERING?

You're certainly already on your way to this one-hour-a-day recommendation of light activity just getting through each day. Getting up in the morning and walking into the kitchen counts. So does walking out for the morning paper and going to your car (sitting in your car driving to work most definitely doesn't count). Walking from the parking lot to your job counts. Taking the stairs instead of the elevator certainly counts, and the three-block walk to the deli for

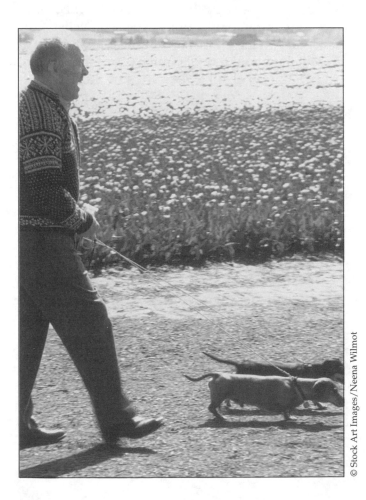

© Stock Art Images/Neena Wilmot

lunch. Mowing the lawn in the evening after work counts, and playing catch with the kids, vacuuming, and walking the dog. Alas, although standing at the kitchen sink washing the dishes is better than sitting in front of the TV, it still doesn't entirely count, although it definitely seems like work. The bottom line when it comes to puttering about is moving the entire body.

But none of this activity need be continuous, remember. What you are looking for is an accumulation of activity throughout the day totaling about one hour. Most of us are awake about 16 hours a day, so that one hour of puttering about represents only four minutes every waking hour, or eight minutes every other hour, or 12 minutes every three hours.

However, it's likely most of us will have to make a conscious effort to add a few minutes of puttering around periodically throughout the day to achieve that total. Although four minutes an hour doesn't sound like much, labor-saving devices, television, and communities organized around automobiles, not walkers or cyclists, all conspire to make sedentary living almost inevitable. Thus it's easy to go for hours at a stretch without moving much of anything but fingers on a keyboard or a thumb on a TV remote control.

HOW MUCH ARE YOU PUTTERING?

Before you know how far you have to go to achieve your Stage One goal, you will need to know where you are now—how much you are on your feet and moving around in a typical day. This will tell you what you need to change.

Estimates of how much time men and women in various occupations spend on their feet paint a rather discouraging picture. A Japanese study, for example, found that most Japanese adults spend much less than an hour a day on their feet moving about.[1] Retired men, the study observed, spend less than 30 minutes each day up and about on their feet; housewives spend more—not surprisingly—but not quite an hour; only elementary and high school teachers and office clerks manage to be up on their feet an hour each day. As the Japanese in general walk much more than we Americans and depend much more on public transportation and less on the automobile, chances are that those in corresponding occupations in the United States spend even less time on their feet.

How can you tell if you spend at least an hour a day on your feet moving about? The most direct way is to keep a record of the time you are in motion, like the one on page 271. Because you have already begun keeping a record as you work to develop the habit of activity, you may have started doing this and may already have an idea how much time you do spend on your feet. And you've probably also discovered that such record keeping is no easy task, if not an outright nuisance (see the daily activity diary). Who wants to be bothered with checking their stopwatch every time they get up to get a drink of water or take out the trash?

The Japanese researchers came up with a simple, no-hassle way to find out with reasonable accuracy how active you are throughout

Daily Activity Diary
(155 pound 40-something manager)

Time	Activity	Steps/stage
6:30-6:40	rise, shower	50/Stage One
6:40-6:50	dress	50/Stage One
6:50-7:30	fix and eat breakfast	250/Stage One
7:30-7:45	brush teeth, pack briefcase	150/Stage One
7:45-9:15	drive to work	
9:15-9:25	walk to office from lot, take stairs	1,000/Stage One
9:30-10:45	work at desk, some moving about	100/Stage One
10:45-11:00	break (walk to lunch room)	150/Stage One
11:00-1:00	work at desk, some moving about	100/Stage One
1:00-2:00	walk to lunch, lunch, walk back	100/Stage One
2:00-3:30	work at desk, some moving about	100/Stage One
3:30-3:45	break (walk to lunch room)	150/Stage One
3:45-5:30	meetings (walk to conference room)	150/Stage One
5:30-6:00	work at desk	
6:00-6:10	walk to lot	1,000/Stage One
6:10-7:25	drive home	
7:30-8:00	change, brisk walk	3,750/Stage Two
8:00-8:30	shower, change	100/Stage One
8:30-9:00	dinner	100/Stage One
9:00-9:30	help clean kitchen, put food away	300/Stage One
9:30-10:30	read, watch evening news	100/Stage One
total kcals: 140*		total steps: 3,950/Stage One
total kcals: 160**		3,750/Stage Two

* Figure a 155-pound man or woman expends about 210 kcals in an hour of Stage One activity, or about 3.5 kcals per minute, or about 3.5 kcals per 100 steps.

To figure exactly how many kcals you expend at your weight, multiply your weight in kilograms (lb/2.2) times 3 (METs of Stage One activity). That is, if you weigh 185 pounds, that's 84kg × 3, or 252 kcals per hour, or 4.2 kcals per minute, or per 100 steps.

** To figure kcals in Stage Two: weight in kg × METs (4.5 or more) × time. A 155-pound (70kg) individual walking briskly for 30 minutes expends 70 × 4.5 × .5 = 157.5 kcals the day—they use a pedometer. Clip it to your belt when you get up in the morning, and check for the day's total before you go to bed. The pedometer counts every step you take (most pedometers automatically convert steps into distance traveled; you'll want to find a pedometer that gives you the option of recording steps taken).

The average adult will take about 100 steps in a minute puttering around in nonvigorous activities. (More vigorous effort, incidentally, increases the number of steps per minute.) To achieve a minimum of an hour a day of puttering around, then, one needs to take about 6,000 steps. (The Japanese researchers call for a minimum of 10,000 steps daily for optimal health; at a leisurely level of effort, this 10,000 steps amounts to about an hour and a half a day. If you have the time, and if for any reason you can't engage in Stage Two activities, this amount of activity will provide significant health benefits, as discussed in chapter 2.

If you're shorter or taller than average, the number of steps you take in an hour of light Stage One activity will vary. To find out

MEASURES OF WALKING

Energy Expenditure for Walking Rates

	Slow walking	Moderate walking	Fast walking
Step rate	100 steps/min	110 steps/min	125+ steps/min
Intensity	3.0 METs	4.5 METs	5.0 METs

Total Amount of Walking Steps in a Day of Workers of Various Kinds

Office clerks	5,800
Technical workers	4,600
Administrators	4,490
Elementary school teachers	6,730
High school teachers	6,075
Translators/copywriters	4,650
Retired men	2,800
Houswives	4,500
Workers at home on holidays	2,930

Data from Yoshiro Hatano article "Use of the Pedometer for Promoting Daily Walking Exercise" in the International Council for Health, Physical Education and Recreation journal.

exactly how many steps you take in an hour of light activity using a pedometer, simply clip it to your belt and go for a leisurely walk for a specific time, say 5 or 10 minutes. It's important to walk at a pace consistent with your pace while shopping in the grocery store or walking from the parking lot to your office. After 5 or 10 minutes, multiply the number of recorded steps by the appropriate amount— 12 or 6—to get an approximate figure for one hour.

A pedometer won't record some activities that count toward either Stage One or Stage Two activities. For example, if you commute to work via bicycle, it certainly counts as Stage One or even Stage Two if you cycle vigorously enough, but your pedometer probably won't record it. Likewise, although exercise machines such as stair-climbing simulators provide excellent exercise, they won't record accurately on a pedometer. Of course, these devices usually have some sort of measuring system attached, such as an odometer or a system for counting flights of stairs climbed, so you can still keep a record of what you do.

WRITE YOUR OWN STAGE ONE PROGRAM

If you find yourself falling short of your Stage One goal, you'll need to intentionally build another few minutes of light activity into your daily life, which isn't that difficult.

In all likelihood, most American women already come close to an hour a day of what we call puttering around, especially if they're homemakers. Despite advances toward equality of the sexes in recent years, American women still do most of the housework, even those who put in an eight-hour day on the job; according to one study, the average husband today does about one-third of the housework (up from a miserly 15 percent in 1965), leaving the other two-thirds to the wife.[2] After retirement, the wife typically remains active, continuing to do the housework, cooking, shopping, and so on, while the husband finishes out his days in the reclining chair, TV remote firmly in hand. Indeed, the fact that American women still do most of the housework may account for at least some of their lower risk of heart disease and superior longevity.

Your long-term LifeFit goal is a lifetime commitment to activity, but you will want to break this into smaller increments. Your daily Stage I goal is an accumulation of at least an hour a day of puttering around. You may want to schedule specific activities for specific times. Write a new program for yourself a week or two weeks at a time, and see how each works for you. Be flexible; over a period of weeks, changing circumstances will require changes in your program.

Perhaps a busy week at the office makes your noon-hour stroll infeasible, or the grandkids are visiting for a week, giving you less time for that morning walk or leisurely shopping (although keeping up with your grandkids can provide plenty of opportunity for being active). But by now you should be experienced in making adjustments.

Next you will want to set goals, keep a record, reward yourself, and reassess to make sure it works.

Set a Goal

Once you know where you are, set out some specific weekly goals for getting from there to an hour a day of Stage One activity. Suppose you find that on a typical weekday, you're on your feet puttering about 30 to 45 minutes. Thus your goal is to increase the time you're on your feet moving about by 15 to 30 minutes. Suppose you walk the dog for 10 minutes each morning. Add another 10 minutes; both your dog and your body will thank you. Or resolve to walk 15 minutes during each lunch hour.

Take a moment to list some of the other things you can do in a week to help you achieve your Stage One goal. Here are a few suggestions:

- Park a few blocks farther from your office and walk. When you go shopping, park in the far corner of the lot and walk to the store.
- Take the stairs rather than the elevator, of course.
- At airports, "carry" yourself and your bags up the stairs; avoid escalators or conveyors.
- During lunch, go for a brief walk around the block. It needn't be strenuous; after all, you'll be wearing your regular clothing, so you won't want to work up a sweat.
- Take a stroll around the neighborhood when you come home from work; it's a good way to build up some minutes puttering around, and it's also a good way to unwind, reflect on the day's events, relieve stress, and build a buffer between work and family life.
- On weekends, build something active into your routine—a bike ride with the family, for example, or a walk in the nearest park, window shopping, a stroll through the neighborhood.
- Be creative; life offers endless opportunities to be active; we simply have to be open to them.

Keep a Record

Whether you do it by jotting down the time you spend on your feet puttering about or by using a pedometer, now's the time to begin a record of Stage One activity. For the time being, count this activity separately from any Stage Two activities in which you might already engage. That is, if you go out for a brisk walk or jog, or any other sustained activity of moderate intensity, don't count it as part of puttering about. For now, you simply want to get an idea of your general level of activities of daily living and how easy or difficult it may be for you to accumulate an hour a day.

Keep a record for an entire week (use the adherence goal chart and performance goal chart). On some days, particularly on weekends, you're likely to be more active than on weekdays; on other days, you

Adherence Goal Chart

Goal: 6,000 steps each day, average
Reward: A John Grisham novel

Week 1 average 6,250	Mon	Tue	Wed	Th	Fri	Sat	Sun
	4,600	5,800	6,900	3,350	5,850	10,000	7,250

Week 2 average 5,820	Mon	Tue	Wed	Th	Fri	Sat	Sun
	5,650	6,250	4,300	7,100	4,950	7,000	5,500

Performance Goal Chart

Goal: 3 30-minute, Stage Two, 3 weeks
Reward: Buy a pound of chocolate mint truffles

Week 1	Mon	Tue	Wed	Th	Fri	Sat	Sun
	walk, brisk	cycle (20 min)	walk (10) cycle (20)			walk	jog (20)

Week 2	Mon	Tue	Wed	Th	Fri	Sat	Sun
		walk (40 min)		jog (15) walk (20)		mow lawn walk (15 min)	

Week 2	Mon	Tue	Wed	Th	Fri	Sat	Sun
Well done! (Buy 2 pounds)	jog (15) cycle (15)	walk (20)	walk (30)		cycle (30)	walk (15) jog (10) cycle (15)	

may not be very active at all. You want to get a picture of a typical week's worth of activities. This will give you a pretty good idea what you have to change, if anything, to achieve and maintain your Stage One goal.

Reward Yourself

Treat yourself when you've reached a specific goal, whether it's a week, two weeks, or more of consistent Stage One activity. Ideally, rewards should be connected in some way to your active life: a new T-shirt or walking shorts, new shoes, a health magazine, a visit to a health spa for a steam bath and massage. Or you can literally treat yourself with treats, but be aware that if you hope to lose weight, the calories in a chocolate fudge brownie—if that's your pleasure—can easily undo much of what you've achieved in a week in terms of energy expenditure.

Is It Working?

After a week or two, you should have an idea whether the plan you've created for yourself is convenient and enjoyable. If you find you're having difficulty accumulating a total of seven hours a week of Stage One activity, it's time to reassess and readjust your program. If job or family commitments interfere, maybe it's time to ask for the cooperation of friends, family, and colleagues; are there ways they can support you in your effort to become and remain more active? If you do most of the cooking, for example, perhaps your spouse or children can take on some of the preparation work and free you for a 10- or 15-minute walk before dinner. Or better yet, you can enlist them in cleanup while you go for a walk after dinner. Many employ-ers allow flex-time schedules, so perhaps there's a way you can adjust your work schedule to allow more free time for activity in the morning, midday, or evening.

An hour a day of puttering around will be optimal and will build a foundation for moderately vigorous Stage Two activities and beyond. If you've been resolutely sedentary for years, you should not attempt to add Stage Two activities to your weekly routine until you've been consistently active in Stage One activities and can walk comfortably at a leisurely pace for about 30 uninterrupted minutes.

PLANNING STAGE TWO ACTIVITIES

Having become accustomed to a more active life over several weeks of consistent, light activity for a total of about an hour a day, your next goal toward optimal health should be to increase the intensity of effort now and then, so that over time you work up to 30 minutes, three times a week, of at least moderately vigorous physical activity. This activity should involve the large muscle groups such as the legs in walking, jogging, or cycling or the arms and back, as in swimming. For best results, these 30-minute or longer sessions of moderately vigorous activity should be sustained effort.

If you engage in 30 minutes of moderately vigorous physical activity (measured as 4.5 METs or more) three times a week, you'll burn approximately 300 kilocalories per hour for a total of 1.5 hours a week, or a total of 450 to 500 kilocalories (if you are of average weight, about 155 pounds). Add these to the 1,400 kilocalories you've already expended puttering around each week and you have a total of about 1,900 kilocalories, essentially the target level of weekly energy expenditure necessary for optimal health and longevity.

Remember, the benefits of physical activity, whether Stage One or Stage Two, increase most rapidly at the lowest levels of effort as we move from sedentary to even moderately active; anything you can do to be up on your feet is going to help.

HOW TO JUDGE

What is "moderately vigorous"? These activities are more strenuous than, for example, bowling or golfing with an electric cart. As mentioned previously, moderately vigorous activities are those that are intense enough to

- elevate the heart rate,
- increase your rate of breathing, and
- bring sweat to your brow.

These are the three most obvious markers of moderate activity, and of course, they'll vary a bit from individual to individual. Some of us, for example, may sweat heavily with even a little exertion, and most of us will sweat heavily in Atlanta or Miami in August, no matter what we're doing, which needs to be taken into account.

If your heart rate isn't elevated somewhat, if your breathing isn't heavy enough to interfere somewhat with normal conversation, if there isn't at least a bit of sheen on your forehead, you probably aren't engaged in moderate physical activity and you aren't getting the health benefits you should (of course, and we can't emphasize this too much, you will nonetheless gain significant benefits from even this light activity). You might want to refer to the activity characteristics chart in chapter 9 again for a list of activities by MET or intensity level; the higher the MET level, the more intense an activity. Generally speaking, activities of 4.5 METs or more provide the most health benefits for time spent.

On the other hand, keep in mind that moderate activities are just that—moderate. They aren't so intense that you end up on your hands and knees writhing in exhaustion; nor are they activities that leave you so sore you can barely get out of bed the next day. And they're definitely not the sorts of activities like running marathons every other weekend that the exercise gurus of 20 years ago main-

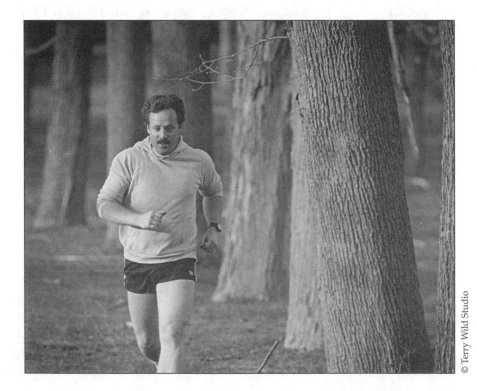

tained you absolutely had to do if you expected to live a long and productive life.[3] Rather they are activities that are somewhat more strenuous than leisurely strolls; they get the sweat flowing, to be sure, but they are well within your comfort zone if you've worked up to them.

Counting Your Heart Rate

One way to judge what is moderate activity for you is to measure your heart rate. Although this is perhaps a more accurate approach to gauging your effort, it's also more of a nuisance if you happen to be one of those who has a hard time finding a pulse to count. In any case, moderate activity is activity intense enough to elevate your heart rate to at least 50 percent of your maximum heart rate (60 to 70 percent is better). You can calculate your rough maximum heart rate by subtracting your age from 220. Thus, if you're 45, your theoretical maximum heart rate will be 175. Fifty percent of this would be only 88 beats per minute. (While exercising, stop and count your pulse for 10 seconds, then multiply by six.) You should measure your heart rate during the sustained effort portion of your workout, not during the beginning warm-up period or the later cool-down, as these measurements won't be as indicative of your true effort. Also, if you're very out of shape, counting your heart rate won't give you a true indication of the intensity of your effort, for reasons we'll discuss shortly.

Counting Steps

If you've been using a pedometer that counts your steps to estimate your puttering around, you can also use the pedometer along with a watch to estimate your intensity of effort, at least while walking or running. As discussed earlier, you'll probably take about 100 steps in a minute of puttering about in daily activities. If you increase your rate to 110 or more steps a minute, and if you can maintain that pace over 30 minutes or so, you will have entered the realm of moderate activity.[4]

Relative Versus Absolute Effort

Of course, if you've been sedentary for years, are overweight, or have any health conditions that have compromised your cardiovascular system, you'll find that even those activities rated as light, such as strolling from gallery to gallery through the Museum of Modern Art, is perhaps enough to get your heart rate up and bring sweat to your brow. But does this mean that you are working at a moderate or even heavy level and thus getting the health benefits of activity at that level of effort?

Well, not quite, but you are getting the health benefits of puttering around, even if it feels as if you're on the brink of exhaustion. And you certainly are laying the groundwork for more intense effort.

But how can this be? Aren't sweating, breathing hard, and a thumping heart the markers of moderate Stage Two exercise as defined above? That depends.

There's a difference between "relative" effort and "absolute" effort, and this is where physiology and common sense seem to part company. When the intensity of activity is measured in terms of METs, this measurement refers to an absolute level of intensity of effort that's completely independent of how you might feel while doing it. Two individuals of the same age, height, and weight, one who has been resolutely sedentary for years, the other a fitness fanatic, could walk a mile at a two-mile-an-hour pace (about 2 METs), and although they'll both be covering the same distance at the same pace, and will expend about the same number of calories, they'll have completely different experiences.

For the sedentary fellow, that mile may seem like a death march. He'll finish up—if he finishes at all—with his heart thumping around in his chest like a beached trout. And if someone—a researcher with an interest in such things, for example—were to come along just then and ask, the sedentary fellow would probably rate his effort, once he caught his breath, as *very* strong, close to his maximum, say at 17 to 19 on the Borg scale (the top of a scale of *perceived* exertion, which researchers who ask such questions like to use for estimating how intense an activity feels) (see table 10.1). On the other hand, that same mile will seem to be barely a warm-up for the other fellow; he might rate the same activity as a 6 (weak) on the Borg scale.

Although it seems as if the sedentary fellow is consuming more oxygen and expending more energy because he is so obviously working harder, in fact, both men are consuming about the same amount of oxygen, both are expending about the same amount of energy, both are exercising at the same low intensity, however different their experiences may be. It seems counterintuitive and, from the perspective of the hard-working former couch potato, downright unfair.

Table 10.1	The Borg Scale Rating of Perceived Exertion (RPE)

6 — no exertion at all

7

8 — extremely light

9 — very light

10

11 — light

12

13 — somewhat hard

14

15 — hard

16

17 — very hard

18

19 — extremely hard

20 — maximal exertion

Reprinted, by permission, from G. Borg, 1985, An introduction to Borg's RPE-scale (Ithaka, N.Y.: Mouvement Publications).

The fact is, because the sedentary fellow is out of shape, it takes more effort for him to perform the same amount of work; but for all that huffing and puffing, he's not getting any more work completed (work defined as moving mass through a specific distance) than the athlete who has yet to break a sweat. The unfit individual's cardiovascular system simply isn't accustomed to the effort; it hasn't been called on for months, perhaps years, to provide more than the minimal amount of oxygen to the working muscles because the muscles haven't been working. Because the cardiovascular system is "out of shape," it has to work near its comparatively low limit to provide adequate oxygen, even at relatively low levels of effort. Even though the unfit walker is huffing and puffing, and his heart is thumping desperately, his still-inefficient cardiovascular system is providing no more oxygen than the finely tuned cardiovascular system of the fit individual (actually, the out-of-shape fellow probably *is* expending somewhat more energy because he probably moves less efficiently than someone who is accustomed to moving, but the difference is not that great).

When just getting started in an exercise program, keep in mind that even very light Stage One activity may seem extremely intense because your body isn't used to the effort. For purposes of estimating where you are on the road to optimal health, you are not quite there, but you are well on your way, and it will be important at this stage to gently push yourself through the mental and physical barriers created by this discomfort. Much of the discomfort you'll face early on results from the fact your body simply isn't accustomed to the effort, but very quickly, probably within a few days, you'll find that you can walk that mile much more rapidly with what seems to be the same or even less effort.

Over a longer period, if you remain consistently active, more profound physiological changes will begin to take place, including increased vascularization of the working muscles, increased muscle strength, and improved cardiac function. You'll be able to perform more work with the same perceived effort, and you'll also be much healthier.

WRITE YOUR OWN STAGE TWO PROGRAM

Your long-term goal, again, is three 30-minute sessions per week of moderate activity (4.5 METs or more). To achieve that goal, you'll want to set some intermediate goals along the way, keep a record, reward yourself, and reassess your program periodically to make sure it works.

Set a Goal

As you approach Stage Two activities, increases in amount and intensity of effort should come prudently. Perhaps the safest approach is to add a brief period of sustained and moderate activity— enough to elevate your heart rate and breathing and bring sweat to your brow—every other day, say for 10 minutes at a time to start. It's important that these "Stage Two" days alternate with "easy" days. This allows the body enough time to recover (for more on rest, recovery, and injury prevention, see chapter 11).

The next week, add a minute or two to each session, and perhaps a bit more than that the week after, and so on. Obviously, you can increase at this modest rate only so long; early on, your ability to increase your effort will develop rapidly, but as you reach your performance limits, at some point, increases in workload will come much less rapidly and will eventually plateau. In all, it should probably take you about three months of steady, gradual progress to move from completely sedentary to the basic level of physical activity combined in Stage One and Stage Two. More rapid increases can lead to injury or burnout, and we'll discuss this at greater length in the next chapter.

Any activity will do for Stage Two, as long as it is sustained and elevates your heart rate. At the end of this chapter, you will find a detailed discussion of the most common Stage Two activities. Feel free to "mix and match." You already have an idea what types of activities you like, what suits your body and temperament, and what's most convenient.

- You might want to walk briskly each Stage Two day; or walk one day, cycle the next, and swim the third. Anything goes.

- Or if you have the facilities, you might walk a few minutes, jump on your bike for a few more, then dive into the pool for some laps.

- You can even turn Stage One activities into Stage Two activities by increasing intensity and sustaining the effort. For example, increasing the pace at which you push your grocery cart while shopping can take you into the realm of Stage Two, if you can avoid running into your more sedate fellow shoppers. Cutting the grass with a push mower is already intense enough (6.0 METs) to qualify it as a Stage Two activity; all you need is a big enough lawn to allow you to sustain the activity. Or volunteer to mow your neighbor's lawn while you're at it. Or mix and match—mow your lawn, then go for a brisk walk immediately after to get in the time you want. Again, anything goes.

Write out your intermediate goals at the beginning of each week. Literally schedule your activity into your day; write exercise into your daily calendar or appointment book, just as you would any other important meeting.

Keep a Record

Use the adherence goal chart and performance goal chart to record your activities throughout a week. Note anything that's relevant: what you did—walking, weight training, cycling, or whatever—and the time or distance spent walking or running, the laps or yards of swimming, and so on. Also, note how you feel and any other observations that might be relevant to you and that might offer some insights into what you should or can be doing. For example, you might note that walking after dinner is a great way to unwind, or that cycling before work is an exercise in terror, given all the traffic at that hour. These sorts of notes will help you determine what comes next and what works best.

Reward Yourself

Reward yourself when you reach specific goals. For example, if your goal is to walk briskly for 10 minutes on Monday, Wednesday, and Friday for the first week, treat yourself if you achieve that goal.

Is It Working?

After a week or two, you should have an idea whether the plan you've created works. If you're having trouble achieving your intermediate goals, examine why and decide what you can change to make it easier to stick to the plan.

• Lack of time, of course, is the most common barrier, so look for ways to readjust your schedule if you're having problems, as you may have done already in achieving your Stage One goals. For example, if you've scheduled your brisk walk before dinner in the evenings but find that other commitments continually interfere, perhaps you need to find a different time. Many find that exercise early in the morning is easier to stick with because they can get in their walk or jog before other commitments get in the way. However, not everyone likes to exercise early in the day, before the body and mind are entirely awake; try it a few times to see how you feel.

• If you find you often simply "don't feel like it," another common reason many of us fail to reach our exercise goals, perhaps it's time to give yourself a pep talk. Review part II of this book to remind yourself of all the benefits you'll achieve if you stay active. Read magazines or books about your chosen activities, get involved in clubs or organizations related to those activities, or enlist friends to exercise with you.

• If you find that after a few weeks it still doesn't feel right, or you're physically very uncomfortable, then perhaps the activity you've chosen really isn't for you and it's time to try something else.

CUSTOMIZING THE PROGRAM

The LifeFit program we've outlined here is only a general guideline, a recommended balance of quantity and intensity for the most benefit with the least effort. But there are other ways to achieve your LifeFit goals; you can create your own balance of Stage One and Stage Two activities that best suits your needs and provides the results *you* want.

For example, suppose you're the 40-something manager we discussed in chapter 9; you have little time for puttering about, and after a few weeks of trying, you find there's simply no way you're going to get in the hour a day you want, and that no matter what you do, the best you can manage is an average of only 30 minutes of Stage One activity each day (about 3,000 steps), half your Stage One goal. On the other hand, you find that brisk walking is an agreeable activity, and that now and then you even break into a slow jog, which you enjoy wholeheartedly. This activity also fits in well with your full schedule.

The solution? Increase your Stage Two activities to make up for your lack of Stage One effort. The good news for the very busy is that you can spend less time in Stage Two activities to gain the same health benefits you'd enjoy if you spent more time in Stage One.

MORE STAGE TWO, LESS STAGE ONE

Substitute 30 minutes of Stage Two activity for one hour of Stage One. Roughly speaking, 30 minutes of sustained Stage Two activity (average of 6 METs), for example, 30 minutes of brisk walking or slow jogging, is equivalent to one hour of accumulated Stage One activities (average 3 METs). More intense activity, for example 30 minutes of running, will be equivalent to even more than an hour of Stage One activity (in the next few pages we'll show you how to figure exactly how much of one activity substitutes for another).

If you can manage only 30 minutes of Stage One activity a day, for a total of 3.5 hours a week, that leaves you another 3.5 hours short of your target total of seven hours. No problem; substitute just 1.75 hours of Stage Two activities (1.75 hours of Stage Two equals 3.5 hours of Stage One). Add this 1.75 to the 1.5 hours of Stage Two activity in which you already engage, and that's about three hours and 15 minutes of Stage Two activity each week.

You can break this down any way you like: say an hour of brisk walking three days, or perhaps 30 minutes of brisk walking on Monday, Wednesday, and Friday, cycling on Tuesday and Thursday, and some weight training on Saturday.

MORE STAGE ONE, LESS STAGE TWO

Substitute one hour of Stage One activity for 30 minutes of Stage Two. Suppose you're the 50-plus retired teacher; you have more time, but you find that you simply don't enjoy moderate activities that work up a sweat. You can still achieve very significant improvements in health if you're willing to spend more time in Stage One puttering about—activities such as working in the garden, for example, or leisurely strolls around town.

As 30 minutes of Stage Two is roughly equivalent to an hour of Stage One, substitute an additional three hours of Stage One activity for 90 minutes of Stage Two activity. This gives you a total of 10 hours of puttering about each week, an accumulation of 1.5 hours a day or about 9,000 steps (100 steps a minute or 6,000 steps an hour).

REFINING YOUR PROGRAM

If you have a calculator and a mathematical inclination, you can further fine-tune your program using the step-by-step plan that follows to find out exactly how much of any Stage Two activity—brisk walking, jogging, running hard uphill, handball, and so on—is equivalent to an hour of Stage One puttering about, or vice versa.

To do this, you'll need to start thinking about energy expenditure in terms of kilocalories expended, not just the time you spend being active:

- First, find your weight in kilograms. To do this, divide your weight in pounds by 2.2. For example, if you weigh 185 pounds, you weigh 84 kilograms. If you weigh 125 pounds, you weigh 57 kilograms.

- Find your LifeFit goal in kilocalories by referring to the chart on page 27 in chapter 2. For example, the 2,000-kilocalorie-per-week goal is for a 70-kilogram (155-pound) individual. If you weigh 185 pounds, or 84 kilograms, your goal will be slightly higher, approximately 2,330 kilocalories. (Remember, this doesn't mean you have to work harder; it simply means that at the same level of effort, larger individuals expend more energy). If you weigh 125 pounds, your goal is about 1,600 kilocalories. The figure corresponding to your weight is your general LifeFit goal as measured in kilocalories expended in Stage One and Stage Two activities combined.

- Now, if you know how much Stage One activity you can manage, say 30 minutes a day, and you want to know exactly how much of a specific Stage Two activity you need to achieve your LifeFit goal, follow these steps:

  1. Multiply your weight in kilograms times 3 METs (the approximate MET value for all Stage One activities) times hours in Stage One activities per week (kilograms × METs × time = kilocalories in Stage One). If you weigh 84 kilograms and you manage 30 minutes a day (3.5 hours a week), then this equals: 84 × 3 × 3.5 = 880 (this is approximate; it's okay to round off, as all of these figures are estimates).

  2. Subtract this from your goal of 2,330 (2,330 − 880 = 1,450). This means you have to expend 1,450 kilocalories in Stage Two activity to achieve your LifeFit goal. How much time does this take?

  3. Suppose very brisk walking and slow jogging are your chosen activities; these are both rated at around 6 METs. To find out how much time you need to spend each week at these activities, multiply your weight (84 kilograms) times 6 METs = 504. This is how much energy you expend in one hour measured at this level of intensity.

  4. Because your goal is a total of nearly 1,500 kilocalories at this level of intensity, you need three hours a week (1,500/500) of brisk walking and jogging to reach that goal. You can divide that three hours any way you like, say 30 minutes on six days a week, an hour on three days, or any combination that works best for you. (You'll want to be careful not to overwork any one muscle group on consecutive days; see chapter 11.)

  5. Suppose you're more ambitious when it comes to Stage Two, or you have even less time. Suppose, in fact, you swim laps very vigorously. Vigorous laps are rated at 10 METs (see the chart on pages 240-243, chapter 9). To figure how much lap swimming you need: 85 × 10 = 850. Divide your 1,500-kilocalorie Stage Two goal by this answer: 1,500/850 = 1.75 hours. Whereas you need about three hours of brisk walking each week, less than two hours of vigorous laps in the local pool will provide the same benefits.

ADAPTING AS YOU AGE

We noted previously that as you grow older, your LifeFit goals can change. The 2,000-kilocalorie figure is the target goal up to age 59 (and about 70 kilograms in weight). The target for those aged 60 to 74 is 1,500 kilocalories, and for those 75 and older it's 1,000 kilocalories. This means that at these age-specific levels, you'll receive the most benefits for effort expended. But it doesn't mean you shouldn't do more if you're able; as we age, differences between individuals increase, so rigid guidelines for older men and women tend to become less meaningful as the years go by.

You may find that as you age, you have a more difficult time maintaining your original levels of activity; in particular, you may find that it's more difficult to maintain the intensity of Stage Two activities. If that happens, it's okay to cut back on intensity or quantity of Stage Two activities. Most likely, you'll find that you're still able to maintain Stage One activities more easily, so use the formulas above to customize your program accordingly for continuing optimal health.

These formulas provide some basic guidelines for starting out. We don't recommend that you spend much time punching buttons on your calculator, however. Once you know approximately how much time you need to spend in Stage One and Stage Two activities to meet your specific goals, forget about the math and enjoy yourself. And remember, anything you do is better than nothing and more is better than less, at least to a point, which we'll discuss more in the next chapter.

A CLOSER LOOK AT SOME STAGE TWO ACTIVITIES

Most likely, you'll choose your Stage Two activities from a handful of common sports. Brief discussions of some of these follow.

BRISK WALKING

Brisk walking is one of the best activities to start with, particularly if you've been sedentary for a long time. Walking is generally considered a perfect aerobic activity; it doesn't require any particular skills or talents; it provides adequate aerobic benefits; because one foot is always on the ground, walking is relatively easy on the joints; it doesn't require any special equipment except a decent pair of shoes; and you can walk just about anywhere, any time. There are few excuses *not* to walk, in fact, unless you're troubled by darkness, bad weather, or the fact that so many of our communities are oriented for automobiles and thus lack sidewalks or at least pleasant, unpolluted areas in which to stroll. But in this era of suburban megamalls, mall walking in the comfort and safety of a well-lit, dry, air-conditioned shopping complex removes even these barriers.

Walking works the major muscles of the legs and lower back and, to a lesser extent, the upper body, particularly if you swing your arms and carry light hand weights.

ENERGY EXPENDUTURE: BRISK WALKING

If you walk 3.5 mph (4.0 METs) for one hour, you'll expend the following energy:

If you weigh	95 lb	125 lb	155 lb	185 lb	215 lb	245 lb
	170 kcals	228 kcals	280 kcals	336 kcals	390 kcals	444 kcals

If you walk 4.0 mph (4.5 METs) for one hour, you'll expend the following energy:

If you weigh	95 lb	125 lb	155 lb	185 lb	215 lb	245 lb
	194 kcals	260 kcals	315 kcals	380 kcals	440 kcals	500 kcals

JOGGING OR RUNNING

Jogging or running (the difference seems to be in the eye of the beholder) offer most of the same advantages of walking—simple, nothing to learn, can be done anywhere—with the additional benefit of increased intensity; you can pack more work into and burn more calories during a limited amount of time. Running may also provide psychological benefits that walking doesn't, at least for the more hard-driving among us, who may feel the need to get from here to there as quickly as possible and that anything less is a violation of the American work ethic. Running works the lower body, like walking, and provides excellent conditioning for the cardiovascular system.

The disadvantage with running is that both feet are off the ground during part of each stride, which means more impact—roughly eight times body weight with each footstrike. This tends to magnify any muscular or skeletal imbalances, increasing the risk of injury; certainly if you're overweight, or suffering from joint problems such as arthritis in the knees, running may not be a good idea, at least not right away. Because of the increased impact, it is also more important to have shoes that are appropriate for your particular body type or footstrike, which in some cases means more expense. In any case, you should experiment with running only after you've been walking for several weeks and are able to walk briskly for at least 30 minutes without discomfort.

ENERGY EXPENDUTURE: JOGGING

If you jog at 6 mph (10 METs) for one hour, you'll expend the following energy:

If you weigh	95 lb	125 lb	155 lb	185 lb	215 lb	245 lb
	430 kcals	570 kcals	700 kcals	840 kcals	980 kcals	1,110 kcals

CYCLING

Because your weight is supported by the bike, you can elevate your heart rate without the pounding associated with activities such as jogging. Thus cycling is an excellent activity for anyone just getting started or anyone with injuries that might make walking or running difficult or painful. Cycling works all of the muscles of the lower body, particularly the thighs. This makes cycling a good complement to running or walking, which tend to work the hamstrings (the muscles in the back of the legs) more. The improved muscle-strength balance that results tends to reduce the risk of injury, particularly to the knees (see chapter 11 for more on the value of "cross-training" or combining activities).

Some disadvantages of cycling are that you have to buy a bike and you have to know how to ride it, how to change gears effectively, how to work the brakes properly, and how to keep it in good repair. If you're a tinkerer at heart, you'll love cycling. But bikes are relatively simple, and even if you are all thumbs, bike maintenance probably won't be beyond your abilities. These are small barriers, however, and learning is part of the fun.

A major downside is that while riding, you'll have to contend with automobiles and the drivers of same, not all of whom are entirely watchful. As noted earlier, most American roadways are not designed to accommodate either bikes or pedestrians, which means sharing the road with sometimes oblivious drivers while riding as close to the shoulder of the road as possible, through all the litter of broken bottles, pieces of old cars, beer cans, unlucky pets, and all the other refuse of a careless civilization; the risk of accident is ever-present. However, there's a workable alternative if you are concerned about safety, and that's a stationary exercise bike. Stationary cycling isn't necessarily the most engaging activity; the scenery doesn't change, so it's easy to get bored. But you can read while you cycle, if you can keep the sweat out of your eyes, or watch TV or listen to the radio (which means making sure you buy a cycle that's quiet).

ENERGY EXPENDUTURE: CYCLING						
If you ride a bike (6-10 METs) for one hour, you'll expend the following energy:						
If you weigh	**95 lb**	**125 lb**	**155 lb**	**185 lb**	**215 lb**	**245 lb**
Leisurely (6 mph)	260 kcals	340 kcals	420 kcals	500 kcals	590 kcals	666 kcals
Moderate (8 mph)	345 kcals	455 kcals	560 kcals	670 kcals	780 kcals	888 kcals
Vigorous (10 mph)	430 kcals	570 kcals	700 kcals	840 kcals	980 kcals	1,110 kcals

SWIMMING

Having said that walking is a perfect aerobic activity, in truth, swimming is probably even more perfect, as long as you know how to swim and have access to a nearby pool that isn't overcrowded when you need it (swimming isn't so perfect as part of your LifeFit program if the inconvenience prevents you from being consistent).

Swimming provides sustained aerobic activity that works the entire body; it is particularly good for upper body development, and it's excellent for anyone who has joint problems, particularly foot, knee, or low-back problems that make walking or running painful. The very overweight and very sedentary will probably find that swimming is a much more "user-friendly" activity for starting out.

The downside, again, is that you need to know how to swim and you need a pool. Of course, just about anyone can learn to swim, and learning a complex motor skill, as noted in part II, seems to build neural connectivity, improving cognitive performance and at the same time building a skill that's good for general health.

As discussed in chapter 4, if weight loss is one of your long-term goals, you should be aware that swimming may not be as effective a means of losing weight as walking, jogging, or other activities done out of the water. The reason? To review briefly, water does such a good job of dissipating body heat that swimming doesn't elevate your core body temperature or metabolism as significantly, and it's this elevation of metabolism that results in an increased expenditure of calories for hours *after* exercise. Whereas you'll expend the same number of calories walking or jogging a mile as you will swimming approximately a quarter mile, you'll probably continue to expend more calories longer after the jog than you will after the walk or swim because your core body temperature and metabolism will remain higher longer after the jog.[5] This continued postactivity metabolic boost, as we've seen, plays a significant role in effective weight loss.

Another aquatic exercise that has a lot of advantages for aging bodies is water aerobics. The resistance the water provides as you move through it helps strengthen your muscles. When most of your body is under water, you don't have to worry about how you look

ENERGY EXPENDUTURE: SWIMMING

If you swim laps (6-10 METs) for one hour, you'll expend the following energy:

If you weigh	95 lb	125 lb	155 lb	185 lb	215 lb	245 lb
Light laps	260 kcals	340 kcals	420 kcals	500 kcals	590 kcals	666 kcals
Hard laps	430 kcals	570 kcals	700 kcals	840 kcals	980 kcals	1,110 kcals

as you exercise. The buoyancy of the water also provides great benefits, especially for those with aching joints. When you are submerged to shoulder depth, the water supports almost 90 percent of your body weight. If you weigh 200 pounds, your bones, joints, and muscles are supporting only 20 pounds of your body's weight when you exercise in water. And water aerobics provides the same cardiovascular advantages that other aerobic exercises do.

AEROBICS

The term *aerobics* has now been almost completely absorbed by what used to be called "aerobic dance," "dance exercise," "dancercize," or some variation on the basic theme of exercise to music, usually with a heavy, repetitive beat, in a mirror-lined room of the local Y or health club. A good aerobics class can offer a total-body workout that develops endurance, strength, and flexibility in a relatively safe package. A good aerobics leader or instructor will take the class through a warm-up into a period of sustained aerobic work in combination with exercises that develop strength and flexibility, followed by a cool-down. Low-impact aerobics classes minimize jumping and the resulting pounding and bouncing that can increase the risk of injury. Newer variations on the theme include stepping up and down on raised platforms for increased work, and routines that use light weights or other forms of light resistance to increase strength.

An aerobics class offers ample opportunities—more than walking or jogging, for example—for social connectedness, and as we've seen in part II, social connections may be one of the most important factors in promoting good health and longevity.

One drawback of aerobics is that you have to live or work near an aerobics class, and then you have to fit the class schedule into your own, two barriers that can provide excuses to "sit one out." Another drawback can be the music and its often maddening, thumping beat. And aerobics classes can be expensive. If you happen to be self-conscious, perhaps the most serious drawback is the mirrors and the unavoidable, perhaps somewhat disheartening, reflections of your-self (or maybe this will further motivate you to do something about your image and posture).

One solution is to do aerobics at home using any of the scores of video workouts on the market. Most of these videos offer the same basic routine of warm-up, exercise, and cool-down, but as a general rule of thumb, it's probably wise to steer clear of celebrity workout videos; these usually feature this or that young (or in the case of Jane Fonda, not so young) starlet bouncing around and smiling—lots of white teeth, in other words, but not always sound physiology. Opt for videos put together by men or women who have credentials as trainers or exercise physiologists.

ENERGY EXPENDUTURE: AEROBICS

If you do aerobic dance (5-7 METs) for one hour, you'll expend the following energy:

If you weigh	95 lb	125 lb	155 lb	185 lb	215 lb	245 lb
Low impact	215 kcals	285 kcals	350 kcals	420 kcals	490 kcals	555 kcals
High impact	300 kcals	400 kcals	490 kcals	590 kcals	685 kcals	777 kcals

ROWING AND CROSS-COUNTRY SKIING

We lump these two quite disparate activities together because cross-country—or Nordic—skiers and rowers are considered by many to be the best endurance athletes in the world; the highest oxygen uptakes (a measure of endurance) ever recorded were found among cross-country skiers, for example.

There's no pounding associated with either rowing or Nordic skiing, thus both are excellent for anyone just starting out, anyone who is overweight and bothered by the pounding of walking or jogging, or anyone who is troubled by injuries. Both activities develop the entire body, working the major muscles of the legs, upper back, shoulders, and arms, and both develop strength *and* endurance.

An obvious problem with skiing, of course, is that you need snow as well as a certain amount of technical skill, although cross-country skiing is not particularly complex. For rowing, obviously, you need an expanse of relatively calm water, uncluttered with such things as speed boats, oil tankers, floating garbage, raw sewage discharges, and the like. However, as with cycling, there are options: rowing machines and cross-country ski simulators. As with exercise bikes, though, using these machines can be a bit boring, and whereas reading is possible on a stationary bike, it's difficult if not impossible while using a rowing or skiing machine. Thus TV or music are the only options for easing the boredom (though some TV programming can be worse than simple boredom).

ENERGY EXPENDUTURE: ROWING						
If you row for one hour (9.5-12 METs), you'll expend the following energy:						
If you weigh	**95 lb**	**125 lb**	**155 lb**	**185 lb**	**215 lb**	**245 lb**
Moderately vigorous	410 kcals	540 kcals	665 kcals	800 kcals	930 kcals	1,055 kcals
Vigorous	515 kcals	685 kcals	840 kcals	1,010 kcals	1,175 kcals	1,330 kcals

ENERGY EXPENDUTURE: CROSS-COUNTRY SKIING						
If you ski for one hour (7-9 METs), you'll expend the following energy:						
If you weigh	**95 lb**	**125 lb**	**155 lb**	**185 lb**	**215 lb**	**245 lb**
Moderately vigorous	300 kcals	400 kcals	490 kcals	590 kcals	685 kcals	777 kcals
Vigorous	390 kcals	510 kcals	630 kcals	755 kcals	880 kcals	1,000 kcals

RACQUET (AND OTHER COURT) SPORTS

Tennis, squash, racquetball, and handball can all provide excellent workouts, developing cardiovascular health, flexibility, and strength. However, it may be difficult for beginners to get the full aerobic benefits from any of these activities, as they will probably spend much of their time chasing balls. As a beginner, you can certainly count your time spent on the courts toward your Stage One puttering around, but you probably shouldn't count this time as Stage Two activity until you've become reasonably accomplished and can keep ball chasing to a minimum. However, because squash, racquetball,

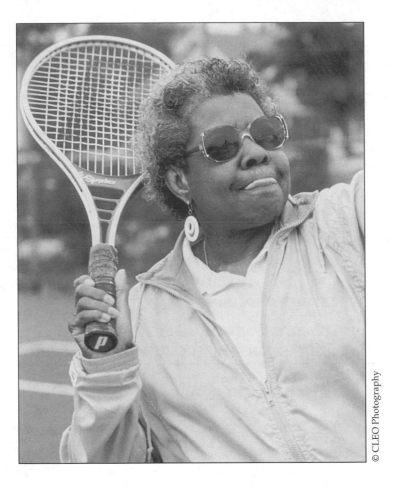

© CLEO Photography

and handball are all played in enclosed courts, it will probably be easier for beginners to get a sustained aerobic workout, even early on, because it's easier to keep the ball in play.

Tennis, squash, and racquetball all tend to develop the body asymmetrically because one arm is used more than the other. Handball uses both hands roughly equally and thus provides a better overall workout. All of these activities involve quite a bit of twisting, which can be hard on the lower back, so keep this in mind when considering any of these activities if you've had previous low-back problems. And they all involve quick, lunging movements that can increase the risk of falls and sprains. If you have chronic knee problems or arthritis in the hands, elbows, or shoulders, you may want to approach these activities with caution. On the other hand this type of training probably helps combat osteoporosis and builds strength and trains the sense of balance to *prevent* falls.

ENERGY EXPENDUTURE: RACQUET SPORTS

If you play tennis (8 METs) or other court sports (7-12 METs) for one hour, you'll expend the following energy:

If you weigh	95 lb	125 lb	155 lb	185 lb	215 lb	245 lb
Singles tennis	345 kcals	455 kcals	560 kcals	670 kcals	785 kcals	888 kcals
Racquetball	300 kcals	400 kcals	490 kcals	590 kcals	685 kcals	777 kcals
Handball	515 kcals	685 kcals	840 kcals	1,008 kcals	1,175 kcals	1,330 kcals

STRENGTH TRAINING

Strength, or resistance, training can seem intimidating at first, particularly if you have been sedentary for years or if you are older. At first glance, a gym filled with weights can seem like the last place you belong, but in fact, it's probably the *best* place you can be, especially if you are getting on in years. As noted earlier, strength training actually becomes more important as we age, not less. Becoming and remaining strong simply make it easier to get about through the day; resistance training builds strength and endurance for whatever you want to do, whether that happens to be carrying in groceries from the car, playing with the kids (or grandkids, or perhaps even great-grandkids), or a hard game of tennis. Strength training enhances your ability to engage in recreational activities and makes it possible to remain vital, functioning, and independent longer. Moreover, the earlier you start a strength training routine, and the more muscle you can build earlier in life, the more reserves of muscle and strength you'll have in old age, delaying frailty even if there is some inevitable loss of strength. (Refer to appendix 2 for more information on strength training.)

Benefits of Strength Training

Strength training increases bone density, reducing the risk of fractures. And improved strength reduces the risk of falls as well as the risk that you'll be injured if you do fall.

Other benefits of strength training include the following:

- As noted in chapter 4, strength training could well be the most effective exercise for weight loss; you can expend more calories during a vigorous strength workout than during most other activities. Strength training also tends to elevate the core body temperature and metabolism more effectively; thus, even after a workout, your body will continue to expend calories at an elevated rate much longer than it would after many other activities. And adding muscle while losing fat will actually rev up your resting metabolism, making it easier to maintain a healthy body weight; muscle is an active tissue that burns energy even at rest. Fat, on the other hand, more or less just sits there.

- Strength training may be the most effective way to make favorable changes in your body image and thus self-esteem; by promoting weight loss, toning old muscles, and creating new muscle tissue, strength training will produce gratifying changes in size and shape in just a few weeks of consistent effort.

- A strong muscle is a more durable muscle; it's less prone to strains and tears or other injuries that can interfere with an active life.

- Strength training for the total body also helps prevent the injury-inducing muscle strength imbalances that can result from a steady diet of any one type of exercise.

- Strength training can develop added strength to prevent weaknesses in specific muscles or muscle groups; for example, weak muscles around the knees can result in knee problems; weak abdominal and lower back muscles can increase the risk of low-back pain, an almost epidemic problem in this country.

- Strength training helps increase endurance, and thus performance, in other recreational activities such as walking, tennis, or golf; a stronger muscle can work at a given level of effort more easily.

- Strength training enhances breathing. About a dozen different muscles around the chest, abdomen, and upper back are used in breathing. When these muscles are strengthened through weight training, breathing becomes more efficient and we're less prone to fatigue.

- Strength training helps maintain proper posture. With fatigue, we begin to slouch; the shoulders round forward, the chest sinks, constricting the lungs and making it more difficult to breathe, which hastens further fatigue. If the muscles of the upper body are strong, we can maintain correct posture longer. Good posture also helps prevent a host of problems including low-back pain.

Women and Strength Training

If anything, strength training is more important for older women because of its beneficial effects on the bones. But one of the primary concerns of women is growth in muscle bulk; whereas most men welcome a few more bulges here and there, if the "here and there" happens to be the arms, shoulders, or other appropriate locations, many women are uncomfortable with the notion of bulky muscles. If you've been sedentary, however, whether a man or woman, you'll find that even a little strength training will produce gratifying strength gains without appreciable gains in muscle size. At some point, of course, a muscle has to grow to become still stronger, but women generally don't gain muscle size as readily as men do, so concerns about significant and unwanted gains in size are unwarranted; generally, when women begin a serious program of weight training, they tend to become much more slender in appearance as body fat is worked off and slack, untrained muscles firm up.[6]

ENERGY EXPENDUTURE: STRENGTH TRAINING					
If you train with weights (6 METs) for one hour (with 30 seconds to two minutes between sets) you'll expend the following energy:					

If you weigh	95 lb	125 lb	155 lb	185 lb	215 lb	245 lb
	260 kcals	340 kcals	420 kcals	500 kcals	590 kcals	666 kcals

TAI CHI CHUAN AND YOGA

Tai chi chuan and yoga may well be two of the most beneficial activities as we grow older. These disciplines have developed over several centuries specifically to promote longevity, and the most advanced practitioners of both seem not to reach their prime until their sixties, seventies, or even later.

Tai chi chuan and yoga are both excellent forms of relaxation for the overstressed, and there's ample research to support the notion that practicing yoga or tai chi is beneficial for general health. For older adults, in particular, tai chi can be enormously valuable as a low-impact form of exercise that works the entire body in slow, rhythmic fashion to develop balance, strength, and flexibility, all essential to the maintenance of an independent, vital life. And in traditional practice settings, parks for example, both tai chi and yoga help develop social connections.

Yoga refers to several disciplines, some of which are strictly philosophical or spiritual. Most commonly here in the West, however, when we think of yoga, we think of that series of postures—*asanas*—breathing exercises, and deep concentration that develop flexibility and strength and focus the mind.

Tai chi chuan (pronounced "tie-jee choowan") literally means "supreme-ultimate system" or "supreme-ultimate fist" (the early practitioners, for all their spiritual development, seem not to have developed a sense of modesty about their art). The practice involves controlled breathing and a series of slow, continuous, and deliberate movements patterned on the movements of animals or other natural phenomena, all of which have a distinctly martial application.

Tai chi chuan is classified as an "internal" martial art in that it emphasizes mental and spiritual development and the development of one's intention and concentration, along with one's *ch'i*—vitality, life force, or internal energy—as well as physical strength, speed, flexibility, and the practice of distinctly combative techniques. Although it's a martial art, one doesn't have to practice it as such, and from the beginning, tai chi has been integrated into an entire system of health based on *Ch'i Gung,* or "energy practice," the purpose of which is to cure or prevent disease by promoting the unobstructed flow of ch'i throughout the body.

Perhaps of most significance to us as we grow older, both yoga and tai chi have as their fundamental goal this cultivation and marshaling of *prana*, as it is called in India, *ch'i (qi)* in Chinese, or *ki* in Japanese—for improved health, vitality, longevity, and at the highest levels of practice, enlightenment. *Prana* and *ch'i* have been variously translated as "life force," "breath," "universal energy," or "human energy field," although none of these translations quite captures the true meaning of these terms. In truth, English doesn't contain an exactly equivalent concept.

Whereas most cultures seem to have some similar concept of a life force or life essence that can be cultivated for improved physical or spiritual health, ours doesn't, perhaps because we tend to divide mind from body. But it has been argued that at the dawn of Western civilization, and even through the Middle Ages and up to the Enlightenment, we also possessed such a concept, and that the light shown radiating from saints in early Christian paintings, for example, is in some ways a representation of high levels of this life force or spiritual power (there are similar images in Asian art).[7-11] The classical Greek term *pneuma*—breath, wind, or spirit, from which we derive words such as *pneumonia*—may be as close an approximation of *ch'i* or *prana* as we have in a Western language.

Whether *ch'i* is simply a useful concept or truly a "substance" like blood or air or a "force" like the bioelectrical activities taking place inside our bodies is open to debate. Skeptics deny that *ch'i* is anything more than a quaint idea. Part of our Western skepticism derives from the fact that *ch'i* hasn't been identified, measured, or controlled in a lab to the satisfaction of many here in the West, which is of small concern to the hundreds of millions of practitioners of these traditional disciplines.

Because aging might ultimately be seen as a decline in life force or vitality, with death the end point of this decline, and because disciplines such as yoga and tai chi work *directly* to cultivate vitality, they might ultimately prove to be among the most valuable resources available to us as we strive for the longest, most vital lives possible.[12,13] (Refer to appendix 2 for more information about tai chi chuan.)

ENERGY EXPENDUTURE: TAI CHI CHUAN AND YOGA

If you practice tai chi chuan or yoga for one hour (4 METs) you'll expend the following energy:

If you weigh	95 lb	125 lb	155 lb	185 lb	215 lb	245 lb
	170 kcals	230 kcals	280 kcals	335 kcals	390 kcals	444 kcals

FLEXIBILITY

Anyone can stretch, and it's easy to work stretching into your daily routine without having to spend much time at it. Spend five minutes or so in the morning doing a few light stretches. Then stretch now and then throughout the day to relieve tension or if you've been sitting or standing in one position for long periods. Before going for a walk or a jog or whatever, spend 5 to 10 minutes stretching all of the body's major muscle groups. This will help you warm up and reduce the risk of injuring cold, stiff muscles. During the cool-down after you've finished, use light stretching to help prevent postexercise soreness and keep the muscles supple and ready for the next day (see appendix 2 for a few basic stretches).

The stretching we're talking about here is different from the sort of stretching many of us learned in school physical education; many of us came of age in an era when physical education teachers taught us to stretch by throwing our bodies about and bouncing for maximum stretching, usually to rhythmic exhortations to "make it hurt, sissies!" Research has shown that not only does this increase the risk of injuries, such "ballistic" stretching is actually counterproductive. Ballistic or excessive stretching activates reflexes that signal the muscles to contract, protecting them from harm; thus you're tightening the very muscles you're trying to loosen. Bob Anderson, author of the excellent how-to guide to stretching, succinctly and appropriately titled *Stretching*, recommends a two-part stretch for the most benefit:

- In the "easy" stretch, go to a point in the stretch where you feel a mild tension, relax, and hold for 10 to 30 seconds. The tension should diminish as you hold the position.

- Then move slowly into the "developmental stretch" by moving a fraction of an inch farther until you again begin to feel a mild tension, then hold for 10 to 30 seconds. Again, you should feel the tension easing off as you hold the stretch.[14]

Why stretch? Flexibility training provides a variety of benefits:

- It delays or prevents the tendency to stiffen with age.
- It helps improve posture.
- The relaxing effect of stretching helps control the harmful effects of stress.

- It prevents injuries that can interfere with one's program of aerobic or strength training, as a tight, inflexible muscle is more prone to strains or tears.

- Stretching is also essential for anyone striving for peak performance, because a flexible muscle can move more easily through its full range of motion.

ENERGY EXPENDUTURE: STRETCHING

If you stretch (4 METs) for one hour, you'll expend the following energy:

If you weigh	95 lb	125 lb	155 lb	185 lb	215 lb	245 lb
	170 kcals	230 kcals	280 kcals	335 kcals	390 kcals	444 kcals

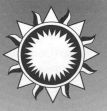

chapter 11

FOR THE LONG HAUL: SENSIBLE TRAINING, SENSIBLE LIVING

The resilience of youth protects us from all sorts of foolishness, including indiscriminate exercise habits. But as we grow older, bad habits can begin to take a toll. With increasing age, the risk of injury increases, and injuries take longer to heal. And if you're hurt or exhausted by inappropriate training, you can't be active and enjoy activity's many benefits. Thus one of the most important factors in sticking with activity is sensible training for the most benefit and least risk. Fortunately, it's easy; it's simply a matter of applying a few basic principles to your activity routine.

Actually, Gail never did show up at the Port Costa 10K, or for Ramos Fizzes afterward, which in retrospect was probably just as well. In truth, there was no bar in Port Costa—a small town across the Bay about 30 miles from San Francisco—that served the best Ramos Fizzes in the world. It was all a ruse. Flory's "airline barroom move," honed to perfection during his years as a navigator, called for an agreement from the intended target to meet first. Explanations would come later. "I figured I'd just tell her the bar must have moved," Flory recalls, "but I never got the chance."

The start of the race was delayed 30 minutes because of an accident and ensuing traffic jam on the Bay Bridge. Because so many participants in the race were from San Francisco, the race director held up the start until more could arrive. But Gail Gustafson never did come, and Flory didn't find out until later that she and a friend were the ones in the accident.

"We were crossing the bridge in a VW Bug. It was a cold, miserable day and the bridge was very slick," Gail recalls. "We spun out, and both of us were thrown from the car. Somehow, I ended up pinned beneath it."

Gail's friend and another driver who'd stopped to help lifted the VW enough to pull Gail free. Both women were bruised and scraped, and Gail had a broken collarbone, but fortunately nothing worse. A few months later, Flory again met Gail—now healed—at another postrace party. One thing, as they say, led to another. "We dated about seven years," Flory recalls, "and finally got married in 1980."

By then, Gail was winning her age division in various 10K races and marathons around the state, and Flory had been putting in several years of 100-mile weeks of training and had already had one knee operation to repair damaged, roughened cartilage.

"That first operation was in 1979," he says. "The surgeon who did the operation told me the knee would never be as good as it had been, but I didn't believe him. I ran my best 10K ever after the operation. I was excited about it, but the problem is, I just didn't know when to quit."

It wasn't until 1991 that Flory and Gail finally ran the Port Costa 10K together, and it was only then that Flory confessed the truth about the Ramos Fizzes. By then, they'd been married ten years, so it probably didn't matter. And by then, both of Flory's knees were a mess. He'd had another operation on his other knee, and as it turned out, the 1991 Port Costa 10K would be Flory's last race, and he'd run his last step.

TESTING THE LIMITS

One of the greatest joys of an active life is that it creates a "space" in which we can probe our physical and mental limits, and no matter how out of shape you are when you take up an activity, once you become active, you'll probably be tempted eventually to see just where your limits lie and how close you can come. And one of the most annoying aspects of the active life is that you can't always determine where your limits are until you've gone beyond them and faced the risk of injury or exhaustion. This can become particularly vexing once you've made the decision to go beyond the LifeFit recommendations for optimal health, once you've set specific performance goals or decided to enter the realm of the competitive master. At this point, determination can much too easily overcome common sense, as airline navigator and marathoner Flory Rodd eventually learned.

For years, Flory would fly five hours from San Francisco to Honolulu, then lay over, and having no responsibilities and plenty of time, he'd run. Then he'd run some more, usually an hour and a half to two hours every day, over 100 miles a week. "As far as I'm concerned," he says, "I couldn't have asked for a better life."

A hearing loss in one ear forced Flory into early retirement from the airlines in 1974. But no problem; he took a job as a radio operator on an oil tanker. He'd been a shipboard radioman during World War II, so it was like coming home, and the move didn't interfere in the least with his training. "My first job back at sea was on a tanker so big it wouldn't even fit in most ports," Flory recalls, "but it was great for training. I'd finish my shift at noon and run laps around the deck—three laps was slightly over a mile. I'd run two hours and seventeen minutes, which would give me time to clean up, eat, rest, and return to my shift. It was great training and great fun. One week I'd be running in the snow, the next in tropical heat. In heavy seas it would be like running up and down hills. When I ran the Boston Marathon in 1974, I hadn't touched land in six months, but I still broke three hours."

But Flory Rodd's training resulted in a chronic injury to his right knee that required the first surgery in 1979, then later a similar operation on his left knee, and then in 1991, Flory had a second operation on the right knee. "That one finished me off," he says. "No more running. Now I walk every day, and I find that's great exercise as well. But I miss the runs. I think if there's any lesson to be learned from my own experience, it's that for each of us, there is clearly an optimal level of exercise. For me, 100 miles a week turned out to be way too much. My advice to anyone starting out in an exercise program, particularly anyone who's getting on in years, is to take it easy. You can do too much, just as you can do too little."

KEYS TO SENSIBLE TRAINING

There are three key issues when it comes to sensible training in your own LifeFit program:

1. How rapidly you approach your particular exercise goals, including the exercise recommendations set forth by the LifeFit program

2. The degree to which you choose to go beyond these goals and how rapidly you do so

3. How persistent you are, even when your body is telling you— or pleading with you—to take a break or back off

If you push toward your LifeFit goal or any exercise goal too rapidly, increasing the intensity of exercise or the duration of effort, or both, without allowing your body adequate time to adapt to these increases, you run the risk of injury or discouragement. But there's no easy answer as to what is "too rapidly" or "too much." Although we can come up with a reasonably precise prescription for the least amount of activity for the most gain that works for all, what is "too rapidly" or "too much" for *you* depends on a host of individual factors ranging from your fundamental genetic endowments to the general health of your joints, the presence of previous disease or injury, and the peculiarities of your stride; from your body weight to local climatic conditions to the local terrain; from the amount of stress you may be under at the office to other demands on your time at home. All of these factors can affect how your body responds to exercise.

In this chapter, we'll consider the basics of sensible training and of sensible living for the long haul.

LIFEFIT PRINCIPLES

- One of the supreme joys of an active life is probing your physical and mental limits; unfortunately, you often won't find out where those limits are until you've gone past them, into the realm of exhaustion, discouragement, and even injury.

- You'll learn where your limits lie only after experience and careful experimentation with activity.

- Become an "athlete" in the game of life, and like any athlete, become ever watchful of how your body and mind cope with your activities.

- Pay attention to your pain—the vague sensations, discomforts, and occasional pains associated with physical activity are valuable messages that tell us when to back off, rest, or change our routines.

CROSS-TRAINING IS BALANCED TRAINING

As we get older, it becomes increasingly important to strive for balance in everything we do, literally and figuratively. As the risk of injury increases with age, and the time it takes to recover lengthens, our activity programs need to be designed around the goal of staying active and avoiding anything that can keep us from that goal. Thus a well-rounded active life will balance exertion with rest, light activities with more intense activities, and a probing of limits with sensible training. Above all, a well-rounded active life incorporates a balance of various activities that together develop and maintain all the components of health and fitness. These include

- endurance through aerobic activities such as walking, jogging, swimming, and so on for improved general health;
- strength through resistance training for improved functioning and independence and a reduced risk of injury or falls;

- flexibility through stretching for improved functioning and independence and a reduced risk of injury due to stiff muscles;
- and, literally, balance through any activities that have us up on our feet for improved functioning and reduced risk of injury, particularly falls.

BENEFITS OF CROSS-TRAINING

Perhaps the best general approach is to "cross-train"; that is, to combine several activities into your daily or weekly exercise routine. Cross-training has many benefits:

- *Total-body fitness:* With the possible exception of activities such as rowing and Nordic skiing, no single sport will provide a total-body workout. A steady diet of walking or running is great for the legs, great for the cardiovascular system, and certainly beneficial for overall health but doesn't do much for the arms, for example. Swimming is great for the upper body but doesn't have much to offer the lower body. Put walking or running together with swimming, however, or swimming with cycling, and you're working all of the body's major muscle groups for optimal health and greatly improved overall muscular fitness.

- *Improved cardiovascular fitness:* Cross-training allows you to tax your cardiovascular system more thoroughly than is likely with any single activity, and do it with less risk of injury. For example, you can walk or jog only a certain amount of time before your legs get tired and your feet start to complain. But you could run until your feet tell you you've had enough, then hop on your bike or into the pool and continue to exercise your cardiovascular system while "resting" the muscles you used while walking or running. This is a particularly effective way of exercising for those of us plagued by old injuries or arthritic problems.

- *Injury prevention:* Cross-training helps prevent injuries in several ways. First, by cross-training, you're spreading the physical stress of exercise over a greater area of the body, so you're less likely to overwork any single joint, muscle, or muscle group. For example, suppose you walk briskly for 30 minutes, three times a week; you'll gain all the health benefits provided by this type of activity, but if you're particularly heavy, or have some inherent weaknesses in your knees or feet, then a steady diet of walking could lead to injury, or at least to overtraining or discouragement. If you walked one day, cycled the second, and swam the third, however, you'd still be gaining the significant health benefits of aerobic activity but with much less chance of injury.

Cross-training also helps prevent the muscle strength imbalances that can develop from single sports; for example, combining walking or jogging with cycling develops more balance between the muscles of the front and back of the legs.

• *Increased variety:* Cross-training provides more training opportunities and more variety, helping to combat boredom or burnout. One symptom of overtraining, and perhaps one of the earliest, is a loss of interest in exercise. That loss of interest not only means that you may be bored, but that you may be pushing your body's limits. If you're bored with walking, however, you might find new incentives in swimming or cycling while giving your feet a rest. Likewise, when the weather is too raw to walk, you can always swim, if there's an indoor pool handy, or take an aerobics class or do some weight training. If the weather's too cold to swim, perhaps you can walk. And so on.

CREATING YOUR OWN CROSS-TRAINING ROUTINE

You can approach a cross-training routine in a virtually endless variety of ways. You can devise a routine around a single day or across an entire week. And you can build a cross-training program around either Stage One or Stage Two activities, or both, although typically, cross-training involves primarily Stage Two activities. Whatever you do, though, remember that your routine should include all the components of activity outlined earlier.

• *A daily routine:* A daily routine might begin with light stretching at the beginning of activity, then five minutes of leisurely walking to warm up, with a gradually increasing pace until you've entered the realm of Stage Two intensity. Maintain this for 5 or 10 minutes, then move on to something else that works another set of muscles. For example, you might hop onto a bike, if one is handy, and cycle for 10 minutes; or if you have the luxury of a nearby pool, swim laps for 10 minutes or so; or do a series of resistance exercises for 10 minutes. Then follow with 5 or 10 minutes of stretching or leisurely walking. The entire routine can be done in 30 to 40 minutes, and you will have worked all of the major muscle groups and developed all aspects of fitness.

You don't need to do everything at one session, though. If you have the time and inclination, you can break your cross-training routine into pieces throughout the day: stretching in the morning and a brisk walk or resistance training in the evening.

Of course, a daily cross-training routine can require access to the right facilities and equipment. If you have a well-equipped home gym, that's no problem. Joining a gym that has a variety of stationary bikes, stair climbers, rowing machines, weights, and the like is a viable option. But you don't really need lots of "stuff" to cross-train at home—just your feet, perhaps a bike, and a set of weights will do.

• *A weekly routine*: A cross-training routine planned across a week is probably more realistic for most of us, especially if you don't have the equipment or facilities close at hand to make a daily routine possible. Over a week, a typical cross-training routine might include walking or jogging on Monday, cycling or weight training on Wednesday, and swimming on Friday, with leisurely walking on the off days or on weekends. Each exercise session would begin and end with some gentle stretching, of course, and a brief period of leisurely walking for a cool-down.

FIVE PRINCIPLES FOR WORKOUT SUCCESS

However you decide to fit activity into your daily or weekly routine, you can employ some basic strategies to help you exercise safely while you explore your own limits. Applying these five principles in your active life will reduce your risk of injury, burnout, and discouragement.

RULE 1: INCREASE YOUR WORKLOAD NO MORE THAN 10 PERCENT PER WEEK

This 10 percent rule of thumb is only a general recommendation, particularly in Stage One of your LifeFit program. At this level, you'll probably find that once you've made the move from sedentary to even a little more active, and after the initial muscle soreness, if any, has worn off, you can increase your workload much more rapidly, at least for the first few weeks. The 10 percent rule becomes more important as you move on to more intense Stage Two activities and the risk of overdoing it increases.

If you walk briskly for 20 minutes, three times a week, for example, and you want to increase to 30 minutes, add a few minutes to each walk for the next five weeks. Or you can increase the intensity of that 20-minute walk while keeping the time the same. If you walk 1.5 miles in that 20 minutes, a 10 percent increase would mean adding about an eighth of a mile to the distance covered in the same period. If you're keeping track of your steps, apply the same 10 percent rule to the number of steps you take in a given period to increase intensity, or to the total number of steps you take to increase the time you are active.

This 10 percent rule applies only during that period when you are trying to increase the amount or intensity of your activity toward your LifeFit or other goals. At some point, you'll begin to level off, and additional increases will become smaller.

RULE 2: DON'T WORK OUT HARD MORE THAN THREE TIMES A WEEK

Of course, what is "hard" is highly individual and refers to whatever level of effort elevates your heart rate, brings on a slight sweat, and deepens your breathing. If you're prone to injuries, limit these sessions to no more than three a week, at least for the first several weeks, until your body becomes accustomed to the effort; there's good evidence that the risk of injury increases as you work out hard more than three times a week. If you're cross-training, however, you'll have more latitude in this regard if you alternate activities that work the upper and lower body.

RULE 3: DON'T WORK HARD ON CONSECUTIVE DAYS

The "hard/easy" rule has by now been carved in metaphorical stone of the training canon. It takes time for the body to recover from a hard workout, and for most of us, 48 hours is the minimum. And bear in mind that as we age, it can take even longer than 48 hours. A hard day should be followed by a day of relative rest with comparatively light Stage One exercise. If you're cross-training, a "legs" day—running or cycling for example—can be followed by an "arms" day—swimming. This cross-training routine allows you to exercise more intensely, more often, while still respecting the hard/easy rule.

You may find you're much more active on weekends than you are on weekdays; most of us probably are because we save the yard work, the family outings, and maybe even much of the shopping for the weekends. But don't try to do a week's worth of activity over the weekend. "Cramming" doesn't work. During a week of relative inactivity, your body becomes accustomed to being sedentary, making it harder for your system to be more active during the weekends. Abrupt and radical changes of activity patterns can increase the risk of injury and even the risk of heart attack. And the metabolism tends to slow with lack of activity, making it much more likely that what you eat on any given day during a week of relative inactivity will be stored around your midsection. Thus it's much more helpful to be active *regularly* throughout the week, particularly in Stage Two activities, with the hard workouts spaced out and easy days between them.

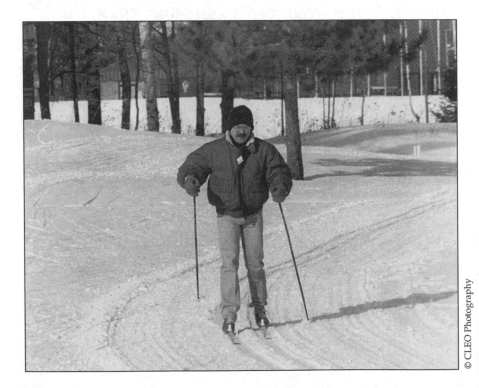

RULE 4: WARM UP THOROUGHLY BEFORE BEGINNING A WORKOUT

You should never go directly from rest into intense effort; a "cold" muscle is prone to injury, and this also puts stress on the heart. Stretch gently before beginning any moderate activity. Allow yourself at least 10 minutes to warm up; walk relatively slowly before increasing the pace to brisk; if you are going to run, walk first at an increasingly brisk pace, then break into a slow jog before increasing your running pace.

RULE 5: LISTEN TO YOUR BODY

Ultimately, the key to success in an active life is to be mindful before, during, and immediately after a workout to note any symptoms that may indicate impending injury, burnout, or other potentially more serious problems, and then to take appropriate action. You need to "listen" to your body, in other words.

WHAT TO WATCH FOR

The muscles and skeleton are constantly sending out messages in the form of aches, mild pains, signals of fatigue, or other sensations, and it's important that you be aware of these messages and know what they mean. You have to be able to interpret signs such as tightness in the chest, pain in a joint during or after a run, or changes in sleep or eating habits, all clear messages from your body that perhaps you are not training sensibly. Then, having interpreted these messages, you have to know how to respond.

OVERTRAINING

By far the most common cause of injury, discouragement, and finally dropping out of an active life is overtraining, typically a result of violating one or more of the rules just listed. You're at risk of overtraining when you don't get enough rest, when you try to do too much, too intensely, too soon. Other factors that contribute to the risk of overtraining include a nutritionally inadequate diet—including not taking in enough fluids—and unresolved biomechanical

TO AVOID PAIN, DON'T OVERTRAIN

Typical Causes of Overtraining and Overuse

- Increasing activity too quickly or not cutting back to accommodate changes in routine or brief layoffs
- Inadequate rest
- Hard training on too many consecutive days
- Inappropriate workload for the conditions, such as training too hard in the heat
- Improper technique
- Stress of life events
- Biomechanical problems aggravated by inappropriate training
- Problems with equipment, such as excessively worn shoes

Tissues Prone to Overuse Injuries

- Stress fractures to the bone
- Soreness in the joints, particularly in the knees in walkers and joggers and the shoulders in swimmers
- Stiffness and soreness in the muscles
- Inflammations of the tendons and ligaments

problems, old injuries, or inappropriate equipment such as poorly fitting or excessively worn shoes.

And in particular, you're at risk of overtraining when you don't pay close attention to what your body is "telling" you.

Symptoms

Overtraining involves a complex of symptoms—some physical, some psychological—that result when we overextend the body's ability to adapt to increases in workload. The most obvious and unmistakable symptom of overtraining is pain, perhaps from an impending overuse injury such as an inflamed, tender knee or sore feet, and we'll have more to say about these particular symptoms later.

But overtraining doesn't always result in an injury to a single body part. Overtraining may result in a more pervasive, systemic malaise, a generalized sense of fatigue and discouragement. But this malaise often precedes some more acute injury when it's not heeded. Fortunately, it takes hard work to reach a point where you are overtrained, and the body does send out ample messages that it's time to back off, get some rest, and give your body time to recover. All you have to do is listen to the messages:

- Mood changes: If you find yourself becoming short-tempered, angry, or depressed, it could mean you're pushing yourself too hard
- Generalized fatigue, a feeling of being "heavy-legged"
- Lack of interest in training
- Declining performance
- Generalized listlessness
- Loss of appetite
- Loss of libido
- Trouble sleeping
- Headaches
- Increased frequency of colds or influenza, or worsening allergies
- Increase in resting pulse
- Swelling of the lymph glands
- Amenorrhea (absence or suppression of menses) in premenopausal women

Try keeping a training log that includes not only performance data, but also such physiological markers as resting pulse, plus more subjective items such as general mood. This is a good way of spotting patterns indicating possible problems before an injury or illness occurs.

Overtraining and Stress

Interestingly, most of these symptoms of overtraining are also the symptoms associated with chronic, unrelieved stress from any source; in fact, overtraining is simply another source of stress, like job stress, the stress of buying a home, or even of taking a long-awaited cruise in the South Pacific.

Change is the key here. As we saw in chapter 7, any change can cause stress, and any change that taxes our ability to adapt, whether physically or psychologically, can cause the classic symptoms of stress, particularly as we grow older and perhaps become somewhat less able to adapt easily. Likewise, other changes besides an increasing workload can put us at greater risk of overtraining. For example, temperature extremes—a heat wave or cold snap—can present new challenges to which our bodies have to adapt, and trying to maintain our usual workload under such circumstances can lead to trouble. When we add new walking or jogging routes that take us over new terrain, for example, or when we change running or walking shoes or buy a new bike without giving our bodies time to adapt, our risk of injury and discouragement increases. Likewise, new stresses on the job or at home, when added to the stress of training, can increase the risk of overtraining.

Thus, if you find yourself under stress on the job or in other areas of your life, you'll want to be particularly careful not to add still more stress by overtraining. Whenever you encounter change in your life, in your training or otherwise, you need to be particularly sensitive to the messages your body is sending out then be willing to allow your body more time to rest and adapt.[1]

Tim Noakes, author of *The Lore of Running*, offers the interesting view that overtraining has an upside. He theorizes that the overtraining syndrome is "a positive response of an exhausted body. Rather than suffer additional damage that would result if the body were allowed to continue training in this depleted state, the body responds by making training impossible. We must learn to respect the messages that our bodies give us when they are trying to tell us they have done too much."[2]

Too Much of a Good Thing?

We've seen that the health benefits of physical activity climb steadily with increasing activity from sedentary to about 2,000 to 2,500 kilocalories a week, at which point the benefits appear to level out. Beyond this, more activity doesn't seem to confer additional health benefits, although as noted earlier, more activity will provide improved fitness and many emotional and cognitive benefits. And as noted, at very high levels of activity (about 3,500 kilocalories or more), the risk of premature mortality appears to take a *slight* upturn (although among the alumni, at least, there are some confounding factors at work; but a variety of other studies do support the observation of a slight upturn in risk). This higher risk is still well below the risk of being sedentary, of course, but higher than the risk among those alumni who spent less time and effort working out, suggesting that extremely active individuals of any age may be somehow putting themselves at a slightly greater risk of early mortality compared with their somewhat less active peers.[3]

But don't be alarmed; this doesn't mean that heavy exercise *kills* (imagine the headlines). Rather, heavy exercise may add to the stresses on a system already stressed by hypertension, for example, or atherosclerosis, on-the-job stresses, or lack of rest, thus contributing to an overall increased risk.

What Does This Mean for You?

Clearly, for each of us, at some point exercise becomes too much of a good thing, increasing not just the risk of injury but even the risk of premature mortality. Some of us are probably able to absorb and benefit from truly gargantuan workloads; others appear to be more vulnerable. You'll learn where your limits lie only after some experience and experimentation with an active life, noting how your body responds to different types and intensities of exercise. But each of us does have limits; our bodies simply aren't designed to withstand excessive levels of exertion, although what's excessive is a matter of wide individual variation and is subject to continually changing circumstances. For Flory Rodd, for example, truly gargantuan training loads didn't seem to be excessive for several years, but as he grew older, hard training combined with biomechanical weaknesses in his knees and stride to create serious problems.

William Rowe, writing in *The Lancet* and referring to the work of Boyd Eaton and Melvin Konner, notes that "primitive hunting societies follow a 'Paleolithic rhythm' of 1 or 2 days of hunting, 6 to 8 hours a day, followed by 1 or 2 days of rest."[4] It seems that our bodies have evolved for that particular rhythm, and we deviate from it at our risk. Rowe hypothesizes that heavy exercise and insufficient rest can actually damage the heart, a notion supported by a study of heart attack and stroke in British adults that found a steady decline in risk until, at the most vigorous levels, risk of both heart attack and stroke climbed slightly, particularly in older men.[5-8]

Heavy training also clearly increases the risk of amenorrhea in young women, with an increased risk of osteoporosis, although it's not certain what effect heavy training has on older women. And a variety of studies have documented a decline in the immune system and infection-fighting T-cells in heavy exercisers. This decline in immune function probably increases the risk of infectious diseases and perhaps even some cancers. The findings help explain the experiences of elite athletes, who seem prone to colds or the flu after major competitions for which they've been training heavily.[9,10]

SUDDEN DEATH DURING EXERCISE

Ever since the legendary Athenian soldier Phidipides dropped dead after running some 20 miles from the plains of Marathon to Athens to bring the news that the Athenians had defeated the Persians, the idea that exercise kills has been lodged firmly—perhaps too firmly—in our cultural psyche. (Incidentally, in some accounts, Phidipides had already put in a hundred miles the day before, which may account for his sudden demise after "only" 20 miles on the day in question.) Of course, the case of Jim Fixx, the fitness advocate who died while jogging, continues to keep alive fears about sudden death from exercise, as do periodic newspaper accounts of this or that suburbanite who dies suddenly while shoveling snow or playing in his company's once-a-year Labor Day softball game.

What Are the Chances?

The risks of an active life in general have been overemphasized in the popular press. After all, hundreds of thousands or millions of men and women avoiding heart attack through exercise aren't a story; one 60-something runner collapsing in the middle of a major marathon is. As you pursue your LifeFit program, you'll want to be careful not to let such occasional but sensational accounts frighten you from pursuing an active life.

Although exercise *can* precipitate what in the literature is called "sudden cardiac death," or SCD—and the more intense the exercise, the greater the risk—in fact, the risk is very low, especially compared with the risks of remaining sedentary.

Those most at risk of SCD during exercise are sedentary men and women who only intermittently work up a sweat. In a study of Finns, for example, Illka Vuori found that among the sedentary, there was a 56-fold increase in risk of SCD during exercise compared with only a 5-fold increase in risk among the habitually active (see figure 11.1). It's the sedentary individual who goes out to shovel the walk after the first snow of the season who is most likely to suffer SCD.[11,12] The overall risk of SCD, at rest or during exercise, was of course much lower among the active.

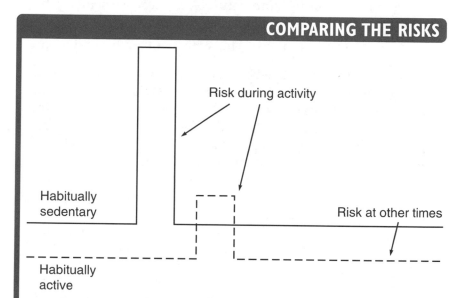

COMPARING THE RISKS

Figure 11.1 Here, the relative risks of death *during* exercise are compared with risks at other times for both the habitually active (dotted line) and the habitually sedentary (solid line). Even with the "spikes" in risk *during* exercise, the *overall* risk of death from heart disease is considerably lower among the habitually active. If you're sedentary, your total overall risk of sudden cardiac death—your risk during activity and all other times as well—is more than three times higher than the risk of more active men and women. And those spikes of increased risk during exertion by the habitually active are much lower than corresponding spikes among the sedentary who, for whatever reason—to shovel snow for example—find themselves suddenly working up a sweat.

In other words, the benefits of activity far outweigh the risks. More important, you can reduce your already low risk of SCD if you learn to "listen" to your body, heed its warning signals, and act appropriately.

Risk Factors

In addition to intermittent participation in physical activity, other activities, habits, or conditions that can increase your risk of SCD during exercise include

- cigarette smoking,
- excessive alcohol consumption,
- chronic stress,
- hypertension,
- physical exertion in temperature extremes, particularly heat, and
- exercise at levels of intensity for which you aren't prepared.

All these factors are well within your control, but your genetic predisposition toward heart disease, of course, is not. Those with a family history of heart disease may be at greater risk of SCD; thus, if you have a family history of heart disease, it's especially important that you eliminate those risk factors that are within your control and heed the warning signs of impending problems.

Although SCD during exercise has a variety of causes, not all of them well known, by far the most common cause appears to be atherosclerosis—obstruction of the coronary arteries. But sudden cardiac death is something of a misnomer. According to one follow-up study of SCD, 50 percent of those who died "suddenly" during exercise had reported beforehand—to spouses most often—that they had some new, perhaps vague symptoms associated with physical activity: excessive tiredness, pains in the neck, shoulder, or chest, a feeling of fullness in the throat, or gastric discomfort.

WARNING SIGNS OF HEART PROBLEMS

If you have these symptoms during exercise, they might signal a heart problem.

- Tightness in the chest (not necessarily pain)
- Chest pain or pain in the arm or jaw (often on the left side)
- Palpitations
- Gastric discomfort
- Unusual fatigue
- Unusual shortness of breath
- Brief loss of consciousness

Indeed, it appears that one of the more typical reactions to symptoms of heart trouble such as tightness in the chest or shortness of breath, among men at least, is a good hard run to prove there's absolutely nothing wrong, that it's perhaps just a bit of indigestion, a pulled muscle in the chest, a bit of a cold, but nothing, of course, to worry about.[13]

PAIN: WHY IT HURTS, WHAT IT MEANS

As an athlete, you'll find that pain, oddly enough, may be the most important training aid you have. Pain is a message and a warning. Pain tells us when to pull our hands away from a hot griddle, for example, and most of us wouldn't have made it to adulthood to read this book and become walkers, joggers, cyclists, or whatever without a pain reflex to protect us from harm. As an athlete, you can apply the rules for sensible training, but you'll find that pain, or the vague sensations and discomforts that sometimes warn of pain to come, tell you when you're breaking those rules.

And this information provides the key to training sensibly. Pain tells you when to slow down, take some time off, change routines, buy new shoes perhaps, or when to see a sports medicine specialist or physical therapist.

WHAT IS PAIN?

The word *pain* comes from the Latin *peona*, which, rather freely translated, means "punishment." (We're using the word *pain* rather loosely to include all the vague sensations, discomforts, and twinges that some wouldn't call pain at all, as well as the unmistakable, teeth-gritting, eye-scrunching aches we all agree is pain.) In many cases, when we don't pay attention to our pain, it can certainly become punishment. To remain unhurt so you can get all the benefits of an active life, you need to listen to your pain, become a connoisseur of pain, as it were, and understand the differences between the types of pains you may feel before, during, and after a workout. You need to know what the pains are "telling" you, which pains warn of damage and which are simply the residue of fatigue, and then respond appropriately.

In the strict clinical sense, pain is what we feel when certain specialized receptors in the skin, muscles, and other tissues are stimulated. Different receptors respond to different types of stimuli—there are heat receptors, cold receptors, pressure receptors, "chemoreceptors," and so on—and the intensity of the feeling, whether pain or otherwise, depends on how many of these receptors are stimulated and how frequently.

But it's all much more complicated than that. We actually feel pain only after the pain receptors send their messages to the brain, where the information is processed and interpreted. *How* we interpret a sensation—as pain or a nagging "not quite pain" or even pleasure—depends very much on our mental landscape. Pain is really a complex of physical and emotional reactions, and the two can never be entirely separated.

Your mood can affect the way you feel and interpret pain. If you're angry or under stress, you're likely to be much more sensitive to pain than if you're in a good mood and relaxed. Thus relaxation exercises are one of the most effective treatments for chronic pain. Your sense of control over the source of pain is also a factor in how you perceive the pain. Thus the pain of a grueling session of "tummy crunches" in an aerobics class might be perceived as tolerable, and even necessary or pleasurable, because you can always stop with the assurance that the pain will quickly diminish. But a toothache that's actually no more intense might seem excruciating because it's beyond your control to make the pain go away—until you've seen the dentist, at least.

Motivation is also a key factor in how we perceive pain. The same qualities of determination and dedication to goals that allow us to push ourselves to be active and train consistently are the very qualities that can lead us to push through pain to injury; exploring one's physical and mental limits can be one of the supreme joys of physical activity, but it's also one of it's greatest dangers.

THE FOUR DEGREES OF PAIN

The challenge, then, is learning to distinguish the normal or "good" pain of exertion from more worrisome types of pain that indicate trouble. Fortunately, there are clear signs that, when heeded, tell us when we're pushing the limits, when we're crossing that sometimes indefinite line separating the "good" ache of a quality workout from the more troubling pain of impending injury. It means paying attention not just to the types of pain you feel, but to the pattern of sensations—painful and otherwise—during and after a workout. Indeed, given the subjectivity of pain, it's the pattern of sensation rather than the quality that for the athlete is perhaps most telling. This pattern can be divided into four distinct degrees representing a continuum from the normal sensations, aches, and pains of exertion and fatigue to the pains accompanying outright injury.[14]

First-Degree Pain

Without doubt, there is a certain amount of discomfort—some might call it pain—associated with physical activity. You'll probably experience some normal muscle tenderness—the pain of "getting

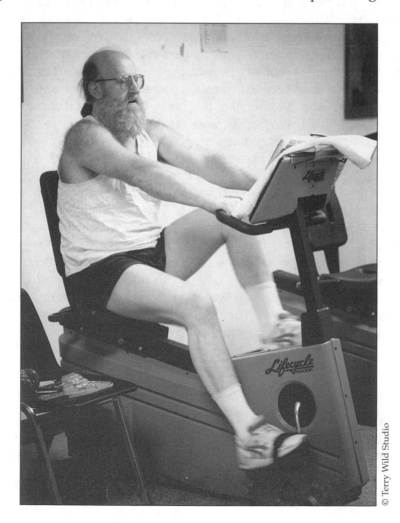

© Terry Wild Studio

into shape"—that appears when you start out on an exercise program, or as you change your routine or suddenly increase the duration or intensity of your training. This type of discomfort usually appears a few hours after you've finished your activity and can leave you feeling a bit stiff and sore. It's quite normal and harmless, however.

This type of tenderness results from several factors, including microscopic tears (microtears) in the muscles and connective tissues and the swelling that results following unfamiliar activity; it lasts a day or so after a workout, and episodes of such discomfort cease once the body becomes more accustomed to the workload.

When you begin a workout, you may also feel dull aches as blood flows to the muscles, causing the tissues to swell, literally pressing on and stimulating "mechanoreceptors." At the same time, the working muscles begin to produce several enzymes that stimulate chemoreceptors, which can be interpreted as discomfort or pain. As you warm up and the tissues relax, however, this discomfort soon passes. Also, during exercise, the body begins to produce endorphins, the body's own painkillers that counteract the pain messages being sent by other enzymes.

Fatigue also causes first-degree pain. The continued release of enzymes throughout exercise leads to accumulations of these chemicals in the tissues, increasing the stimulation of chemoreceptors and increasing the discomfort. The more intense the activity, the more rapidly these chemicals accumulate and the more intense the discomfort or pain, which is why most of us take to relatively low-intensity endurance activities such as walking, swimming, or cycling rather than sprinting, where the intense pain of anaerobic fatigue is a routine part of a workout. Fortunately, such pain is not an indication of any specific damage. It simply hurts and lets you know you're approaching the limits of your ability to perform; the pain dissipates within a few minutes with rest.

You may experience some normal discomfort after exercise as well, depending on the intensity of the workout. This discomfort, the result of residues of lactic acid and other chemical by-products of exertion, usually only lasts for a few hours.

Action: Relax and don't worry. The discomfort will go away. Rest is appropriate, of course. To speed the recovery process or ease the discomfort, gentle massage and heat will help, as will an over-the-counter analgesic such as aspirin or a nonaspirin substitute.

Second-Degree Pain

This pain, which tends to come on more immediately after a workout, is longer lasting. It's pain that's more localized, say in an arm or leg—with more discreet tenderness—rather than more diffuse, as in the case of first-degree pain. This type of pain is an indication that you are pushing up against some physical limit, that perhaps it's time to just "coast" without increasing the amount of work, simply maintaining until your body becomes accustomed to the new level of effort. Second-degree pain may also be the first hint of muscle strength imbalances or biomechanical problems, aggravated by increased workload, that presage an overuse injury. The key sign at this point is increasing localization of the pain.

Action: You might want to cut back on your training, or at least go into a "holding pattern" without increasing your activity level or changing your routine. Wait a few days to see what becomes of the tenderness. Make sure your shoes aren't excessively worn, and check other equipment for wear or other factors that may be affecting your biomechanics. You may have to begin exploring the possibility of biomechanical problems that need to be addressed. Rest, gentle massage, heat, and over-the-counter analgesics are all appropriate.

Third-Degree Pain

Now we're clearly into the realm of flashing red warning lights. Third-degree pain comes on in the middle of activity, say two miles into a brisk three-mile walk. At this stage, pain may interfere with activity. There's more "point tenderness" than with first- or second-degree pain, and after a workout, you may see some swelling at the site; this is a sign that some tissue—muscle, tendon, or bone—is not coping well with the load you've put on it.

Action: Third-degree pain is clearly an indication that it's time to cut back, take some time off, or find an alternative activity; rest and recovery are very important at this point.

Apply ice to the point of tenderness to reduce swelling that may increase the discomfort. Elevation and compression also help reduce swelling and stiffness. Think of the mnemonic RICE—rest, ice, compression, elevation. Once the initial swelling and tenderness have subsided, apply heat or gentle massage to speed healing.

Persistent third-degree pain may clearly indicate a biomechanical or equipment problem that needs to be corrected before you go further. If you repeatedly feel third-degree pain in your knees during or after walking, for example, it may be time to consult a sports medicine specialist, physical therapist, or other movement specialist who can analyze your gait, shoes, and other factors.

Fourth-Degree Pain

This is pain that comes on at the beginning of the workout and doesn't go away; or pain that has lingered from exercise the day before, through the night, and into today's activities. It is sharp and increasingly localized, with holdover swelling and tenderness from the day before, and impedes motion and performance. At this stage, you've moved beyond the normal pain of exertion into the realm of overuse syndrome.

Action: Rest is imperative. Stop doing whatever causes the pain, *but don't quit being active.* This is important. You want to stay active, but without causing additional irritation to the tissues that have been injured. If you have pain in your knee from running, for example, perhaps you can swim. If you have pain in a shoulder from tennis, perhaps cycling or brisk walking will be a good substitute. This is called "relative rest"; you're resting what needs to be rested while staying active.

While you rest, explore what may be causing the pain and ways of correcting the cause(s). At this point, you may want to seek professional advice from a sports medicine specialist. Apply RICE and analgesics, then heat and gentle massage. Physical therapy may be appropriate.

A PATTERN OF PAIN

The pattern to watch for here is the movement from delayed, diffuse, dull sensations that are a normal part of any good workout through a continuum toward more immediate, localized, and sharp pain, otherwise known as acute pain.

Acute Pain

The telling characteristics of acute pain are that it is sharp and very localized. You can literally put your finger on acute pain. Acute pain comes from sources other than too much exercise, of course. Drop a frying pan on your toe, for example, and the pain you experience is acute pain. You know precisely where the pain is, and the message is unequivocal: Don't drop another one, or move your foot if you do. Likewise, the athlete who enters the realm of fourth-degree pain that is localized and sharp is in a good position to do something about it by changing routines, resting, and identifying and correcting biomechanical problems.[15]

If acute pain is disregarded too long, though, you enter the realm of chronic pain, the treatment of which is much more complex and involved.

Chronic Pain

When the sharp, localized pains are ignored, they tend to spread out with time as more tissues become inflamed. The original site of the injury is now surrounded by swollen, irritated tissues, and it becomes more difficult to put your finger on the site of pain. In many cases, chronic pain seems to be located deeper in the tissues than acute pain; thus it's often much more difficult to determine the source of chronic pain and much more difficult to treat and cure it. And chronic pain is just that—*chronic*; it's persistent, always lingering on the edge of consciousness, if not intruding. Chronic pain can be a sign of serious damage to bones, muscles, or nerves.

Sometimes chronic pain can begin to create "feedback" loops; because of the pain, we begin to favor one leg, perhaps throwing our stride out of balance, perhaps creating new sites for other injuries. The muscles around the site can weaken, perhaps leading to the risk of further injury. It's a vicious cycle of pain and disability leading to still more pain and disability, too often ending with a return to sedentary living.

The treatment for chronic pain is much more involved. It usually takes much longer to relieve, and it's vitally important that the cause is found and corrected; "working through" chronic pain can lead to a lifetime of problems, particularly later arthritic changes in sites of particular wear and tear, such as the knees, as Flory Rodd discovered to his dismay.

SPECIAL CONSIDERATIONS

Not all pain follows the four-stage pattern, however, and it's important to be aware of the following types as well.

Heart Attack

The classic symptoms of heart attack include pain anywhere from the head to the hips, not just the typical pain in the chest or left arm. But pain isn't the only symptom, and sometimes a heart attack can begin without pain at all. Shortness of breath, palpitations, sensations similar to gastric upset, the feeling of a heavy weight on the chest, and overwhelming fatigue can also indicate coronary insufficiency and impending trouble. These symptoms, alone or in combination, require immediate attention from a physician. Under no circumstances should you try to work through this pain.

Referred Pain

Referred pain results when a nerve is irritated or injured. When this happens, often the entire length of the nerve communicates pain signals to the brain, even though the actual injury site is limited. A common example is sciatica caused by pressure on the sciatic nerve from a low-back injury such as a bulging or herniated disk. Although the injury site is in the lower back, the victim feels pain down the outside of one or both legs, often to the toes. This pain is usually a burning sensation, perhaps accompanied by tingling.

Herniated or bulging disks aren't the only cause of sciatica; sometimes a muscle spasm or excessive tightness in the lower back or buttocks can irritate the sciatic nerve, causing referred pain down a leg. In either case, this type of pain indicates pressure on the nerve, and you should consult with your physician. If it's accompanied by muscle weakness, loss of feeling, or bowel or bladder problems, it's a sign of potentially very serious injury and should be looked at *immediately*.

Arthritic changes in the vertebrae of the neck are another common source of referred pain; often the pain is manifested in the arm, or even the hand or fingers.

Pain in the Morning

Pain from arthritic changes or prearthritic conditions doesn't always follow the pattern discussed above. If you have arthritis or prearthritic inflammations in your knees, for example, you may feel pain in the morning that dissipates—at least in the early stages—once you get out of bed and start moving around. Heel spurs and plantar fasciitis (inflammation of the fibrous bands along the bottom of the feet) also tend to follow this pattern. Because the pain may go away once you're up and moving about, these types of injuries are particularly easy to ignore and thus make worse. Note how you feel the next morning after a workout. If the pain's back and is worse than the day before, you've done too much.

Stitches

Stitches are sudden, sharp pains in the upper abdomen. No athlete is immune to them, and their cause is still a matter of debate, although the consensus is that they're caused by cramps in the diaphragm, the large muscle that aids in breathing. These cramps are probably caused by blocked blood flow to the diaphragm or upper abdominal viscera, perhaps due to spasm of the arteries, or by pressure from intestinal gas, eating too soon before exercise, milk intolerance, or weakness in the abdominal muscles. To prevent stitches, don't eat before you exercise and avoid foods that cause gas. Some hypothesize that exercises such as "crunches" or bent-knee sit-ups are effective in preventing stitches, but these exercises are so helpful for posture and for protecting the lower back from injury that they're a good idea whether you have stitches or not.

Muscle Cramps

Cramps occur when all of the fibers in a muscle contract at once. They usually last for a few moments and vary in intensity from mild flutterings of the muscle to severe spasms. Cramps are generally caused by low levels of minerals in the body, dehydration, an injury, or obstruction of blood flow to the working muscle. Muscle cramps, most commonly in the legs, may result from peripheral vascular disease in which the vessels supplying blood to the working muscles are narrowed by atherosclerosis (angina pectoris, that biting or crushing chest pain that plagues millions of Americans, is essentially a cramp in the heart muscle resulting from the same cause, narrowing of the coronary arteries).

SENSIBLE TRAINING FOR YOUR KNEES AND BACK

The two areas of the body that are perhaps most vulnerable to overtraining and thus to injury are the knees and the lower back.

Almost every American has suffered or is now suffering from low-back pain; and by some estimates, 50 million Americans have had or now suffer from knee pain or injury. And as we age, the risks increase; thus, as you pursue an active life, it's very important to do everything you can to prevent knee and low-back problems.

THE WOUNDED KNEE

It should come as no surprise that many of us have knee problems; structurally speaking, the knee is little more than a ball sitting on a flat tabletop, more or less (and too often less) held in place by four elastic bands. Considering the inherent instability of the human knee and all the strange things we do to it, the amazing thing is not how many of us have ruined ours but that more of us haven't.

How It Happens

Most often we get into trouble when we upset the balance between the structure of our knees and the amount and type of training we do. The classic orthopedic patient with knee trouble is someone who has been walking or running 10 or 20 pain-free miles a week for months or years, then one day goes to Hawaii on vacation and decides to jog around the big island, or maybe just a half mile. Next thing you know, the vacationer is nursing a swollen, aching knee.

A fundamental problem is the repetitiveness of many of the most popular aerobic activities such as walking, cycling, or running. In these activities, certain tissues are stressed repeatedly, and although the stress may not be that great, this repetitiveness can magnify what, under normal circumstances, are minor and largely harmless misalignments. And thus the key to avoiding knee problems is to understand how the interplay between knee structure and training habits can contribute to knee problems, or cure them once they've occurred.

Most knee problems occur at the interface of the patella (kneecap) and the femur (thighbone). When the leg is flexed and straightened, as in walking, running, or cycling, the patella slides up and down a groove in the end of the femur. Anything that can affect the way the patella tracks along the groove can increase friction, irritate the articular cartilage lining the underside of the kneecap, and result in knee pain.

The most common cause of maltracking of the patella is over- or underpronation of the feet, which causes excessive heel motion and twisting of the leg that's transmitted to the knee. To determine whether you overpronate, place an older pair of shoes that you wear for walking or running side by side on a flat surface, say a tabletop, and view them from the rear. If you have a normal footstrike, your shoes should be slightly worn on the outside edges. If you overpronate, however, the inside edges of your shoes will be very worn and the tops of the shoes will tilt inward toward each other. Excessive wear on the outside edge of the shoes indicates underpronation. Worn shoes, muscle strength imbalances, or tightness in the muscles around the knee can all aggravate over- or underpronation.

When the problem is ignored, "runner's knee" can progress to the point where the articular cartilage is not only inflamed but has begun to roughen and degenerate. Because articular cartilage does not regenerate well, it's very important to listen to the warning signs of pain and swelling; if you have an inflammation of the knee and you keep running anyway, you can do permanent damage.

Prevention

Because most knee problems result from the interplay of training habits and any inherent structural problems in the knee, the key to prevention is to make sure your training is appropriate for your particular knees. But what is appropriate can change almost daily based on fatigue, the presence of previous injuries, even the durability of one's shoes.

Here are some basic principles to help you keep your knees healthy.

• Apply the 10-percent-per-week principle during periods of increasing effort. Also, if you make any changes in your routine, for example, changing your walking or jogging routine, taking a new route over an unfamiliar surface, or buying a new pair of shoes, you should reduce your mileage slightly. If you have to lay off for a few days due to a cold or other reasons, you'll lose about 3 percent of your conditioning every day that you don't exercise, so make appropriate cutbacks in your mileage when you resume training.

• Apply the hard/easy principle to your training. Sufficient rest is an important part of appropriate training for the knees; fatigued muscles can't stabilize the knee and keep the patella tracking properly. If you are troubled by misalignment of the knees due to overpronation or other causes, adequate rest is particularly important.

• Use cross-training that includes walking, running, cycling, or swimming, all of which help build or maintain aerobic fitness while strengthening the muscles that protect the knees. If you cycle, though, be sure your bike fits properly; the seat should be high enough that the leg is almost extended when the pedal is down. Pedaling while sitting on a seat that's too low can actually aggravate knee problems.

• Worn shoes, which often exaggerate any inherent misalignment, can be the culprit in knee pain. Keep shoes in good repair. It's wise to have two or more pairs of your favorite shoes and alternate them to spread the wear over a longer period.

• The ideal surface is predictable, with a little "give" to it. A tartan or cinder track or a walking trail with wood chips, fine gravel, or packed sand are ideal. Less ideal are concrete and asphalt. In any case, it's important to vary the surfaces and terrain on which you travel. The body tolerates variety better than constant repetition. Rolling terrain and varying surfaces present forces to the body from different directions rather than one constant strain. Walkers or runners who train on good dirt roads or mountain trails and golf courses usually have fewer knee problems. Approach hills with caution. Going downhill exerts a great deal of force on the knees (and just about every other joint, for that matter). If you walk or jog regularly on a track, change direction from time to time. This may mean you'll be going against the flow sometimes, as most track habitues tend to run the same direction. A few indignant looks, however, are probably preferable to sore knees. If you walk or jog on crowned roads facing traffic (and for safety, you should always face traffic), you'll always have your left leg on the downhill side; to avoid trouble, you might consider wearing a wedge under the outside edge of the downhill foot. Of course, the best solution is to simply avoid crowned roads.

• Learn to distinguish the "good" pain of a quality workout from the more troublesome pain of an injury, as described above and heed the difference, an important step in avoiding serious knee problems.[16,17]

THE ATHLETIC BACK

The good news is that if you exercise regularly, you're less likely to suffer low-back pain from strained muscles or weakened, bulging, or ruptured disks between the vertebrae. Low-back pain is rare or nonexistent in cultures where people tend to be leaner, walk more, and don't spend as much time sitting behind a desk trying to cope with all the pressures of modern life. Our present epidemic of back pain is really the result of our sedentary habits; the typical back pain sufferer is usually a somewhat overweight, out-of-shape, middle-aged man (or a woman, although guys are more likely to suffer low-back pain) with a bit of a paunch who suddenly decides to do something physically demanding, such as agreeing to help his brother-in-law move a refrigerator one weekend. Because our typical back pain sufferer is out of shape, the muscles of his lower back and abdomen, which help support the spine and protect it from injury, are weak and more prone to injury, thus he ends up pulling a muscle or even tearing an intervertebral disk (tough cushioning pads between the vertebrae).

When someone who is regularly active and fit ends up with back pain, the injury often resulted from something *other* than exercise, and now the pain is interfering with his or her training. But inappropriate exercise itself can cause some problems; gait problems, for example, can increase the risk of low-back trouble, particularly muscle strains.

Overtraining

By far the most common cause of low-back pain among athletes is overtraining. The typical "athletic back" is an overuse syndrome, usually resulting when the lower back muscles become fatigued. Fatigued muscles can go into spasm, and these spasms cause pain, which may cause more spasms, and so on.

Vertical Loading

Sometimes, low-back pain can have its source in the feet. When we walk or run, we experience a shock with each footstrike that travels up from the ground through our bodies. A jogger running on level ground might experience several hundreds of pounds of shock each time his foot hits the surface; running downhill can increase this force many times over. A certain amount of this shock—what the orthopedists refer to as "vertical load"—is absorbed by the feet and ankles. More of this vertical load is absorbed by the muscles of the legs and hips, and ideally very little shock makes its way to the lower back and spine.

Misalignments such as excessive pronation or underpronation can increase the shock traveling up to the spine. The result of increased vertical loading during a walk or run is repeated, small shocks to the spine and an increased risk of muscle spasm as the muscles around the spine grow fatigued trying to absorb these shocks. This increased shock also can increase the risk of swollen or ruptured disks in those who may be prone to the problem.

An intervertebral disk is rather like a stale jelly-filled donut: It consists of a tough outer layer (the annulus) with a soft jelly-like interior. Disks are incredibly durable, but there are limits to the abuse they can take. Disks rarely go bad all at once, however. Rather, poor posture, pushing the joints past their range, lifting heavy objects carelessly, excessive rotating movements, and repeated shocks to the spine create microscopic tears in the fibers of the annulus. Over time, these tears accumulate and the annulus weakens and begins to bulge or even tears completely, pressing on the root of nerves where they leave the spinal cord. Thus older adults are more prone to disk disease than younger adults because they've had more time for these microtears to accumulate.

The symptoms of a bulging or ruptured disk in the lower back include low backaches accompanied by sciatica. Sciatica occurs when the disk presses on the root of the long sciatic nerves running down the backs of both legs. In the most severe cases, the pressure on the sciatic nerve can damage the nerve, causing numbness, weakness, and permanent neurologic impairment.

Lordosis

One of most common causes of low-back pain results from lordosis, or swayback—extreme inward curvature of the lower back. Excessive lordosis can affect the lower back in several ways: It can increase the risk of muscle fatigue and spasms. It can put added pressure on the disks, increasing the risk of microtears (imagine pressing your hand straight down on a jelly-filled donut; it can absorb that pressure evenly throughout, but if you press harder on one edge, the jelly is more likely to squirt out the other side). And excessive lordosis can cause inflammation of the facet joints of the vertebrae.

Being overweight is probably the most common cause of lordosis when much of the weight has collected around the abdomen. A protruding gut tends to pull on the lower back. Weight loss and appropriate exercises, particularly those that strengthen the abdominal muscles and stretch tight muscles, will decrease lordosis. Shortening your stride when you walk or jog may also help. And if you do speed work, make sure you're thoroughly stretched beforehand.

Prevention

Whether you have a history of back trouble or simply want to avoid it, there are some simple things you can do to improve your chances of pain-free activity:

- Make abdominal exercises part of your fitness routine. Strong back and abdominal muscles are less likely to fatigue and go into spasm, and they help protect the spine and disks. Crunch-type sit-ups are excellent. Avoid leg-raisers and straight-leg sit-ups, as these put strain on the lower back.

- Stretch well before you exercise; tight muscles create gait abnormalities and put extra strain on the tissues of and around the spine.

- When you run or walk, do so with control; when you come to hills, take it easy, especially if you're new to rolling terrain. Be especially cautious running downhill, and try not to lean back.

- Don't make abrupt changes in training. The good old 10 percent rule applies, and of course, let pain or signs of overtraining be your ultimate guide.

- Keep your weight under control.

- If you sit for long periods on the job, take a break every 15 minutes or so and stand and stretch. Make sure your chair is adjusted properly and fits you; the angle between your upper and lower leg should be 90 degrees, and there should be good lumbar (low back) support. Armrests should support your arms comfortably, without forcing your shoulders upward. Your head should be upright, and if you work on a computer, the screen should be high enough that you look straight ahead, not up or down.

- If you stand for long periods, put one foot up; this flattens the curve of the lower back and takes the strain off the tissues there.

- Use good sense when lifting (tell your brother-in-law sorry, you have another engagement the day he wants to move that refrigerator). Never bend over at the waist when lifting. Rather, keep your back as straight as possible, bend at the knees, get a firm grip on the object, and use the strong muscles of your thighs to do the lifting. Keep the object being lifted at waist level and as close to your body as possible.

- Vary your fitness routine. Swim, cycle, and lift weights regularly if you can fit them in. These help strengthen all the muscles of the torso and lower back, affording an extra level of protection from injury and pain.

- Never exercise with back pain. If you feel any pain in your back during activity, slow down, or if that doesn't work, stop what you're doing. Change your routine and do something that doesn't cause pain. Use the standard remedies of rest, ice, gentle stretching, and anti-inflammatory medications for pain relief. If the pain persists after a week, or if you experience neurological symptoms such as numbness, tingling, or weakness in one or both legs, it's time to seek professional help.[18,19]

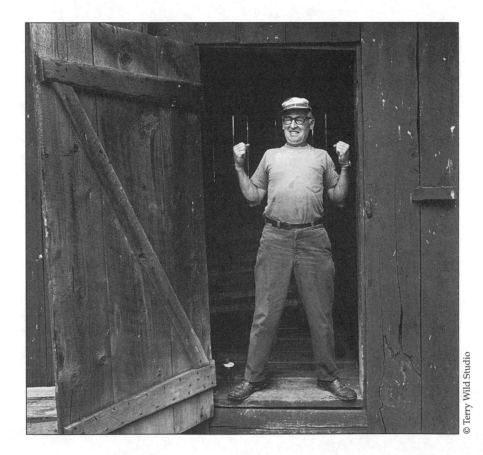

© Terry Wild Studio

THE GAME OF LIFE, REVISITED

Remember, it's not too late to take up an active life and develop your own program for optimal health and longevity. But activity is only part of living "the good life." Moderation and common sense are essential—a balance between activity and rest, between types of activities, between the physical, mental, and even spiritual aspects of existence becomes especially important as we get older. In chapter 9, we suggested that each of us is an athlete in the ultimate competition—the "game of life" as George Leonard calls it. In becoming and remaining active throughout our lives, we achieve a sort of victory every time we take a step. Granted, as we grow older, the steps may come a bit slower, with a bit more effort, but if anything, the victory becomes even sweeter.

TRAINING PRINCIPLES FOR THE GAME OF LIFE

1. Exercise regularly for a total of 2,000 kilocalories a week in activities that combine an hour a day of puttering around with 30 minutes, three times a week, in activities that will elevate the heart rate, deepen breathing, and bring sweat to the brow.

2. Eat "low on the food pyramid"—plenty of fruits, grains, and vegetables and a minimum of refined foods, simple sugars, animal fat, and hydrogenated vegetable oils.

3. Get ample rest.

4. Practice techniques for stress reduction and relaxation, such as meditation or deep breathing.

5. Stay engaged with life; remember that social connections are a major factor in longevity. Cultivate friendships; get involved in community activities; be a volunteer.

6. Keep the mind active. Continue learning through reading, writing, and coursework in college extension or community programs. Continually try new things; develop new hobbies or intellectual pursuits to keep the mind flexible and growing.

In such a context, then, as athletes in the game of life, everything we do in our lives is part of training for victory in that game. And what more important, rewarding, and at times difficult competition can there be, after all, than the competition against the forces of time and the struggle to live a vital, fulfilling life and to age with grace and verve when so much in our world makes that increasingly difficult? And what greater prize can there be than a long, vital life? What greater victory can there be than to have lived life to the fullest, free of the chronic ailments and mental impairments that result from a sedentary, careless lifestyle?

In the *Laws*, Plato's Athenian asks: "What then is our right course? We should pass our lives in the playing of games, *certain* games— song, dance, making sacrifices—with the result that we gain heaven's grace, and repel our enemies."[20]

appendix I

ISSUES OF SCIENCE

Collecting valuable information about the health benefits and hazards of physical activity requires the methods of epidemiology; that is, the study in human populations of the distributions and dynamics of disease. The key procedures are comparison and contrast, but epidemiological methods used to study physical activity and health often rely on inferential evidence to assess cause-and-effect relations. Through measurement and contrast, the methods aim to determine whether persons who are more physically active experience a lower incidence of disease than do people who are less active; that is, there is an *association* between activity and health. Where such a statistical association is demonstrated, the methods then seek to verify by further evidence, to eliminate confounding influences, to establish collateral circumstances, or to develop optional hypotheses. Often this sum of evidence, inferential though it may be, will support or deny a causative relation.

CAUSE AND EFFECT

The issue of cause and effect nips at the heels of every epidemiological study, ruining the researcher's sleep and occupying a major part of his or her waking hours. If good health were *entirely* a matter of genetics, and if you had the bad luck of having the "wrong" genes, you'd have a higher risk of heart disease and heart attack no matter how much you exercised or didn't, how resolute you were about not smoking, or how much unbuttered whole-wheat bread, nonfat milk, steamed tofu, and brown rice you consumed. There would be no cause-and-effect relation at all, but there could still be an association between health and physical activity. In the case of exercise and health, one of the chief concerns for researchers is the troubling thought that perhaps more active people tend to be healthier and more active because they happen to have the "right" genes. The good luck of having the right parents causes both good health and the ability (or perhaps even the inclination) to be active. In this scheme, activity doesn't *cause* good health. Rather, good health and activity might both be the results—or *effects*, if you will—of a third factor: genes.

Of course, most investigators looking at the health benefits of physical activity, even though their sleep is ruined by fretting over cause-and-effect relations, tend not to let scientific uncertainties get in the way of jogging, swimming, or cycling regularly themselves, and sometimes to the point of downright fanaticism; what they may not be sure of *scientifically* is quite different from what they *know* (or sincerely hope) to be true from their own personal experiences.

Fortunately, through the epidemiological method, cause-and-effect relations can be separated from other associations. To do so, we rely on a number of strategies. Of the many types of epidemiological studies that would show cause-and-effect relations between physical activity (together with other personal characteristics) and disease outcomes, prospective observations are the most reliable. These are designed to follow groups of individuals initially presumed to be free of the disease under study over a period of time and, by using appropriate interview and clinical assessments, to make initial and progressive measurements of the prevalence of physical activity and the incidence (first attacks) of disease. Data on the presumed causes, for instance, the level of physical activity, are collected in advance and independent of the occurrence of the presumed effect; that is, the disease under study. These data are then considered in the context of several epidemiological principles that help establish a cause-and-effect relation between physical activity and risk of developing coronary heart disease. These principles are explained in the following paragraphs.

STATISTICAL ASSOCIATION

In a cause-and-effect relation, there would be a strong statistical association between exercise and reduced risk of disease, and by *association* we mean a change in one characteristic that is followed or accompanied by a change in the other. In the College Study, for example, there is a substantial reduction (by nearly one-half) in deaths from all causes among the more active alumni as compared with deaths among the less active. This reduction is beyond what can be attributed solely to chance.

TEMPORAL SEQUENCE

Epidemiologists also look for a "temporal sequence" when trying to determine if a relation between an observed event and observed outcome is cause and effect; that is, does the presumed cause come *before* the effect? Is the horse before the cart?

This seems straightforward enough, but at first glance, it's not always easy to tell which comes first when looking at associations between lifestyle and disease, particularly when diseases develop very slowly. For example, we know that it is smoking of many years ago that induces the early beginnings of cancer; the disease usually is started by smoking 10, 20, or even 30 years before it becomes clinically manifest, not by the cigarettes smoked yesterday. In the meantime, the smoker or ex-smoker might also have made a variety of lifestyle changes that could confound the findings. Because it's smoking of many years ago that produces a cancer, someone might quit smoking for years and still develop lung cancer, and without some understanding of the biological mechanisms at work, it might appear that not smoking or quitting smoking may cause lung cancer.

In the case of physical activity and heart disease, it's not the fact that someone didn't exercise last week that may cause a heart attack this week; rather, it is a habitual pattern of inactivity over a period of months, years, or decades that appears to relate to disease.

Another question we must ask is: Does a specific lifestyle habit such as sedentariness lead to the disease, or does the disease, perhaps in the early stages, lead to that specific lifestyle habit? For example, perhaps the sedentary seem to have more heart disease because early on they have undiagnosed heart disease that dissuades them from being active. In fact, this probably does occur. In the College Study, in an attempt to deal with this problem, the first few years of observation were "tossed out" to eliminate most of those individuals who might have undiagnosed disease that encouraged a sedentary life. That leaves a presumably healthy population at the start of the follow-up observation that can be followed for a decade or so to see what if any difference appears between the active and inactive subjects. Once we do that (discard the first few years of observation), in the case of exercise and heart disease, the presumed cause—exercise—still does precede the presumed effect, improved health. It's one more link in a chain of circumstantial evidence leading toward the firm conclusion of cause and effect.

CONSISTENCY

For the findings of an epidemiological study to suggest a cause-and-effect relation, they ordinarily would be consistent in terms of demographic characteristics: age, race, sex, occupation, socioeconomic status, geography, and so on. Ordinarily, if a cause-and-effect relation between physical activity and a reduced risk of heart disease is shown for men, it would also be shown for women; if for the old, then for the young; if for whites, then for blacks, and so on. On the other hand, if we observed that exercise seemed to improve health among men, for example, but not among women, we might suspect other, perhaps unknown, factors were at work. Likewise, we'd expect the findings to be consistent geographically; if we saw a relation between activity and health among subjects in California, for instance, but not in New York, we'd begin to suspect other factors. In the case of the college alumni, however, we observe the association between activity and health wherever the alumni happen to be. And we observe it across a range of ages spanning several decades. Other studies, including those exclusively of women and across a variety of ethnicities, show the same broad associations.

PLAUSIBILITY

A cause-and-effect relation should be plausible and logical in terms of common sense, and it should reflect the current understanding of the physiological and pathophysiological circumstances involved. The relation between exercise and health is plausible in this regard because the notion that exercise causes good health is common sense, based on current knowledge. Of course, that's the problem with this particular standard; biological plausibility does depend on what is understood at the time, thus the idea that there was a cause-and-effect link between, say, smoking and lung cancer might not have seemed all that plausible without a good understanding of the nature of cancer and the course of the disease. This may seem like a weak rationale, but any scientist will tend to disbelieve data that defy good judgment, at the same time understanding that breakthroughs often occur when a scientist does explore a hypothesis that defies common sense, or what appears to be prudent and "conventional wisdom."

PERSISTENCE

In a cause-and-effect relation, the findings would be persistent over time as well; that is during successive intervals of time. In the case of the Harvard and Penn alumni, for example, the more active group showed a reduced risk of heart disease in each successive period of follow-up during the past 30 years. The observed association was not a one-time "snapshot" finding but a continuing relation that could be demonstrated again and again as time went on. The importance of such an observation is that it argues against self-selection: that the sedentary individuals did not engage in physical activity because they were unfit or already had impaired cardiac function. The long-term effect fails to support a hypothesis of self-selection.

An analysis of this sort can also gain strength by assessing potential confounders that may have become altered between one interval and another: The influence of changes in cigarette smoking or dietary cholesterol intake may be compared or contrasted with the influence of physical activity on disease risk. If there is a true cause-and-effect relation between exercise and disease risk, it would remain evident with or without any changes in other influences on CHD, unless the mechanism linking activity levels and disease risk is via these other influences.

INDEPENDENCE

In a cause-and-effect relation, we'd expect to see the association between exercise and improved health in both the presence and the absence of other influences. For example, although cigarette smoking is a powerful influence on the risk of sudden death from heart attack, and although most smokers tend not to exercise and most athletes tend not to smoke, in fact, we find the beneficial effects of exercise even among smokers; the beneficial effects of exercise are independent of smoking, in other words. Likewise, these benefits of exercise are independent of hypertension, obesity, and a family history of CHD. If you smoke, if you are overweight, if you have a family history of CHD, even if you have diabetes, by staying active, you will have less risk of heart disease and live longer than sedentary men and women with the same health risks. This persistence and independence of activity, and its seeming ability to counter adverse influences such as smoking, high blood pressure, and obesity, also lend plausibility to the idea that physical activity acts on natural bodily processes, still another link in the chain of evidence leading to cause and effect.

DOSE-RESPONSE RELATION

With increased activity, we'd expect a corresponding reduction in the risk of death from CHD and other causes. And we'd expect an increased risk with a decreased level of activity, if the association between physical activity and disease is in fact one of cause and effect. As we've seen, data from numerous studies all show the same dose-response. This principle is also important in determining the beneficial levels and characteristics of physical activity, since gradient effects have been observed in numerous studies, and this is just what is found among the alumni.

SPECIFICITY

The epidemiologist also looks for what is called "specificity" when trying to determine if an association is cause and effect: Does exercise reduce the risks of some diseases and not others? If exercise reduced the risk of all disease equally, it would seem almost too good to be true, and likely would be. Data from numerous studies of physical activity and health show that most of the increased longevity associated with exercise results specifically from a reduced risk of heart disease; exercise also reduces the risk of some cancers—colon cancer in particular—but not others; exercise reduces the risk of stroke but seems to have no effect on the risk of gall bladder disease, peptic ulcer, and cancer of the pancreas; exercise seems to improve mood and even cognitive functioning but has only a very slight effect, if any, on the risk of Alzheimer's or amyotrophic lateral sclerosis (Lou Gehrig's disease). All of this suggests that exercise has certain specific protective effects, reducing the risk of certain diseases but not others, fitting the hypothesis that the association is a cause-and-effect relation.

REPEATABILITY

Different investigators in different places at different times, and using different study methods on different populations, should tend to come up with similar results if the relation between exercise and health is one of cause and effect, and this has been the case over the years. The British civil servants study, MRFIT, the Framingham Heart Study, studies among Finns, Swedes, Danes, Israelis, the Dutch, Germans, South Africans, New Zealanders, Canadians, and others all find a strong relation between exercise and improved health. Such reiterations of epidemiological results are of particular value for asserting the strength and validity of the circumstantial evidence and inferential reasoning we must rely on for determining the kinds and amounts of physical activity essential for good health. And all of the accumulating data add still more weight to the notion that the relation between fitness and improved health and longevity is one of cause and effect.

CONFIRMATION

Epidemiological findings for physical inactivity leading to higher risk of CHD have seldom sought experimental verification among human subjects in clinic or laboratory settings, such subjects being understandably reluctant to be pricked, prodded, and dissected; however, some confirmation has been obtained from animal studies, usually of the ever-accommodating lab rat. Although one should always be skeptical of generalizing from the experience of lab animals, such confirmation does lend further weight to the argument that the relation between disease risk and activity level is one of cause and effect.

ALTERABILITY

The epidemiologist also asks whether changing the presumed cause results in a corresponding change in the observed effect; if it does, that's yet another piece of evidence on the side of cause and effect. In the College Study, this is exactly what was observed: Alumni who had been active and then dropped the habit had an increased risk of disease. In fact, for reasons discussed previously in *LifeFit*, their risk was slightly greater than that of alumni who had always been sedentary. Alumni who had been sedentary but took up activity enjoyed the same lowered risk of disease as those who had always been active.

This is a particularly important finding when we try to understand the relative influence of genetic and other factors such as lifestyle on disease. In the case of physical activity and disease, the alterability of the association between them suggests a cause-and-effect relation; that is, since genes can't be altered, and if the relation were based entirely or mostly on genetic factors, changing the level of physical activity should have little or no effect on the risk of developing disease.

As noted in chapter 1, the alterability of the relation between activity and disease became obvious early on in the College Study, when we considered college athleticism in the context of disease risk later in life. Alumni who had been varsity athletes in college did not enjoy a reduced risk of disease later in life unless they *remained* active.

We assume that varsity athletes were genetically inclined to good health, strength, speed, and other factors that contributed to their college athleticism. Otherwise, they probably wouldn't have made it onto the varsity squad. Yet if they didn't remain active, if they became sedentary, they had the same high risk of disease as sedentary alumni who weren't athletes in college. We also assume that these alumni, the bookworms in college, tended to be less genetically gifted with the physical tools it takes to make the team. Yet if they became active later in life, they reduced their risk of developing disease. In other words, those alumni who reversed their activity patterns after college likewise reversed their disease risk.

DISCUSSION OF LIFE CURVES

The following lifecurves chart the chances of surviving to any given age, up to age 90, by various activity patterns and health habits, including total energy expenditure, vigorous or nonvigorous sports play, cigarette smoking, and hypertension.

The charts are developed from the experiences of nearly 14,786 college alumni aged 45 to 84 in 1977. They had responded to questionnaires on health habits and health status in the early 1960s and again in 1977. Classified by walking, stair climbing, recreational activities, cigarette habit, and blood pressure status, the alumni were then followed for 12 years, to 1988, for rates of mortality. The experience represents 165,402 man-years of observation, during which 2,343 men died. From these data, it's possible to derive some reasonable conclusions as to the role of exercise, smoking, and hypertension in influencing mortality, at least up to about age 85, beyond which the numbers become too small for meaningful conclusions. Overall, findings reveal lower risks of death with higher levels of each activity pattern in gradient or step-wise fashion, and show that the more active have a significantly better chance of living to any age than the less active.

FIGURE AI.I

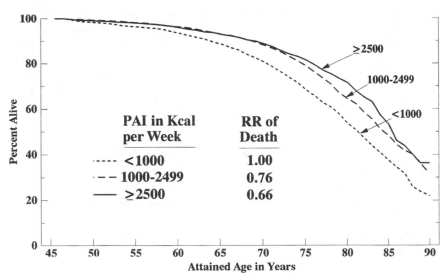

Adapted with permission of American College of Sports Medicine, © 1994, pp. 101-102, *ACSM 40th Anniversary Lectures.*

Figure A1.1 presents survivorship curves to age 90 according to arbitrary levels of activity at less than 1,000 kcal; 1,000 to 2,499 kcal; and 2,500 kcal or more per week, which levels divide the population into roughly equal man-years of follow-up. These curves predict the prolonged survival for the two more active groups as compared with the least active. Figure A1.1 also presents relative risk of death (RR) in the 12 years of follow-up according to these same levels of energy expenditure, using 1,000 kcals per week as the referent (RR of 1.00). Men in the middle group were at 24% lower risk (RR .76), and the most active men were at 34% lower risk (RR .66), compared with the least active.

The curves show the experiences of the least active begin to diverge from those of the most active at the youngest ages, and from that point on, the experiences of the least and most active continue to diverge sharply across the years. The gap or area between the lifecurves of the least active and the two more active groups represents added years of life for the more active; or fewer years of life for the less active.

The lifecurves show that the least active have a significantly lower chance of making it to any given age than the most active. For example, only 81% of the least active can expect to live to the age of

70 compared with 90% of the most active. Only 39% of the least active can expect to live to 85 compared with 52% of the most active. The gap remains wide at every age beyond the median age at death to age 90, at the end of observation. When half of the most active had died (at about the age of 87), they were six years older than the least active, half of whom had died by about the age of 81. Overall, risk of early mortality was one-quarter lower among the intermediate, and one-third lower among the most active men. These add up to big differences in expectation of life.

The meaning of all this? You have a much better chance of living to any given age, up to age 90, if you remain active. We'd expect that beyond age 90, the curves would tend to converge, since few men and women live significantly beyond that age, regardless of their health habits.

FIGURE A1.2

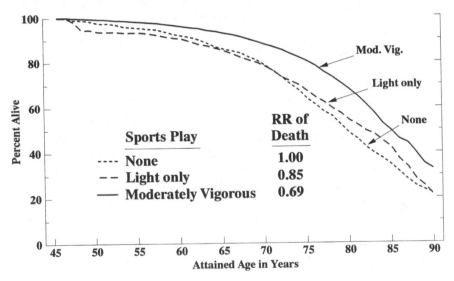

Adapted with permission of American College of Sports Medicine, © 1994, pp. 101-102, *ACSM 40th Anniversary Lectures.*

Figure A1.2 distributes the total population by recreational or sports play, with the absence of participation as referent (RR 1.00). Men who played light sports were at a 15% lower risk of premature mortality. Those playing moderately vigorous sports had a 31% lower risk than non-sports players. The curves predict a prompt and persistent advantage for those involved in both light sports play (less than 4.5 METs) and moderately vigorous recreational activities (4.5 METs or more of intensity).

Ninety percent of those who regularly engaged in moderately vigorous sports play activities can expect to live to age 70, compared with only about 79% of those who never worked up a sweat. Only 31% of those who engaged in no sports play can expect to live to the age of 85, compared with 50% of those who did. Through age 90, the broad gap between the expectations of those who engaged in sports play and those who didn't continues. Any significant increase in survival for less vigorous recreational activities (light sports play) would seem to come only at age 75 and beyond, suggesting that as we get older, some sort of recreational activities, even if they aren't particularly vigorous, are enormously beneficial.

FIGURE AI.3

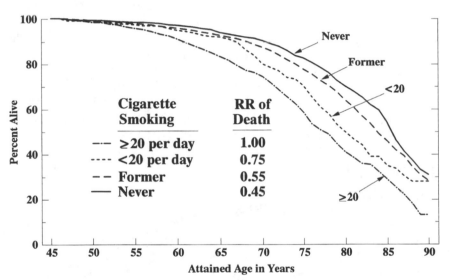

Figure A1.3 charts cigarette habit and all-cause mortality. The dangers of smoking are well-known, and these lifecurves are a stark portrayal of the dangers; the area between the lifecurves of the smokers and nonsmokers is vast, and telling. The likelihood that heavy smokers will make it to any given age begins to fall sharply at the youngest ages and continues its precipitous decline thereafter. Only about 77% of heavy smokers might make it to age 70, compared with about 95% of never smokers. At the age of 85, the difference is apt to be even more striking; only about 30% of smokers might live to age 85, compared with about 51% of never smokers. The curves also show that those who quit smoking can expect to enjoy nearly the same favorable expectation of a long life as the never smokers.

FIGURE A1.4

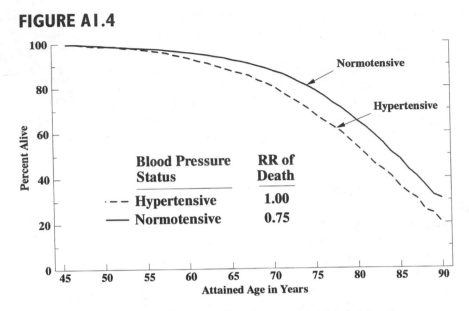

Figure A1.4 presents lifecurves for alumni with high blood pressure and alumni with normal blood pressure. As expected, the normotensive alumni had the lower risk of mortality (RR 0.75) at any given age compared with the hypertensive alumni (RR 1.00).

FIGURE A1.5

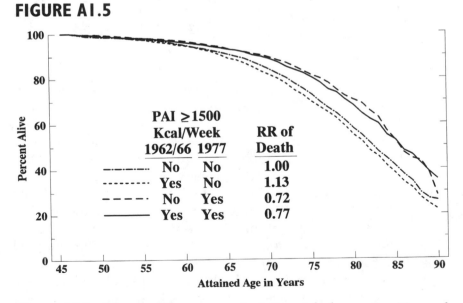

Figure A1.5 addresses lifecurves and relative risks by continuities and changes in physical activity index at the cut point of 1,500 kcals per week. Men are classified as active or not in 1962/1966, and again in 1977.

FIGURE A1.6

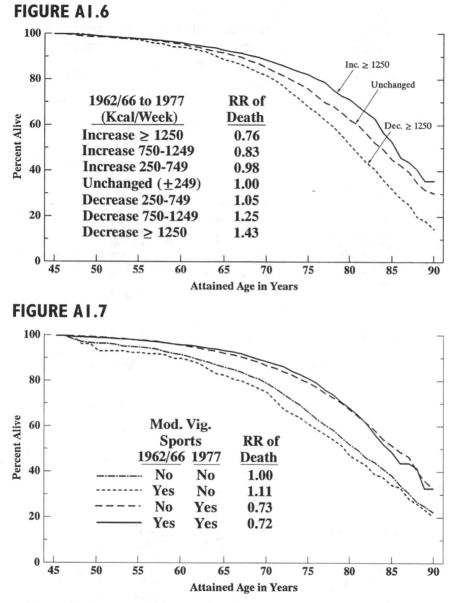

1962/66 to 1977 (Kcal/Week)	RR of Death
Increase ≥ 1250	0.76
Increase 750–1249	0.83
Increase 250–749	0.98
Unchanged (±249)	1.00
Decrease 250–749	1.05
Decrease 750–1249	1.25
Decrease ≥ 1250	1.43

FIGURE A1.7

Mod. Vig. Sports 1962/66	1977	RR of Death
No	No	1.00
Yes	No	1.11
No	Yes	0.73
Yes	Yes	0.72

Alumni who were active at both points of the survey and those who took up activity by the second survey enjoyed nearly the same expectations for a long life as those who were active all along. Those who dropped or decreased activity had a worse experience than those who had not been active in either survey.

Figure A1.6 charts the benefits of increasing activity depending on how much one changes. Again, those who made the greatest increases enjoyed the highest expectation of living to any given age.

Figure A1.7 charts the benefits of adopting moderate sports (4.5 METs or more). The expectations it predicts are very similar to those shown in figure A1.5. It's never too late to benefit from change.

FIGURE AI.8

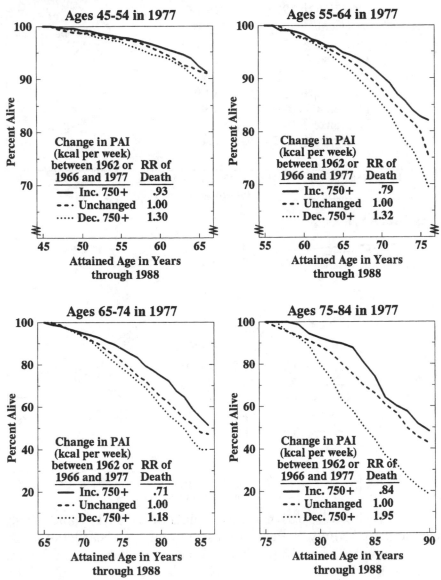

FIGURE A1.9

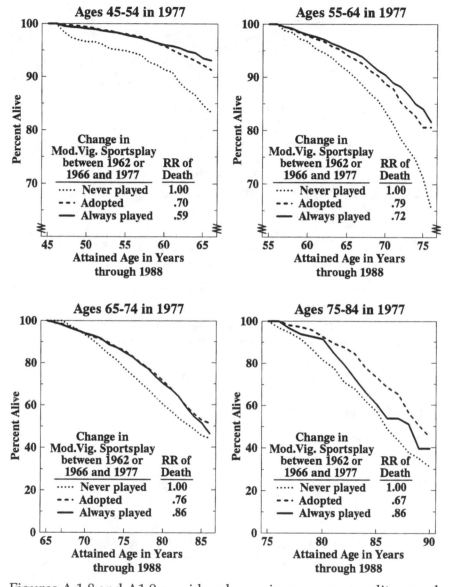

Figures A 1.8 and A1.9 consider change in energy expenditure and sports play by age-specific groups. There's an advantage to increasing physical activity or taking up sports and a disadvantage in decreasing activity or dropping sports at each age group. The most significant differences appeared in the oldest men.

FIGURE A1.10

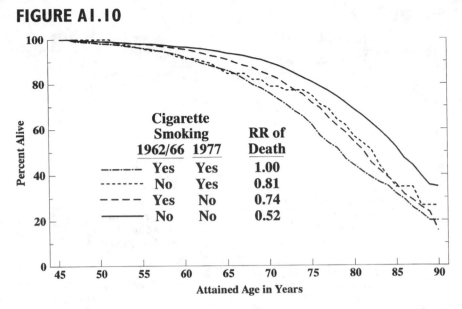

Figure A1.10 compares the experiences of those who always smoked, those who never did, those who quit, and those who took up smoking. Not surprisingly, those who never smoked enjoyed the best expectation of long life (RR .52, or about half the risk of death of the smokers), and those who always smoked, the worst. Those who took up smoking and those quit had expectations of life in between.

FIGURES A1.11

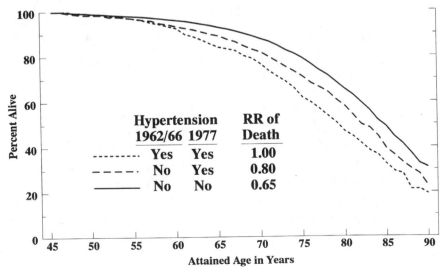

Figure A1.11 presents lifecurves for alumni who had normal blood pressure at both points of the survey, those who became hypertensive, and those who were always hypertensive.

FIGURE AI.12 (TOTAL MORTALITY)

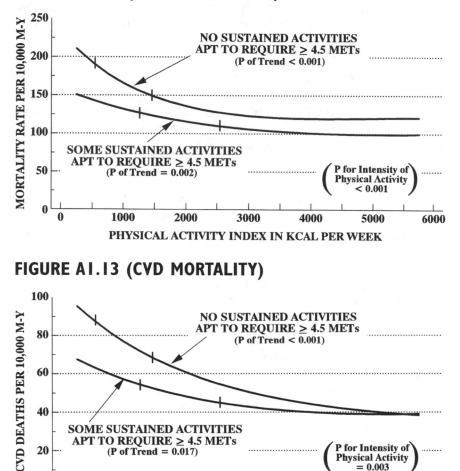

FIGURE AI.13 (CVD MORTALITY)

Adapted with permission of American College of Sports Medicine, © 1994, pp. 101-102, *ACSM 40th Anniversary Lectures.*

Figures A1.12 and A1.13 chart the experiences of alumni based on their participation, or nonparticipation, in moderately vigorous Stage Two activities. For the purposes of analysis, alumni were separated into those whose activities generally required less than 4.5 METs of effort, and those who included some weekly activities requiring 4.5 METs or more. (Vertical ticks on each curve seperate the experience into thirds of man-years.)

Figure A1.12 shows that with increasing levels of energy expenditure both light and moderately vigorous activities are associated with a reduced risk of all-cause mortality, and the greatest reductions occur at the lowest levels — even a little activity is much better than none at all. Weekly outputs greater than about 2,500 kcal confer little further benefit, but at any level of energy expenditure, the risk is significantly lower when some moderately vigorous activities are included. Based on these scales, the mean death rate for the less vigorous was 170 per 10,000 man-years, contrasted with 120 for the more vigorous, or 20 percent less.

In Figure A1.13 (CVD mortality), we see that the lines charting the experiences of the less and more vigorous alumni also show a significantly lower risk among the more vigorous up to about 2,500 kcals of energy expenditure a week, at which point the curves converge and level off, suggesting that at very high levels of energy expenditure, both less and more vigorous physical activity are equally beneficial. This suggests that to achieve the most benefits from non-vigorous activity in terms of CVD risk, you would have to spend a couple of hours a day up on your feet puttering about. The mean death rate for less vigorously active men was 75 per 10,000 man-years; the corresponding death rate among the more vigorous men was 50, or one-third less.

The message? Any physical activity of any kind is beneficial, and enormously preferable to no activity at all, but if optimal health is your goal, that is if you wish to achieve all of the health benefits possible from physical activity, you'll need to combine both low-intensity and moderately vigorous activities in your weekly exercise routine. Low-intensity activities might include anything, from a leisurely stroll around the block, to "puttering" around in the garden, to playing with the kids, to anything at all that gets you up on your feet moving about instead of sitting in front of the TV. Moderately vigorous activity will be intense enough to elevate your breathing and heart rate and bring sweat to your brow, and for optimal health, we believe you should engage in moderately vigorous activity for about 30 continuous minutes, at least three times a week.

Beyond about 2,500 kcals per week, however, additional benefits in terms of physical health and delayed mortality begin to level off, whether you've included nonvigorous or moderately vigorous activities; that is, at this point, in terms of energy expenditure, you apparently have achieved everything you can to delay disease and mortality. This doesn't mean that additional activity beyond this level doesn't have other benefits, however. For example, additional activity, particularly more intense activity, will probably confer additional fitness for improved performance, depending on your genetic makeup. And there may be significant psychological or even philosophical consolations for some of us well beyond the 2,500 kcal level (depending on our desires and goals, or on what demons happen to plague us).

appendix 2

SUGGESTED EXERCISES FOR STRENGTH, FLEXIBILITY, AND RENEWAL

STRENGTH TRAINING

If you're new to the active life, strength training may seem like the last thing you ought to be doing, particularly if you're troubled by old injuries, arthritis, or similar ailments. But a sensible strength training program can be quite safe, and fun.

You don't have to join a gym to train for strength, though gyms have their good points. A good gym has plenty of equipment for variety, and trainers to help teach you proper techniques. And a gym is a great place to meet others of like mind. It's a quite effective motivation to be around others doing what you're doing, with as much enthusiasm.

Gyms can be a bit intimidating at first, but don't be put off. They're fundamentally democratic institutions where everyone is united in the same pursuit of good health (and firm glutes).

EQUIPMENT

You can get a complete strength workout with no equipment at all, or just a few items. Here are some basic pieces of equipment that will serve you well:

- Ankle and wrist weights
- Adjustable dumbbells with a variety of weight plates
- An adjustable barbell (optional)
- A sturdy, comfortable padded bench

A FEW GENERAL RULES OF GYM ETIQUETTE

Here are a few guidelines to follow while exercising in a gym.

- Bring a "workout" towel to keep with you as you work out, to wipe sweat off benches.
- Make sure someone isn't already using a piece equipment before you start to use it yourself. If it is, ask if you can "work in." Or find something that isn't in use.
- Put your weights back when you're through with them.

That's about it. Follow those rules and you'll fit right in.

BASIC WEIGHT-TRAINING RULES

Here are some basic rules to follow while weight training:

- Generally, you should use as much weight as you can lift 10-15 times in one "set." (A "set" is one series of repetitions before you stop to rest.) For a more "aerobic" workout, use lighter weights and higher reps, perhaps 15-20 per set. However, for a "warm-up" set, use much less weight and do many more reps, perhaps 25-30.
- Add weights only when you can complete 10 reps comfortably on your final "set" of any particular exercise. Another way to increase the load is to increase sets, or the number of reps in each set. In a particular exercise, you might do two or three or even more sets, with a minute to two minutes between each one.
- Follow all of the other strategies for sensible training in chapter 11.
- Be consistent. Any strength training is going to help, but lifting only occasionally will make you sore, without doing much to help you build strength. One day a week will help. Two days a

week is better, and you'll see some gains. Ideal is three days a week or more, provided you're getting adequate rest.

GETTING STARTED

We've divided exercises up by body-part. Each exercise consists of one or more sets, each set of 10-15 reps. The following is a beginning program that involves a whole-body workout three times a week. The following routine is based on an at-home workout, but we've included some suggestions if you're in a gym, where it's relevant.

In the very beginning, start with one set using low weights and high reps for each body part. For most exercises, after a couple weeks, or as you begin to feel stronger and more confident, add a set. After a couple more weeks, add a third. Rest between sets for 40 seconds to 2 minutes. Less rest than that won't be sufficient, and with a longer rest, there's a risk your muscles could cool off and tighten, making them prone to injury on the next set. Also, don't forget to warm up thoroughly.

Abdominals
Lie on your back with your knees bent, feet flat on the floor. Fold your hands on your chest, or, for an easier curl, reach forward as you lift your head from the floor, then, as if you're a roll of toothpaste, curl up vertebra-by-vertebra to a sitting position, or as far as you can go. Let yourself back down *slowly*. Don't flop back, or you lose much of the benefit of this exercise. Repeat as many times as you can.

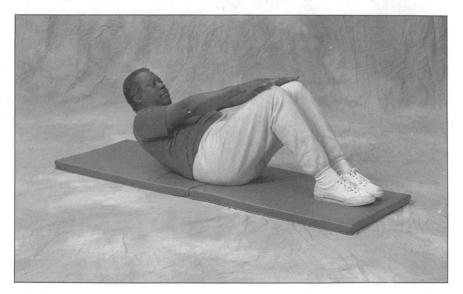

Thighs (Quadriceps)

These are the big muscles on the front of your upper leg. They're important in helping us simply get around, up and out of chair, up stairs, or lifting things.

Put on your ankle weights. Sit on a stool or the edge of a sturdy and secure table or desk. Slowly straighten first one leg, then the other. At the top of each lift, when the leg is straight, pause for a breath or two. Be sure to let each leg back down *slowly*. Keep your back straight. Repeat 10 to 15 times each leg. In a gym, look for the "leg extension machine" for the same workout.

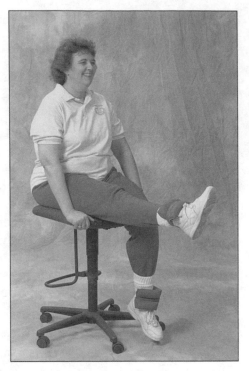

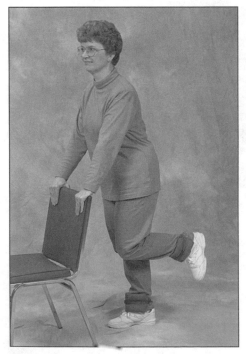

Hamstrings (Back of the Leg)

This is the big muscle opposite the quads. It's also very important in helping you get around.

Stand and hold the back of a chair for balance. First with one leg, then the other, slowly lift your heel toward your buttocks. Hold for a breath or two, lower slowly. Repeat 10 to 15 times, each leg. In a gym, look for the "leg curl" machine.

Chest

With a dumbbell in each hand, lie back on the bench and hold the dumbbells against your chest, palms facing toward your feet. Push up slowly until your arms are extended. Hold a beat, and make sure the small of your back is flat against the bench, or as flat as you can make it. *Don't* arch your back. Lower slowly. Repeat 10 to 15 times. You can do the same exercise using a barbell. In the gym, there are a variety of machines that provide the same workout.

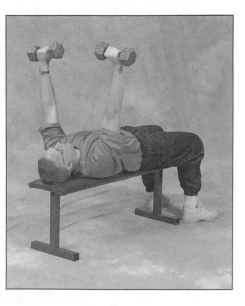

Note, if you use a barbell rather than dumbbells, it is absolutely essential that you have a "spotter." Otherwise, there's a danger of getting trapped under the bar if you fail to complete a lift.

Abdominals

Sitting on the edge of the bench and leaning back slightly on your hands, extend your legs out in front of you, pull back so your heels are near your seat, extend again and repeat as many times as you can.

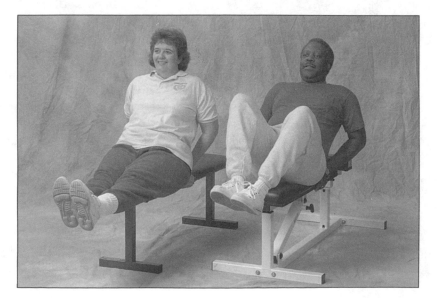

Shoulders

Standing or sitting, hold a dumbbell in each hand at your sides. Then slowly raise your arms, keeping them straight, to shoulder level. Hold a beat, then slowly lower the starting position. Repeat 10 to 15 times.

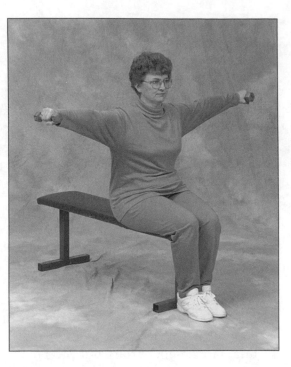

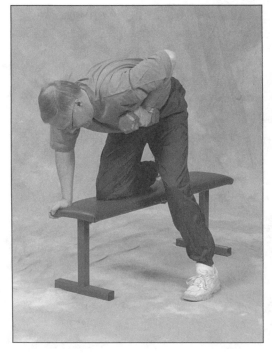

Back

Holding a dumbbell in your right hand, put your left knee on the bench and lean forward on your left hand so your back is roughly parallel with the floor. Let the weight in your right hand hang down toward the floor. Then, slowly pull the weight up as close to your chest as you can, keeping your back level with the floor. Don't arch your back. Lower the weight slowly and repeat 10 to 15 times. Switch hands and repeat. In the gym, look for the "cable row" machine for a similar exercise.

Biceps

Sit on the bench or a chair with a dumbbell in your right hand and your right elbow supported on your thigh. Lean slightly forward and support yourself with your left hand on your left thigh. Start with your right arm extended down, then slowly curl the dumbbell toward your chest. At the top, hold a beat, then slowly lower the weight. Repeat 10 to 15 times. Switch hands and repeat 10 to 15 times.

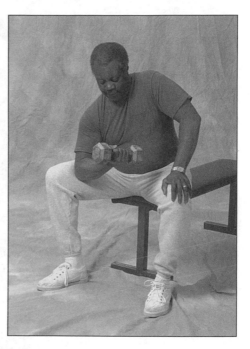

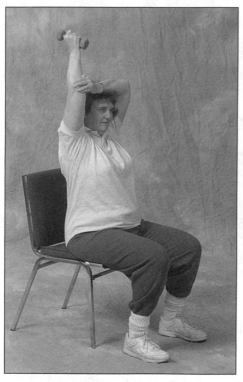

Triceps

Sit on the edge of the bench or a chair with a dumbbell in your right hand. Hold your right arm up so your elbow is by your ear. Let the weight down slowly behind your head, then straighten your arm slowly, until your arm is completely straight and the weight is above your head. As you do so, keep your elbow by your ear. You might want to support the elbow with your other hand. Lower and repeat 10 to 15 times. Switch hands and repeat 10 to 15 times.

Calves

Stand with your toes on a thick phonebook, bricks, or a step, supporting yourself against a wall or railing. Slowly let your heels down as far as you can. Hold a beat and feel the stretch in the backs of your legs. Then rise up on your toes. Hold a beat and lower. Repeat to exhaustion. This can also be used as a stretching exercise by lowering your heels as far as they'll go.

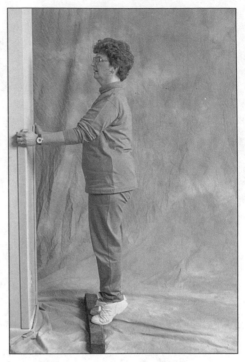

Following is an "advanced beginner" routine, a variation on the "beginning beginner's" routine we just described.

Monday

Bench press — 2-4 sets — 10-15 reps each set
Shoulders — 2-4 sets — 10-15 reps each set
Triceps — 2-4 sets — 10-15 reps each set
Crunches and/or seated abs

Wednesday

Thighs — 2-4 sets — 10-15 reps each set
Hamstrings — 2-4 sets — 10-15 reps each set
Calves — 2-4 sets — 10-15 reps each set
Crunches and/or seated abs

Friday

Bent over row — 2-4 sets — 10-15 reps each set
Arm curl — 2-4 sets — 10-15 reps each set
Crunches and/or seated abs
(Add chest, thighs, hamstrings, or calves from previous days.)

STRETCHING

Here are some simple stretches anyone can do. The whole routine should take five minutes or so. You can do these any time, and as often as you wish. You may find that stretching in the morning upon rising is a nice way to wake up. But since your muscles tend to be "cold" and stiff, stretching then might be more difficult. You may find that stretching in the evening before bed is a relaxing end to the day. If you plan to work stretching into your Stage Two activities, we suggest doing these after your brisk walk, bike ride, or whatever, rather than before. After, your muscles will be warmed up and more relaxed, so you can probably get a more effective stretch.

In each of the following stretches, it's important not to "bounce" into the stretch. Bouncing actually activates reflexes that cause your muscles to tighten, which simply defeats the whole purpose. Rather, slowly sink into the stretch, hold for a breath or two, and relax, then sink a bit further and hold again. Hold for five to 20 seconds, then repeat three to five times. Always breathe slowly and deeply; never hold your breath during these stretches.

Hamstring Stretch

There are three variations on this. You can do them standing, sitting, or lying on your back.

Standing, with your feet shoulder width apart, bend slowly at the waist and reach down to your toes. Hold, sink further, hold again. For a more ambitious stretch, cross your ankles. (Note, if you have a hard time keeping your balance, try one of the following instead.)

Sitting, with your legs straight, reach forward toward your toes.

The third variation is to lie on your back and bring one of your knees to your chest. Clasp your hands behind your knee and then straighten your leg slowly. Hold and repeat. Then switch legs.

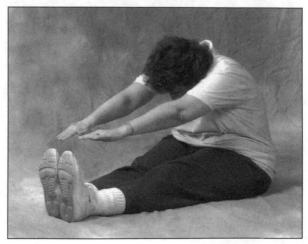

Quad Stretch

Stand on your right foot near a wall. With your left hand, grasp your left ankle and pull it toward your buttocks. Use your free hand to balance yourself. Hold and repeat, then switch legs.

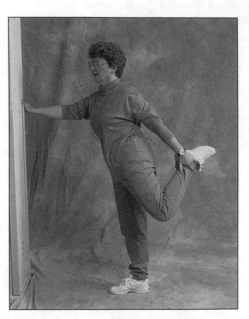

Low-Back Stretch

Lie on your back and pull your knees toward your chest. Grasp the tops of your knees and pull them toward you. For a more intense stretch, raise your head and try to tuck your chin into your chest. Hold and repeat.

A variation of this exercise is to stand with your feet shoulder width apart, your knees bent slightly. Lean forward and put your hands on your thighs just above your knees. Next, try to push your abdomen toward your back, rounding your back. Hold 10 to 20 seconds. Then push your abdomen toward the floor and straighten your arms and look up, pushing your shoulders toward the ceiling. Hold 10 to 20 seconds. Repeat.

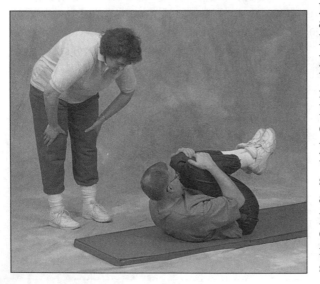

Side Stretch

Stand with your right side toward a wall, about an arm's length from the wall. Cross your left leg over your right, and support yourself against the wall with your right hand. Then slowly let your right hip sink toward the wall. Hold and repeat five or six times, then turn and do the left side.

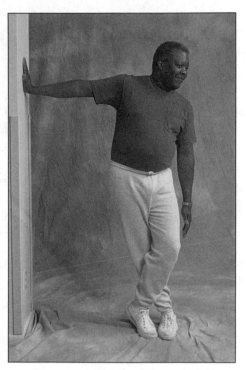

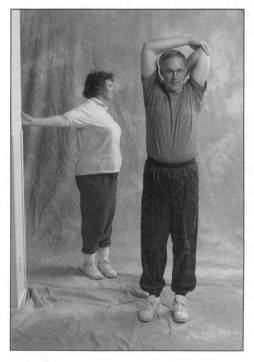

Shoulder Stretch

Grab the corner of a wall or doorframe with your right hand at shoulder level, your arm extended out. Then twist your upper body slowly to the left. You should feel the stretch in your shoulder. Hold and repeat. Then switch to your left side.

A variation of the shoulder stretch is to reach up with your hand and extend your arm back behind your shoulders, as if trying to scratch your upper back. With your other hand, push your elbow back a bit further. Hold and repeat, then switch to your other shoulder.

TAI CHI CHUAN AND CH'I GUNG

Tai chi chuan and *Ch'i Gung* ("energy practice") are closely related disciplines, with many overlapping exercises, and the same underlying principle, the development of *ch'i* for improved health, strength, vitality, and longevity. These are the fundamental practices of the "internal" martial arts as they have developed in Asia. However, as noted in chapter 10, as these practices have evolved over the centuries, they've been fully integrated into the healing arts.

The following exercises derive from both disciplines. They're a good starting point for anyone interested in pursuing this particular approach to optimal health and fitness. They're not intended as a complete substitute for other Stage One or Stage Two activities, but they are a valuable complement, particularly as we get older. These disciplines are especially valuable for older men and women since they specifically help in the maintenance of good balance, flexibility, and strength.

Ideally, we would show the entire tai chi chuan "form" here, a series of 108 movements (or fewer in some styles) that exercise all parts of the body. However, because these are *movements*, it's very difficult to do them justice with still photos. If you have an interest in tai chi, we recommend finding a teacher or a video. The exercises here form a foundation, then, for further practice. However, they are sufficient themselves. We've simply given the technique here. The philosophy and spirit of the form add much to its helpfulness. Again, if you're interested, find a good teacher.

These practices will seem very much like meditation. In truth, *Ch'i Gung* and meditation are very similar in many regards, including breathing and posture. They have somewhat similar goals, too, though not entirely. Meditators are seeking relaxation and calmness at one level, and at a loftier level, a particular state of consciousness or enlightenment, a sense of one's place as part of all existence. *Ch'i Gung* has rather more mundane goals: The cultivation of ch'i for improved health, as well as a certain type of relaxed consciousness, *sung*, and finally the "unlearning" of old habits of posture and movements and a fuller integration of body and mind. Of course, enlightenment is always welcome.

You'll want to wear loose, comfortable clothing. Pleasant surroundings help, a quiet spot in the park or backyard, perhaps under a tree. Indoors, your room should be light and well-ventilated, but free of drafts. The only equipment you'll need are a sturdy chair that is the proper height for you, so that when you sit on it, your upper and lower legs form a 90-degree or right angle.

The following are laid out in the order in which they should be practiced by beginners. However, it's quite OK to change the sequence or otherwise vary the routine to suit what feels best for you.

All of the following photos are of tai chi master Cheung Fong Ha of Berkeley, California, a friend of the authors.

SITTING

Here are the steps to follow to achieve a good sitting position.

- Sit on the edge of a sturdy chair so that your upper and lower legs, and upper body and legs, form right angles.

- Your feet should rest flat on the floor, parallel, and about shoulder width apart.

- Rest your hands lightly on your thighs. Relax your shoulders.

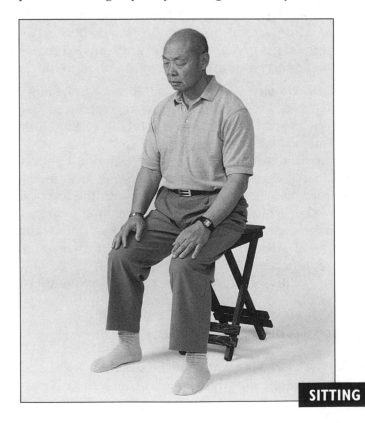

SITTING

- As you sit, gently push the top and back of your head up toward the sky to stretch your spinal column. Imagine that there's a filament of energy running from the base of your spine, up your spine, and through your head, and that your entire spinal column is stretching upward along this filament. Or, imagine a hook attached to the top of your head, in a straight line with your spinal column, and that this hook is attached to a line that is *gently* pulling upwards. As you sit, now and again remind yourself of this filament or line *gently* pulling up on your spinal column and head.

- With your eyes level, gaze off into the distance without focusing on anything in particular for a moment. Then close your eyes.

- At this point, your awareness is probably located behind your eyes. A fundamental principle of this practice is that your *ch'i* tends to concentrate where your awareness is. Now you want to "sink your *ch'i*" by letting your awareness sink down to your *tan tien*, a point about two inches below your navel.

- Breathe regularly and slowly. Let thoughts come and go. Don't try *not* to think. But on the other hand, don't dwell on the thoughts, or grasp at them. Simply acknowledge the thoughts and then return your awareness or attention to the tan tien.

The goal at this point is a quality called *sung* in Chinese. Loosely translated, it means relaxation. Imagine a cat seemingly asleep in the sun, its eyes closed to mere slits. It's totally relaxed, but ready to pounce. This is *sung*.

As you breathe deeply and regularly, play with your awareness now and then. As you inhale, imagine your awareness rising up from your tan tien along your spine and out the top of your head toward the sky. When you inhale, imagine your awareness sinking rapidly back down along your spine, down your legs, and through the bottoms of your feet into the earth. But always return your attention to your tan tien.

Practice this sitting posture for 5 or 10 minutes, or until you feel the desire to stand.

STANDING (*WU CHI CH'I GUNG*)

Stand slowly. Your feet should still be shoulder width and parallel. Bend your knees just slightly, so they are not locked. Next, tuck your pelvis under slightly to flatten the inward curve of the small of your back. Let your hands hang relaxed at your sides. Your head should be upright, your spine elongated along that filament of energy we mentioned. Push the top of your head up slightly, as if it's being pulled gently up by a rope. Your weight should be shifted slightly forward, over the balls of your feet, not back on your heels.

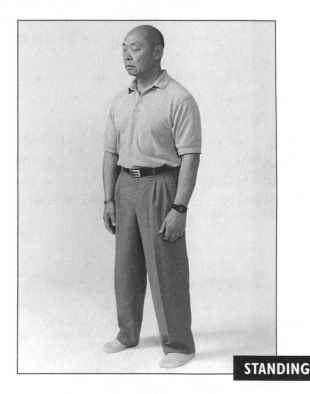

STANDING

Continue to breathe as before, with your awareness on your tan tien. Whenever you feel uncomfortable, sit down for a few moments, again maintaining the same state of sung, or relaxed readiness, your awareness located in your tan tien. It's very important not to force yourself to stand or hold any posture to the point you become uncomfortable and tense.

You should practice the *wu chi* (*wu chi* means "void") posture, with sitting as needed, for 20 to 30 minutes, or longer if you are able. Now and then, "check in" on your posture. Is your pelvis tucked under? Are your knees slightly bent? Is your weight over the balls of your feet? Are you relaxed?

FIRST POSITION

This is the basis for a number of other positions, and it begins to bring us more closely to the realm of the martial arts.

- When you feel relaxed, raise your arms *slowly* to shoulder level. Imagine that *you* aren't raising them, but rather that they are floating up. Try inhaling, and as you do so, imagine you are holding a large beach ball, which fills and lifts your arms.

- Hold your arms as if they are wrapped around that beach ball. Your hands should be relaxed, the fingers slightly spread. There should be no sharp angles in your shoulders, elbows, or wrists.

- Your hands should be spread apart about the width of your shoulders or perhaps a bit less.

- As always, your awareness should be located in your tan tien.

- Don't hold this position so long that you tighten. In the beginning, you may be able to hold this position only a moment or two. When you feel tense, return to wu chi position, or sitting, or go to the second position.

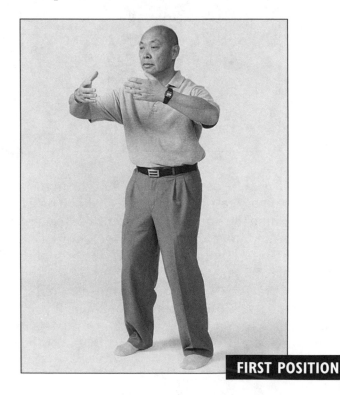

FIRST POSITION

SECOND POSITION

Still "holding the beach ball," rotate your arms around it, until your hands are at about the level of your tan tien. Your palms now should be facing your abdomen. Your fingers are still slightly spread, but relaxed. All of the basic principles of posture, breathing, and awareness still apply.

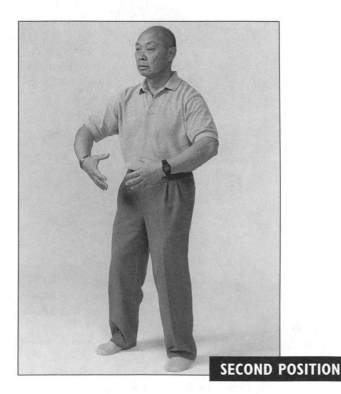

SECOND POSITION

Half Squat

While in the second position, turn your palms toward the floor. Your hands now are still at the level of your abdomen. This particular exercise is great for strengthening the legs and all the joints.

- Your feet should still be shoulder width and parallel, your weight over the balls of your feet, your pelvis tucked under, your posture upright.
- Exhale, and as you do so, sink slightly, bending your knees and lowering your hands to just below your waist. Imagine your hands are floating on water, and that the water level has dropped.

- Inhale, and as you do so, rise slightly, raising your hands back to the level of your tan tien, or a bit higher. Imagine, again, that the water has risen, carrying your hands with it.

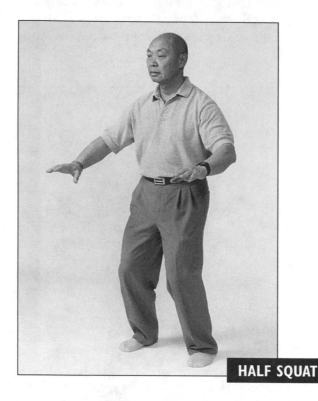

HALF SQUAT

Grasp the Sparrow's Tail

Grasp Sparrow's Tail takes us out of the realm of *Ch'i Gung* into tai chi chuan proper. The series of movements consists of "ward off," "roll back," "press," and "push," with transitional movements as one movement becomes the next. Incidentally, we're starting with the right foot forward, but you can start with the left in front, if you wish. All instructions to follow assume the right foot is forward. With the left foot in front, all the following directions are simply reversed. When you practice Grasp the Sparrow's Tail, you'll want to switch stances periodically, so both legs are worked equally.

Ward Off

While in the standing position, feet shoulder width apart and your right foot slightly forward, inhale. As you exhale, slowly raise your arms as if to the first position in standing, but with a difference. As you do so, extend your right arm just a bit further than the left, with your right palm facing you. At the same time, turn your left palm away.

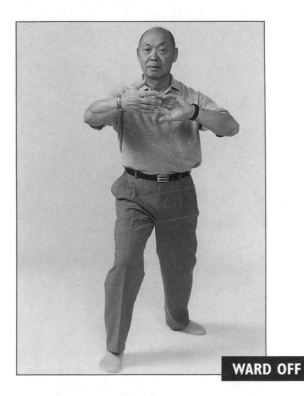

WARD OFF

Your palms should now be facing one another. And unlike the first position, they should be aligned more closely around your centerline, about shoulder or chest high. Hold this position and relax for a few breaths. If you find yourself getting tense, lower your hands, or return to the wu chi or sitting positions.

Transition 1
Inhale and, as you exhale, twist slowly to your right, and as you do so, turn your right palm *away* from you, and your left palm *toward* you. Keep your knees over your feet. Check your posture. Is your pelvis tucked under? Is your spine elongated? Is your head up?

Relax into this position and breathe deeply and slowly for a few breaths.

"Roll back" and as you exhale
- settle your weight back toward your left foot,

- turn your torso back so you are facing forward, and

- at the same time, lower your hands to waist level or a bit below, so that your left hand is now palm-up by your left thigh, and your right is palm-down by your right thigh.

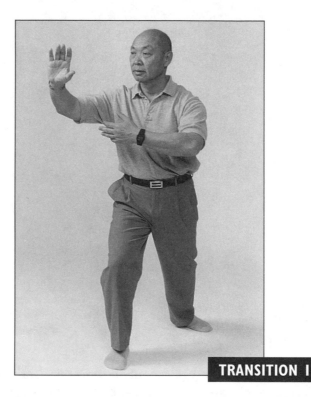

TRANSITION I

Transition 2
Relax into this position a moment, breathing deeply. Check in on your posture, and awareness.

Exhale one more time, and as you inhale turn to your left. As you do so, raise and extend your left arm behind you, to about shoulder height. Open your hips, that is, push your right knee toward the right, and your left toward the left. You should have a sense here that your pelvis is stretching and opening.

At this point, much of your weight should be over your left (rear) foot. Your right hand is still facing palm-down, by your right thigh. This is a transitional position between "Roll back" and "Press."

Following are instructions on how to do the "press."

- Exhale, and as you do so, shift your weight forward and turn so you are facing forward.
- At the same time bring your left arm forward and your right arm up, so both are chest-high.
- Press your left palm against your right wrist. Your arms should still be "rounded" in front of you, as if you are still holding the beach ball.

At this point, your weight should be shifted slightly forward, your left leg almost straight (don't lock your knee). Check to make sure your hips are square, your pelvis is tucked under. Breathe deeply and slowly.

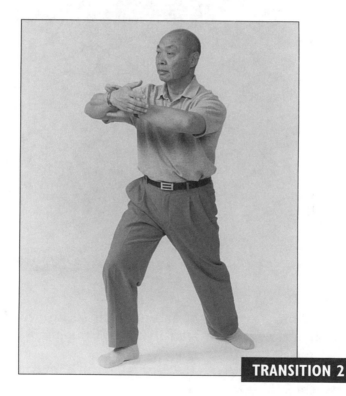

TRANSITION 2

Transition 3

Inhale, and as you do so shift your weight back to your rear foot and separate your hands to shoulder width apart. Simultaneously draw your hands back toward your shoulders. Exhale, sink down on your rear foot and "press" down with your hands toward the ground. Complete this movement of sinking back and down, lowering your hands, and exhaling all at the same time.

Next, inhale, and as you do so, raise your hands to shoulder level, "push," and exhale. Shift your weight toward your front foot, "pushing" forward with your hands, until your arms are nearly extended, but without locking your elbows.

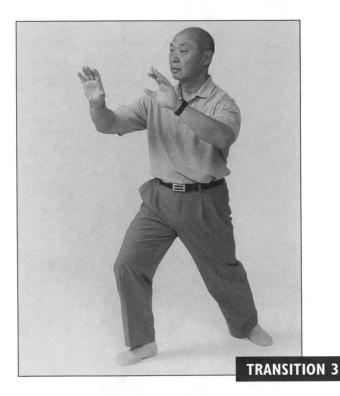

TRANSITION 3

Transition 4

Inhale, and turn to your right, and as you do so, turn you hands into the position described in Transition 1. At this point, you're now ready to repeat Grasp the Sparrow's Tail.

As you get familiar with the form, you can eliminate the pauses and extra breathing between positions, and practice fluidly moving from one to the next, following the pattern of inhalation and exhalation as noted. Practice the complete form a few times first on one side, then switch to the left-foot-forward position and practice an equal number of times.

suggested readings

General Health

Arnot, R. 1992. *The best medicine*. Reading, MA: Addison-Wesley Publishing.

Blair, S.N. 1991. *Living with exercise*. Dallas: American Health Publishing.

Bortz, W.M., II. 1991. *We live too short and die too long*. New York: Bantam.

Brody, J. 1982. *Jane Brody's guide to personal health*. New York: Times Books.

Cooper, K.H. 1968. *Aerobics*. New York: Bantam.

Eaton, B.; Shostak, M; & Konner, M. 1988. *The paleolithic prescription*. New York: Harper and Row.

Farquhar, John W., MD. 1987. *The american way of life need not be hazardous to your health*. Reading, MA: Addison-Wesley Publishing.

Hayflick, L. 1994. *How and why we age*. New York: Ballantine Books.

Johnson, R. & Tulin, B. 1995. *Travel fitness*. Champaign, IL: Human Kinetics.

Nuland, S.B. 1993. *How we die: Reflections on life's final chapter*. New York: Knopf.

Reese, P. & Henderson, J. 1993. *Ten million steps*. Waco, TX: WRS Publishing.

Sapolsky, R.M. 1994. *Why zebras don't get ulcers: A guide to stress, stress related diseases and coping*. New York: W.H. Freeman.

Simon, H. & Levinsohn, S. 1987. *The athlete within*. Boston: Little Brown.

Simon, H.B. 1992. *Staying well. Your complete guide to disease prevention*. Boston: Houghton Mifflin.

Simon, H.B. 1994. *Conquering heart disease*. Boston: Little Brown.

YMCA of the USA, with Sammann, P. 1994. *YMCA healthy back book*. Champaign, IL: Human Kinetics.

Nutrition

Brody, J. 1981. *Jane Brody's nutrition book*. New York: W.W. Norton.

Ornish, D. 1993. *Eat more. Weigh less*. New York: Harper Perennial.

PDR family guide to nutrition and health. 1995. Montvale, NJ: Medical Economics.

Tribole, E. 1992. *Eating on the run*, 2nd ed. Champaign, IL: Human Kinetics.

Running

Fixx, J. 1977. *The complete book of running*. New York: Random House.

Fixx, J. 1980. *Jim Fixx's second book of running*. New York: Random House.

Galloway, J. 1984. *Galloway's book on running*. Bolinas, CA: Shelter Publications.

Noakes, T. 1991. *The lore of running.* Champaign, IL: Human Kinetics.

Strength Training

Pearl, B. & Moran, G.T. 1986. *Getting stronger.* Bolinas, CA: Shelter Publications.

Baechle, T.R. & Earle, R.W. 1995. *Fitness weight training.* Champaign, IL: Human Kinetics.

Stretching

Anderson, B. 1980. *Stretching.* Bolinas, CA: Shelter Publications.

Alter, M. 1990. *SportStretch.* Champaign, IL: Human Kinetics.

Swimming

Sova, R. 1995. *Water fitness after 40.* Champaign, IL: Human Kinetics.

Tai Chi & Ch'i Gung

Diepersloot, J. 1995. *Warriors of stillness.* Walnut Creek, CA: Center for the Healing Arts.

Lee, M.; Lee, E.; & Johnson, J. 1989. *Ride the tiger to the mountain: T'ai chi for health.* Reading, MA: Addison Wesley.

Walking

Fletcher, C. 1973. *The complete walker.* New York: Alfred A. Knopf.

Rippe, J.M. & Ward, A. 1989. *The Rockport walking program.* New York: Prentice Hall.

Rudner, R. 1996. *Walking.* Champaign, IL: Human Kinetics.

Sussman, A. & Goode, R. 1969. *The magic of walking.* New York: Simon and Schuster.

Professional Sources

Dishman, R.K. 1994. *Advances in exercise adherence.* Champaign, IL: Human Kinetics.

Driver, B.L.; Brown, P.J.; & Peterson, G.L., eds. 1991. *Benefits of leisure.* State College, PA: Venture Publishing.

Fries, J.F., & Crapo, L.M. 1981. *Vitality and aging.* San Francisco: W.H. Freeman.

Morris, J.N. 1975. *The uses of epidemiology.* Edinburgh: Churchill Livingston.

Rose, G. 1992. *The strategy of preventive medicine.* Oxford: Oxford University Press.

Shephard, R.J. 1978. *Physical activity and aging.* Chicago: A Croom Helm Book.

Thomas, G.S.; Lee, P.R.; Franks, P.; & Paffenbarger, R.S., Jr. 1981. *Exercise and health: The evidence and the implications.* Cambridge, MA: Oelgeschlager, Gunn & Hain Publishers.

notes

CHAPTER I: AN INTRODUCTION TO CHANGE (pp. 3-12)

1. The title derives from our intent—to give you the information you need to become and remain fit for life as we live it these days in this frenetic, postmodern world, and live as long as possible free of all the debilitating diseases and frailties the conventional wisdom would have us believe are the inevitable result of increasing years.

2. A person-year of observation represents one person observed for one year. A million person-years might represent one person observed for a million years, or a million persons observed for one year, or any combination of persons and years. Man-years and woman-years are the obvious variations. In the College Study, more than 50,000 men and women have been observed over a period of 45 to 80 years, from 1916, when the first men took physical exams at Harvard, or from 1931, when University of Pennsylvania men and women first took them.

3. Walter Bortz, MD introduces the concept of three phases of life in his intriguing book, *We Live Too Short and Die Too Long.* Until recently, he notes, most men and women never made it to the third phase, which begins in his scheme at about the age of 80 (youth is 0 to 40 years, middle age 40 to 80 years).

4. U.S. Department of Health and Human Services. 1992. *Healthy people 2000, national health promotion and disease prevention objectives.* Boston: Jones and Bartlett. The report calls for at least 30 percent of the population to engage regularly in light to moderate physical activity at least 30 minutes a day; the report also calls for half of Americans over the age of 65 to walk, swim, or engage in other appropriate aerobic exercise three times a week.

5. Pate, R.P.; Prat, M.; Blair, S.N.; Haskell, W.L.; Macera, C.A.; Bouchard, C.; Buchner, D.; Ettinger, W.; Heath, G.W.; King, A.C.; Kriska, A.; Leon, A.S.; Marcus, B.H.; Morris, J.; Paffenbarger, R.S.; Patrick, K.; Pollock, M.L.; Rippe, J.M.; Sallis, J.; & Wilmore, J. 1995. Physical activity and public health: A recommendation from the Centers for Disease Control and Prevention and the American College of Sports Medicine. *Journal of the American Medical Association* 273 (5): 402-7.

6. Hewlett, S.A. 1991. *When the Bough Breaks.* New York: Basic Books.

CHAPTER 2: IT'S NEVER TOO LATE (pp. 13-51)

1. The terms *calorie* and *kilocalorie* are used rather indiscriminately to refer to the same measurement of energy. *Kilocalorie* is the more accurate term, thus we use it throughout the book. Keep in mind that one kilocalorie is the same as one calorie in the common usage.

2. Paffenbarger, R.S.; Hyde, R.T.; Wing, A.L.; & Hsieh, C.-C. 1986. Physical activity, all-cause mortality, and longevity of college alumni. *New England Journal of Medicine 314* (10): 605-12.

3. Paffenbarger, R.S.; Hyde, R.T.; Wing, A.L.; Lee, I.-M.; Jung, D.L.; & Kampert, J.B. 1993. The association of changes in physical activity level and other lifestyle characteristics with mortality among men. *New England Journal of Medicine 328* (8): 538-45.

4. Paffenbarger, R.S.; Kampert, J.B.; Lee, I-M.; Hyde, R.T.; Leung, R.W.; & Wing, A.L. 1994. Chronic disease in former college students: LII. Changes in phyical activity and other lifeway patterns influencing longevity. *Medicine and Science in Sports and Exercise 26*: 857-65.

5. Paffenbarger, R.S.; Kampert, J.B.; Lee, I-M.; Hyde, R.T.; Leung, R.W.; & Wing, A.L. 1994. Chronic disease in former college students: LII. Changes in phyical activity and other lifeway patterns influencing longevity. *Medicine and Science in Sports and Exercise 26*: 857-65.

6. Lee, I-M.; Hsieh, C-C.; & Paffenbarger, R.S. 1995. Chronic disease in former college students: LIV. Exercise intensity and longevity in men. *Journal of the American Medical Association 273* (15): 1179-84.

7. Ainsworth, B.; Haskell, W.L.; Leon, A.S.; Jacobs, D.R., Jr.; Montoye, H.J.; Sallis, J.F.; & Paffenbarger, R.S. 1993. Compendium of physical activities: Classification of energy costs of human physical activities. *Medicine and Science in Sports and Exercise, 25*: 71-80.

8. Paffenbarger, R.S.; Kampert, J.B.; Lee, I-M.; Hyde, R.T.; Leung, R.W.; & Wing, A.L. 1994. Chronic disease in former college students: LII. Changes in phyical activity and other lifeway patterns influencing longevity. *Medicine and Science in Sports and Exercise 26*: 857-65.

9. Powell, K.E.; Thompson, P.D.; Caspersen, C.J.; & Kendrick, J.S. 1987. Physical activity and the incidence of coronary heart disease. *Annual Review of Public Health 8*: 253-87.

10. Berlin, J.A., & Colditz, G.A. 1990. A meta-analysis of physical activity in the prevention of coronary heart disease. *American Journal of Epidemiology 132*: 612-28.

11. Blair, S.N. May 1992. Physical activity, fitness, and coronary heart disease. Paper presented at the International Conference on Physical Activity, Fitness and Health, Toronto.

12. Blair, S.N.; Kohl, H.W., III; Paffenbarger, R.S.; Clark, D.G.; Cooper

K.H.; & Gibbons, L.W. 1989. Physical fitness and all-cause mortality: A prospective study of healthy men and women. *Journal of the American Medical Association 262*: 2395-2401.

13. Kaplan, G.A.; Seeman, T.E.; Cohen, R.D.; Knudsen, L.P.; & Guralnik, J. 1987. Mortality among the elderly in the Alameda County Study: Behavioral and demographic risk factors. *American Journal of Public Health 77*: 307-12, 818.

14. Leon, A.S.; Connett, J.; Jacobs, D.R.; & Rauramaa, R. 1987. Leisure-time physical activity levels and risk of coronary heart disease and death: The Multiple Risk Factor Intervention Trial. *Journal of the American Medical Association 258*: 2388-95.

15. Lindsted, K.D.; Tonstad, S.; & Kuzma, J.W. 1991. Self-report of physical activity and patterns of mortality in Seventh-Day Adventist men. *Journal of Clinical Epidemiology 44*: 355-65.

16. Morris, J.N.; Clayton, D.G.; Everitt, M.G.; Semmence, A.M.; & Burgess, E.H. 1990. Exercise in leisure time: Coronary attack and death rates. *British Heart Journal 63*: 325-44.

17. Paffenbarger, R.S.; Hyde, R.T.; Wing, A.L.; & Hsieh, C.-C. 1986. Physical activity, all-cause mortality, and longevity of college alumni. *New England Journal of Medicine 314* (10): 605-12.

18. Pekkanen, J.; Marti, B.; Nissinen, A.; & Tuomilehto, J. 1987. Reduction of premature mortality by high physical activity: A 20-year follow-up of middle-aged Finnish men. *Lancet 1*: 1473-77.

19. Lee, I-M.; Paffenbarger, R.S.; & Hsieh, C-C. 1992. Time trends in physical activity among college alumni, 1962-88. *American Journal of Epidemiology 135* (8): 915-25.

20. Paffenbarger, R.S.; Hyde, R.T.; & Wing, A.L. 1990. Physical activity and physical fitness as determinants of health and longevity. In *Exercise, fitness, and health*, edited by C. Bouchard, R.J. Shephard, T. Stephens, J.R. Sutton, & B.D. McPherson, 33-48. Champaign, IL: Human Kinetics.

21. Bouchard, C.; Shephard, R.; Stephens, T.; Sutton, J.R.; & McPherson, B.D., eds. 1990. *Exercise, fitness, and health: A consensus of current knowledge.* Champaign, IL: Human Kinetics.

22. Bouchard, C., & Shephard, R. 1994. Physical activity, fitness, and health: The model and key concepts. In *Physical activity, fitness, and health*, edited by C. Bouchard, R. Shephard, & T. Stephens, 14-15. Champaign, IL: Human Kinetics.

23. Hein, H.O.; Saudicani, P.; & Gyntelberg, F. 1992. Physical fitness or physical activity as a predictor of ischaemic heart disease? A 17-year follow-up in the Copenhagen Male Study. *Journal of Internal Medicine 232*: 471-79.

24. Paffenbarger, R.S.; Blair, S.N.; Lee, I-M.; & Hyde, R. 1993. Measurement of physical activity to assess health effects in free-living populations. *Medicine and Science in Sports and Exercise 25*: 60-70.

CHAPTER 3: NOT JUST MORE YEARS, BUT BETTER YEARS (pp. 53-78)

1. Bortz, W.M., II. 1991. *We live too short and die too long.* New York: Bantam.

2. Fries, J.F., & Crapo, L. 1981. *Vitality and aging.* San Francisco: W.H. Freeman.

3. Fries, J.F., & Crapo, L. 1981. *Vitality and aging.* San Francisco: W.H. Freeman.

4. Olshansky, S.J.; Carnes, B.A.; & Cassel, C.K. 1993. The aging of the human species. *Scientific American 268* (4): 51.

5. Smith, T. 1992, November 21. Of flies and men. *British Medical Journal. 305:* 1242.

6. Statistics about the average length of life from one generation to the next include everyone, from infants who die at birth to young children killed by childhood diseases for which we now have effective immunization. Once past the considerable dangers of birth and childhood, adults of previous generations could expect to live a reasonably long time, even without the benefits of such modernities as indoor plumbing, automobiles, ample food supplies, and prime-time news.

7. *Life span* refers to the length of life of a given species; the human life span seems to be about 85, give or take five years, although there are some widely diverging opinions on this. *Longevity* refers to average length of life. Thus a population of humans with a life span of 85 years might nonetheless have an average longevity of only 40 or 50 years due to famine, warfare, infection, pollution, or other factors.

8. Montagu, J.D. 1994. Length of life in the ancient world: Controlled study. *Journal of the Royal Society of Medicine 87:* 25-26.

9. Sagan, L.A. 1987. *The health of nations: True causes of sickness and well-being.* New York: Basic Books.

10. Olshansky, S.J.; Carnes, B.A.; & Cassel, C.K. 1993. The aging of the human species. *Scientific American 268* (4): 46-52.

11. Olshansky, S.J.; Carnes, B.A.; & Cassel, C.K. 1990, November 2. In search of Methusalah: Estimating the upper limits to human longevity. *Science 250:* 634-40.

12. Interestingly, some anthropologists think that gruel, or to use the somewhat more palatable-sounding British term *porridge,* made civilization possible. It was the boiling of cereal in a cooking pot that enabled Stone Age women to double their lifetime fertility.

13. Fries, J.F., & Crapo, L. 1981. *Vitality and aging.* San Francisco: W.H. Freeman.

14. Bortz, W.M., II. 1991. *We live too short and die too long.* New York: Bantam.

15. Olshansky, S.J.; Carnes, B.A.; & Cassel, C.K. 1990, November 2. In search of Methusalah: Estimating the upper limits to human longevity. *Science 250*: 634-40.

16. Shephard, R. 1978. *Physical activity and aging.* Chicago: Croom Helm.

17. Moore, T.J. 1993. *Lifespan: Who lives longer and why.* New York: Simon and Schuster.

18. R.J. Shephard, MD, PhD, professor of applied physiology in the Department of Preventive Medicine at the University of Toronto, suggests that the maximum human life span is around 112 to 114 years. Moore writes: "The finality with which the curtain falls on humans at 115 years hints at a biological clock whose time has run out." Bortz believes that the human animal is meant to live 120 years.

19. Vildik, A. 1992, October 17-20. Can the aging process be challenged? Presented at Aging, Life, Fitness symposium, Copenhagen.

20. Leonard Hayflick. 1994. *How and why we age.* New York: Ballentine.

21. Barinaga, M. 1991, November 15. How long is the human lifespan? *Science 254*: 936-38.

22. Bortz, W.M., II. 1991. *We live too short and die too long.* New York: Bantam.

23. Olshansky, S.J.; Carnes, B.A.; & Cassel, C.K. 1993. The aging of the human species. *Scientific American 268* (4): 46-52.

24. Kirkwood, T.B.L., & Rose, M.R. 1991, April 29. Evolution of senescence: Late survival sacrificed for reproduction. *Philosophical Transactions of the Royal Society of London 332*: 15-24.

25. Comfort, A. 1973. Theories of aging. In *Textbook of geriatric medicine & gerontology,* edited by J.C. Brocklehurst. Edinburgh, Scotland: Churchill Livingstone.

26. Pelletier, K.R. 1981. *Longevity, fulfilling our biological potential.* New York: Delacorte Press/Lawrence.

27. Foreman, J. 1992, September 28. Longer life, the next frontier. *Boston Globe*: 37-41.

28. Rusting, R.L. 1992, December. Why do we age? *Scientific American.* 131-41.

29. Shephard, R. 1978. *Physical activity and aging.* Chicago: Croom Helm.

30. Rusting, R.L. 1992, December. Why do we age? *Scientific American.* 131-41.

31. Alpha-Tocopherol, Beta Carotene Cancer Prevention Study Group. 1994, April 14. The effect of vitamin E and beta carotene on the incidence of lung cancer and other cancers in male smokers. *New England Journal of Medicine 330*: 1029-35.

32. This study of smokers in Finland found no protective effect from antioxidant vitamins, news that caused something of a stir. But bear in mind that this was a study of smokers, most of whom were elderly and suffering from all the health problems typical of smokers. It's likely that nothing would have helped these men as long as they continued to smoke.

33. Shephard, R. 1978. *Physical activity and aging.* Chicago: Croom Helm.

34. Virgil. Eclogues IX, line 51.

35. Wilson, J.Q. 1993. *The moral sense.* New York: Free Press.

36. Fries, J.F., & Crapo, L. 1981. *Vitality and aging.* San Francisco: W.H. Freeman.

37. Bortz, W.M., II. 1994, March 31. *Successful Aging.* From a talk at the 50+ Fitness Association annual meeting. Stanford University.

38. Bortz suggests that a decline in functioning of about 0.5 percent per year from about age 30 or 40 is normal and healthy aging, and he notes that declines of about 2 percent per year are more typical of the sedentary American adult. The difference, he says, is amenable to change and intervention.

CHAPTER 4: FORM AND FUNCTION (pp. 81-136)

1. Spirduso, W., & Macrae, P.G. 1991. Physical activity and quality of life in the frail elderly. In *The concept and measurement of quality of life in the frail elderly,* edited by J.E. Birren, J.E. Lubben, J.C. Rowe, & D.E. Deutchman. San Diego: Academic Press.

2. Kuczmarski, R.J.; Flegal, K.M.; Campbell, S.M.; & Johnson, C.L. 1994, July 20. Increasing prevalence of overweight among U.S. adults: The National Health and Nutrition Examination Surveys, 1960-1991. *Journal of the American Medical Association, 272*: 205-211.

3. Manson, J.E.; Colditz, G.A.; & Stampfer, M.J. 1994, June 8. Parity, ponderosity, and the paradox of a weight-preoccupied society. *Journal of the American Medical Association 271*: 1788-90.

4. Wilmore, J. 1994, May. Exercise, obesity, and weight control. In *Physical Activity and Fitness Research Digest,* edited by C. Corbin and B. Pangrazi. *1(6):* 1-6.

5. Lee, I-M.; Manson, J.E.; Hennekens, C.H.; & Paffenbarger, R.S., Jr. 1993, December 15. Chronic disease in former college students: LVI. Body weight and mortality: A 27-year follow-up of middle-aged men. *Journal of the American Medical Association 270*: 2823-28.

6. U.S. Public Health Service. 1988. *Disease prevention, health promotion.* Palo Alto, CA: Bull.

7. Harvard Medical School. 1994, March. Losing weight: A new attitude emerges. *Harvard Health Letter 4:* 1-6.

8. Hamermesh, D.S., & Biddle, J.E. 1994, December. Beauty and the labor market. *American Journal of Economics 85*: 1174-94.

9. Harvard Medical School. 1994, March. Losing weight: A new attitude emerges. *Harvard Health Letter 4:* 1-6.

10. Lee, I-M.; Manson, J.E.; Hennekens, C.H.; & Paffenbarger, R.S., Jr. 1993, December 15. Chronic disease in former college students: LVI. Body weight and mortality: A 27-year follow-up of middle-aged men. *Journal of the American Medical Association 270*: 2823-28.

11. Willett, W.C.; Manson, J.E.; Stampfer, M.J.; Colditz, G.A., Rosher, B.; Spelzar, F.E.; & Hennekens, C.H. 1995, February 8. Weight, weight change, and coronary heart disease in women: Risk within the "normal" weight range. *Journal of the American Medical Association 273*: 461-65.

12. Manson, J.E.; Colditz, G.A.; & Stampfer, M.J. 1994, June 8. Parity, ponderosity, and the paradox of a weight-preoccupied society. *Journal of the American Medical Association 271*: 1788-90.

13. Mayo Foundation for Medical Education and Research. 1994, June. Weight control: What works and why. *Mayo Clinic Health Letter 12* (Suppl.): 1-8.

14. Harvard Medical School. 1994, March. Losing weight: A new attitude emerges. *Harvard Health Letter 4:* 1-6.

15. Paffenbarger, R.S.; Hyde, R.T.; Wing, A.L.; & Hsieh, C.-C. 1986, March. Physical activity, all-cause mortality, and longevity of college alumni. *New England Journal of Medicine 314* (10): 605-12.

16. Leibel, R.L.; Rosenbaum, M.; & Hirsch, J. 1995, March 9. Changes in energy expenditure resulting from altered body weight. *New England Journal of Medicine 332*: 621-28.

17. Molé, P.A. 1990. Impact of energy intake and exercise on resting metabolic rate. *Sports Medicine 10*: 72-87.

18. Molé, P.A.; Stern, J.S.; Schultz, C.L.; Bernauer, E.M.; & Holcomb, B.J. 1989. Exercise reverses depressed metabolic rate produced by severe caloric restriction. *Medicine and Science in Sports and Exercise 21*: 29-33.

19. Poehlman, E.T. 1989. A review: Exercise and its influence on resting energy metabolism in man. *Medicine and Science in Sports and Exercise 21*: 515-25.

20. Poehlman, E.T., & Horton, E.S. 1990. Regulation of energy expenditure in aging humans. *Annual Review of Nutrition 10*: 255-75.

21. Lee I-M., & Paffenbarger, R.S., Jr. 1992. Chronic disease in former college students: LI. Change in body weight and longevity. *Journal of the American Medical Association 268*: 2045-49.

22. Lissner, L.; Odell, P.M.; D'Agostino, R.B.; Stokes, J.; Kreger, B.E.; Belanger, A.J.; & Brownell, K.D. 1991. Variability of body weight and health

outcomes in the Framingham population. *New England Journal of Medicine* 324: 1839-44.

23. Also see National Task Force on the Prevention and Treatment of Obesity. 1994. Weight cycling. *Journal of the American Medical Association 272:* 1196-1202.

24. Poehlman, E.T. 1989. A review: Exercise and its influence on resting energy metabolism in man. *Medicine and Science in Sports and Exercise 21:* 515-25.

25. Wood, P.D. & Haskell, W.L. 1979. The effect of exercise on plasma high-density lipoproteins. *Lipids 14:* 417-27.

26. Wood, P.D.; Stefanick, M.L.; Dreon, D.M.; Frey-Hewitt, B.; Garay, S.C.; Williams, P.T. 1988. Changes in plasma lipids and lipoproteins in overweight men during weight loss through dieting as compared with exercise. *New England Journal of Medicine 319:* 1173-79.

27. Wood, P.D.; Stefanick, M.L.; Williams, P.T.; & Haskell, W.L. 1991. The effects on plasma lipoproteins of a prudent weight-reducing diet, with or without exercise, in overweight men and women. *New England Journal of Medicine 325:* 461-66.

28. Stefanick, M.L. 1993. Exercise and weight control. In J.O. Holloszy, ed., *Exercise and Sport Sciences Reviews 21:* 363-96.

29. Wood, P.D.; Stefanick, M.L.; Dreon, D.M.; Frey-Hewitt, B.; Garay, S.C.; Williams, P.T. 1988. Changes in plasma lipids and lipoproteins in overweight men during weight loss through dieting as compared with exercise. *New England Journal of Medicine 319:* 1173-79.

30. Wood, P.D.; Stefanick, M.L.; Williams, P.T.; & Haskell, W.L. 1991. The effects on plasma lipoproteins of a prudent weight-reducing diet, with or without exercise, in overweight men and women. *New England Journal of Medicine 325:* 461-66.

31. Willett, W. 1993, June. From the Langmuir Lecture at the 1993 EIS Conference, reported in *EIS Bulletin.*

32. Olsen, E. 1980, January. Eat, and run better. *The Runner,* pp. 56-67.

33. Ornish, D. 1993. *Eat more, weigh less: Dr. Dean Ornish's Life Choice Program for losing weight safely while eating abundantly.* New York: HarperCollins.

34. Willett, W.; Stampfer, M.J.; Colditz, G.A.; Rosner, B.A.; & Speizer, F.E. 1990, December. Relation of meat, fat, and fiber intake to the risk of colon cancer in a prospective study among women. *New England Journal of Medicine 323* (24): 1664-72.

35. Harvard Medical School. 1994, July. Trans-fatty acids: The new enemy. *Harvard Heart Letter 4:* 1-3.

36. Willett, W.; Stampfer, M.J.; Colditz, G.A.; Rosner, B.A.; & Speizer, F.E. 1990. Relation of meat, fat, and fiber intake to the risk of colon cancer in a

prospective study among women. *New England Journal of Medicine 323* (24): 1664-72.

37. Fenton, M., & Lesch Kelly, A. 1994, July / August. The real truth about burning fat. *Walking Magazine:* 42-44, 93-94.

38. Molé, P.A. 1990. Impact of energy intake and exercise on resting metabolic rate. *Sports Medicine 10:* 72-87.

39. Poehlman, E.T. 1989. A review: Exercise and its influence on resting energy metabolism in man. *Medicine and Science in Sports and Exercise 21:* 515-25.

40. Wilmore, J. 1994. Interview with E. Olsen (coauthor), American College of Sports Medicine Conference, Indianapolis, IN.

41. Work, J. 1989, November. Strength training: A bridge to independence for the elderly. *The Physician and Sportsmedicine 17:* 134-40.

42. Fiatarone, M.A.; Marks, E.C.; Ryan, N.D.; Meredith, C.N.; Lipsitz, L.A.; & Evans, W.J. June 13, 1990. High-intensity strength training in nonagenarians: Effects on skeletal muscle. *Journal of the American Medical Association 263:* 3029-34.

43. Work, J. 1989, November. Strength training: A bridge to independence for the elderly. *The Physician and Sportsmedicine 17:* 134-40.

44. Beck, M. 1992, December 7. The new middle age (baby boom generation approaches middle age). *Newsweek 120,* 50-55.

45. Bouchard, C. & Shephard, R.J. 1994. Physical activity, fitness, and health: The model and key concepts. In *Physical Activity, Fitness, and Health* edited by C. Bouchard, R.J. Shephard, & T. Stephens. Champaign, IL: Human Kinetics.

46. Shephard, R. 1978. *Physical activity and aging.* Chicago: Croom Helm.

47. Work, J. 1989, November. Strength training: A bridge to independence for the elderly. *The Physician and Sportsmedicine 17:* 134-140.

48. Frontera, W.R., Meredith, C.; O'Reilly, K.; Knuttgen, H.; & Evans, W. 1988. Strength conditioning in older men: Skeletal muscle hypertrophy and improved function. *Journal of Applied Physiology 64:* 1038-44.

49. Fiatarone, M.A.; Marks, E.C.; Ryan, N.D.; Meredith, C.N.; Lipsitz, L.A.; & Evans, W.J. 1990, June 13. High-intensity strength training in nonagenarians: Effects on skeletal muscle. *Journal of the American Medical Association 263:* 3029-34.

50. Foreman, J. 1992, September 28. Longer life, the next frontier. *Boston Globe,* pp. 37-41.

51. Work, J. 1989, November. Strength training: A bridge to independence for the elderly. *The Physician and Sportsmedicine 17:* 134-40.

52. Wright, J.E. 1992, September. Build your body to live a longer and happier life. *Muscle & Fitness,* pp. 130-31, 243-44.

53. Åstrand, P-O., & Rodahl, K. 1977. *Textbook of work physiology.* New York: McGraw-Hill.

54. Petit, C. 1993, February 19. Surge in hip fractures feared. *San Francisco Chronicle.*

55. Simon, H.B. 1992. *Staying well. Your complete guide to disease prevention* (346-49, 419). Boston: Houghton Mifflin.

56. *Tufts University Diet and Nutrition Letter.* 1994, June. pp. 3-6.

57. Shephard, R. 1978. *Physical activity and aging.* Chicago: Croom Helm.

58. Shephard, R. 1978. *Physical activity and aging.* Chicago: Croom Helm.

59. Simon, H.B. 1992. *Staying well. Your complete guide to disease prevention* (346-49, 419). Boston: Houghton Mifflin.

60. Åstrand, P-O. 1992. Why exercise? *Medicine and Science in Sports and Exercise.* (24).

61. Smith, E.L.; Smith, K.A.; & Gilligan, C. 1990. Exercise, fitness, osteoarthritis, and osteoporosis. In *Exercise, fitness, and health,* edited by C. Bouchard, R.J. Shephard, T. Stephens, J.R. Sutton, & B.D. McPherson. Champaign, IL: Human Kinetics.

62. Fiatarone, M.A.; Marks, E.C.; Ryan, N.D.; Meredith, C.N.; Lipsitz, L.A.; & Evans, W.J. 1990, June 13. High-intensity strength training in nonagenarians: Effects on skeletal muscle. *Journal of the American Medical Association 263*: 3029-34.

63. *The PDR Family Guide to Nutrition and Health.* 1995. Montvale, NJ: Medical Economics. 400.

64. *Tufts University Diet and Nutrition Letter.* 1994, June. pp. 3-6.

65. Samples, P. 1990, January. Exercise encouraged for people with arthritis. *The Physician and Sportsmedicine 18*: 122-26.

CHAPTER 5: THE HEART OF THE MATTER (pp. 137-165)

1. Åstrand, P-O., & Rodahl, K. 1977. *Textbook of work physiology.* New York: McGraw-Hill.

2. Saltin, B. 1990. Cardiovascular and pulmonary adaptation to physical activity. In *Exercise, fitness, and health,* edited by C. Bouchard, R.J. Shephard, T. Stephens, J.R. Sutton, & B.D. McPherson. Champaign, IL: Human Kinetics.

3. Jackson, A.; Beard, E.F.; Wier, L.T.; Ross, R.M.; Stuteville, J.E.; & Blair, S.N. 1995. Changes in aerobic power of men, ages 25-70. *Medicine and Science in Sports and Exercise 27*: 113-20.

4. U.S. Department of Health and Human Services. 1992. *Healthy people 2000, national health promotion and disease prevention objectives.* Boston: Jones and Bartlett.

5. American Heart Association. 1992, July 1. Press release.

6. Manson, J.E.; Tosteson H.; Ridker, P.M.; Satterfield S.; Hebert P.; O'Connor, G.T.; Burning, J.F.; & Hennekens, C.H. 1992, May 21. The primary prevention of myocardial infarction. *New England Journal of Medicine 326*: 1406-16.

7. Wannamethee, G., & Shaper, A.G. 1992, March 7. Physical activity and stroke in British middle-aged men. *British Medical Journal 304*: 597-601.

8. Simon, H.B. 1992. *Staying well. Your complete guide to disease prevention* (207). Boston: Houghton Mifflin.

9. *The PDR Family Guide to Nutrition and Health*. 1995. Montvale, NJ: Medical Economics. 400.

10. U.S. Public Health Service. 1988. *Disease prevention, health promotion*. Palo Alto, CA: Bull.

11. Eaton, B.; Konner, M.; & Shostak, M. 1988. *The Paleolithic prescription*. New York: Harper & Row.

12. For more on this notion, also see Montagu, J.D. 1994. Length of life in the ancient world: Controlled study. *Journal of the Royal Society of Medicine 87*: 25-26.

13. Eaton, B.; Konner, M.; & Shostak, M. 1988: *The Paleolithic prescription*. New York: Harper & Row, p. 5.

14. Berlin, J.A., & Colditz, G.A. 1990. A meta-analysis of physical activity in the prevention of coronary heart disease. *American Journal of Epidemiology 132*: 612-28.

15. Blair, S.N.; Kohl, H.W., III; Paffenbarger, R.S.; Clark, D.G.; Cooper K.H.; & Gibbons, L.W. 1989, November 3. Physical fitness and all-cause mortality: A prospective study of healthy men and women. *Journal of the American Medical Association 262*: 2395-2401.

16. Kannel, W.B.; Belanger, A.; D'Agostino, R.; & Israel, I. 1986. Physical activity and physical demand on the job and risk of cardiovascular disease and death: The Framingham Study. *American Heart Journal 112*: 820-25.

17. Leon, A.S.; Connett, J.; Jacobs, D.R.; & Rauramaa, R. 1987. Leisure-time physical activity levels and risk of coronary heart disease and death: The Multiple Risk Factor Intervention Trial. *Journal of the American Medical Association 258*: 2388-95.

18. Powell, K.E.; Thompson, P.D.; Caspersen, C.J.; & Kendrick, J.S. 1987. Physical activity and the incidence of coronary heart disease. *Annual Review of Public Health 8*: 253-87.

19. Such findings have been repeated in numerous studies worldwide among very diverse populations, including studies of farmers and nonfarmers; American letter carriers and mail clerks; American Cancer Society volunteers; American and Italian railroad trackmen and clerks; Israeli kibbutzim workers in various occupations; San Francisco

longshoremen, cargo handlers, and warehousemen; insurers of the Health Insurance Plan of New York; Japanese and Japanese-Americans in Hawaii and San Francisco; residents of various regions of Finland, Norway, Sweden, Denmark, Holland, and New Zealand, among other countries. Among the most significant are the following.

MRFIT—The Multiple Risk Factor Intervention Trial (MRFIT) looked at over 12,000 men at high risk for heart disease and found that the most active of them had a 20 percent lower rate of heart disease during an eight-year follow-up than did the least active.

The Framingham Study—A group of 5,000 men and women in Framingham, Massachusetts, 30 to 62 years of age, who were free of any evidence of heart disease at the outset of the study were followed for decades, and investigators found that heart disease was significantly more common among those men and women who were sedentary

The Cooper Clinic—At the Cooper Institute for Aerobics Research in Dallas, Texas, Steven N. Blair and colleagues used a treadmill to quantify physical fitness and, in a study of 3,000 men, found that those who trained to improve their aerobic fitness—that is, their ability to perform endurance exercise, in this case, specifically running on a treadmill—improved their blood lipid profiles, had lower diastolic blood pressure, reduced their body weight, and showed several other changes associated with decreased risk of heart disease. Observations from a similar study of women ran parallel to those of the men.

20. Helmrich, S.P.; Ragland, D.R.; Leung, R.W.; & Paffenbarger, R.S. 1991. Chronic disease in former college students: XLII. Physical activity and reduced occurrence of non-insulin-dependent diabetes mellitus. *New England Journal of Medicine 325*: 147-52.

21. Manson, J.E.; Rimm, E.B.; Stampfer, M.J.; Colditz, G.A.; Willett, W.C.; Krolewski, A.S.; Rosner, B.; Hennekens, C.H.; & Speizer, F.E. 1991, Sept. 28. Physical activity and incidence of non-insulin-dependent diabetes mellitus in women. *Lancet 338*, 774-78.

22. Paffenbarger, R.S.; Hyde, R.T.; Wing, A.L.; & Hsieh, C.-C. 1986. Physical activity, all-cause mortality, and longevity of college alumni. *New England Journal of Medicine 314* (10): 605-12.

23. Blair, S.N.; Kohl, H.W., III; Gordon, N.F.; Paffenbarger, R.S., Jr. 1992. How much physical activity is good for health? *Annual Review of Public Health. 13*: 99-126.

24. Paffenbarger, R.S. & Hyde, R.T. 1980, May 1. Exercise as protection against heart attack, *New England Journal of Medicine 302*: 1026-27.

25. Rauramaa, R.; Salonen, J.T.; Seppanen, K.; Salonen, R.; Venalainen, J.M.; Ihanaien, M.; & Rissanen, V. 1986. Inhibition of platelet aggregability by moderate-intensity physical exercise: A randomized clinical trial in overweight men. *Circulation 74*: 939-44.

26. Williams, R.S.; Logue, E.E.; Lewis, J.L.; Barton, T.; Stead, N.W.; Wallace, A.G.; & Pizzo, S.V. 1980. Physical conditioning augments the fibrinolytic response to venous occlusion in healthy adults. *New England Journal of Medicine 302*: 987-91.

27. Barndt, R.; Blankenhorn, D.H.; Crawford, D.W. 1972, August. Regression and progression of early femoral atherosclerosis in treated hyperlipoproteinemic patients. *Annals of Internal Medicine 86*: 139-46.

28. Blankenhorn, D.H.; Johnson, R.L.; & Elzein, H.A. 1988. Dietary fat influences human coronary lesion formation. *Circulation 78* (Suppl. II): 11.

29. Ornish, D.; Brown, S.E.; Scherwitz, L.W.; Billings, J.H.; Armstrong, W.T.; Ports, T.A.; McLanahan, S.M.; Kirkfeeide, R.L.; Brand, R.J.; & Gould, K.L. 1990, July 21. Can lifestyle changes reverse coronary heart disease? *The Lancet, 336*: 129-33.

30. Wood, P.D. & Haskell, W.L. 1979. The effect of exercise on plasma high-density lipoproteins. *Lipids 14*: 417-27.

31. Wood, P.D.; Stefanick, M.L.; Williams, P.T.; & Haskell, W.L. 1991. The effects on plasma lipoproteins of a prudent weight-reducing diet, with or without exercise, in overweight men and women. *New England Journal of Medicine 325*: 461-66.

32. Hagberg, J.M. 1990. Exercise, fitness, and hypertension. In *Exercise, fitness, and health*, edited by C. Bouchard, R.J. Shephard, T. Stephens, J.R. Sutton, & B.D. McPhersen, 455-66. Champaign, IL: Human Kinetics.

33. Blair, S.N.; Kohl, H.W., III; Paffenbarger, R.S.; Clark, D.G.; Cooper K.H.; & Gibbons, L.W. 1989, November 3. Physical fitness and all-cause mortality: A prospective study of healthy men and women. *Journal of the American Medical Association 262*: 2395-2401.

34. Blair, S.N.; Goodyear, N.N.; Gibbons, L.W.; & Cooper, K.H. 1984. Physical fitness and incidence of hypertension in healthy normotensive men and women. *Journal of the American Medical Association 252*: 487-90.

35. Hagberg, J.M.; Blair, S.N.; Ehsani, A.A.; Gordon, N.F.; Kaplan, N.; Tipton, C.M.; & Zanbraski, E.J. 1993. Physical activity, physical fitness, and hypertension (American College of Sports Medicine Position Statement). *Medicine and Science in Sports and Exercise 25*: i-x.

36. Paffenbarger, R.S.; Hyde, R.T.; Wing, A.L.; & Hsieh, C.-C. 1986. Physical activity, all-cause mortality, and longevity of college alumni. *New England Journal of Medicine 314* (10): 605-12.

37. Seals, D.R., & Hagberg, J.M. 1984. The effect of exercise training on human hypertension: A review. *Medicine and Science in Sports and Exercise 16*: 207-15.

38. Tipton, C.M. 1991. Exercise training and hypertension: An update. In J.O. Holloszy, ed., *Exercise and Sport Sciences Reviews 19*: 447-505.

CHAPTER 6: CANCER PREVENTION AND PHYSICAL ACTIVITY (pp. 167-182)

1. Boring, C.C.; Squires, T.S.; & Tong, T. 1992. *Cancer Statistics 42*: 19-38.

2. U.S. Department of Health and Human Services. 1992. *Healthy people 2000, national health promotion and disease prevention objectives.* Boston: Jones and Bartlett.

3. Davis, D.L.; Dinse, G.E.; & Hoel, D.G. 1994, February 9. Decreasing cardiovascular disease and increasing cancer among whites in the United States from 1973 through 1987: Good news and bad news. *Journal of the American Medical Association 271*: 431-37.

4. Davis, D.L.; Dinse, G.E.; & Hoel, D.G. 1994, February 9. Decreasing cardiovascular disease and increasing cancer among whites in the United States from 1973 through 1987: Good news and bad news. *Journal of the American Medical Association 271*: 431-37.

5. Doll, R. 1991. Progress against cancer: An epidemiological assessment. *American Journal of Epidemiology 134*: 675-88.

6. Lee, I-M. 1994. Physical activity, fitness, and cancer. In *Physical activity, fitness, and health,* edited by C. Bouchard, R. Shephard, & T. Stephens, 814-31. Champaign, IL: Human Kinetics.

7. Paffenbarger, R.S., Jr.; Hyde, R.T.; & Wing, A.L. 1987. Physical activity and incidence of cancer in diverse populations: A preliminary report. *American Journal of Clinical Nutrition 45*: 312-17.

8. Blair, S.N.; Kohl, H.W., III; Paffenbarger, R.S.; Clark, D.G.; Cooper K.H.; & Gibbons, L.W. 1989, November 3. Physical fitness and all-cause mortality: A prospective study of healthy men and women. *Journal of the American Medical Association 262*: 2395-2401.

9. Garabrant, D.H.; Peters, J.M.; Mack, T.M.; & Bernstein, L. 1984. Job activity and colon cancer risk. *American Journal of Epidemiology 119*: 1004-14.

10. Gerhardsson, M.; Steineck, G.; Hagman, U.; Rieger, A.; & Norell, S.E. 1990. Physical activity and colon cancer: A case-referent study in Stockholm. *International Journal of Cancer 46*: 985.

11. Gerhardsson, M.; Floderus, B.; & Norell, S.E. 1988. Physical activity and colon cancer risk. *International Journal of Epidemiology 17*: 743.

12. Paffenbarger, R.S., Jr.; Hyde, R.T.; & Wing, A.L. 1987. Physical activity and incidence of cancer in diverse populations: A preliminary report. *American Journal of Clinical Nutrition 45*: 312-17.

13. Vena, J.E.; Graham, S.; Zielezny, M.; Swanson, M.K.; Barnes, R.E.; & Nolan, J. 1985. Lifetime occupational exercise and colon cancer. *American Journal of Epidemiology 122*: 357.

14. Vena, J.E.; Graham, S.; Zielezny, M.; Brasure, J.; & Swanson, M.K.

1987. Occupational exercise and risk of cancer. *American Journal of Clinical Nutrition 45*: 318-27.

15. Wu, A.H.; Paganini-Hill, A.; Ross, R.K.; & Henderson, B.E. 1987. Alcohol, physical activity, and other risk factors for colorectal cancer: A prospective study. *British Journal of Cancer 55*: 687-94.

16. Relative risks were 1.00 for less than 1,000 kilocalories; 0.52 for 1,000 to 2,499 kilocalories; 0.50 for 2,500 or more kilocalories. The relative risks of change were increased physical activity, 0.87; decreased physical activity, 1.02. Paffenbarger, R.S., & Lee, I-M. 1992. The influence of physical activity on the incidence of site-specific cancers in college alumni. In *Exercise, calories, fat, and cancer*, edited by M.M. Jacobs, 7-15. New York: Plenum Press.

17. Walter Willett, of Harvard, says dietary fat is perhaps not a factor, according to findings from his nurses' study.

18. Colditz, G.A.; Hankinson, S.E.; Hunter, D.J.; Willett, W.C.; Stampfer, M.J.; Hennekens, C.; Rosner, B.; & Speizer, F.E. 1995, June 15. The use of estrogens and progestins and the risk of breast cancer in postmenopausal women. *New England Journal of Medicine 332*: 1589-93.

19. Frisch, R.E.; Wyshak, G.; Albright, N.L.; Albright, T.E.; Schiff, I.; Witschi, J.; & Marguglio, M. 1987. Lower lifetime occurrence of breast cancer and cancers of the reproductive system among former college athletes. *American Journal of Clinical Nutrition 45*: 328-35.

20. Caspersen, C.J.; Heath, G.W.; DiPietro, L.; & Yeager, K. 1991. Health effects of physical activity and exercise. Manuscript of American College of Sports Medicine position stand, 5.

21. Some data suggest that leanness is associated with lower risk before menopause, but obesity is associated with lower risk after menopause.

22. Vena, J.E.; Graham, S.; Zielezny, M.; Brasure, J.; & Swanson, M.K. 1987. Occupational exercise and risk of cancer. *American Journal of Clinical Nutrition 45*: 318-27.

23. U.S. Public Health Service. 1988. *Disease prevention, health promotion.* Palo Alto, CA: Bull.

24. Lee, I-M; Paffenbarger, R.S., Jr.; & Hsieh, C-C. 1993. Chronic disease in former college students: XLVI. Physical activity and risk of prostatic cancer among college alumni. *American Journal of Epidemiology 135*: 169-79.

25. The relative risks were 1.00 for less than 1,000 kilocalories; 1.08 for 1,000 to 3,999 kilocalories; 0.53 for greater than 4,000 kilocalories. Paffenbarger, R.S., & Lee, I-M. 1992. The influence of physical activity on the incidence of site-specific cancers in college alumni. In *Exercise, calories, fat, and cancer*, edited by M.M. Jacobs, 7-15. New York: Plenum Press.

26. Whittemore, A.S.; Paffenbarger, R.S., Jr.; Anderson, K.; & Lee, J. 1985. Chronic disease in former college students: XXVII. Early precursors of

site-specific cancers in college men and women. *Journal of the National Cancer Institute 74*: 43.

27. Albanes, D.; Blair, A.; & Taylor, P.R. 1989. Physical activity and risk of cancer in the NHANES I population. *American Journal of Public Health, 79*: 744-50.

28. Paffenbarger, R.S., Jr.; Hyde, R.T.; & Wing, A.L. 1987. Physical activity and incidence of cancer in diverse populations: A preliminary report. *American Journal of Clinical Nutrition 45*: 312-17.

29. Severson, R.K.; Nomura, A.M.Y.; Grove, J.S.; & Stemmermann, G.N. 1989. A prospective analysis of physical activity and cancer. *American Journal of Epidemiology 130*: 522-29.

30. The relative risks were 1.00 for less than 1,000 kilocalories; 0.79 for 1,000 to 2,499 kilocalories; and 0.39 for 2,500 or more kilocalories. From Lee, I-M., & Paffenbarger, R.S., Jr. 1994. Chronic disease in former college students: XLIX. Physical activity and its relation to cancer risk: A prospective study of college alumni. *Medicine and Science in Sports and Exercise 26*: 831-37.

31. Frisch, R.E.; Wyshak, G.; Albright, N.L.; Albright, T.E.; Schiff, I.; Jones, K.P.; Witschi, J.; Shiang, E.; Koff, E.; & Marguglio, M. 1985. Lower prevalence of breast cancer and cancers of the reproductive system among former college athletes compared to non-athletes. *British Journal of Cancer 52*: 885-91.

32. Levi, F.; La Vecchia, C.; Negri, E.; & Franceschi, S. 1993. Selected physical activites and risk of endometrial cancer. *British Journal of Cancer 67*: 846-51.

33. United Kingdom Testicular Cancer Study Group. 1994. Aetiology of testicular cancer: Association with congenital abnormalities, age at puberty, infertility, and exercise. *British Medical Journal 308*: 1393-99.

34. Nieman, D.C. 1994. Exercise, upper respiratory infection, and the immune system. *Medicine and Science in Sports and Exercise 26*: 128-39.

35. Pedersen, B.K., & Ullum, H. 1994. NK cell response to physical activity: Possible mechanisms of action. *Medicine and Science in Sports and Exercise 26*: 140-46.

36. Shephard, R.J. 1991. Physical activity and the immune system. *Canadian Journal of Sports Science. 16*: 169-85.

37. Woods, J.A., & Davis, J.M. 1994. Exercise, monocyte/macrophage function, and cancer. *Medicine and Science in Sports and Exercise 26*: 147-56.

38. Calabrese, L. 1990. Exercise, immunity, cancer, and infection. In *Exercise, fitness, and health*, edited by C. Bouchard, R.J. Shephard, T. Stephens, J.R. Sutton, & B.D. McPherson, 574. Champaign, IL: Human Kinetics.

39. Nieman, D.C. 1994. Exercise, upper respiratory infection, and the immune system. *Medicine and Science in Sports and Exercise 26*: 128-39.

40. Nieman, D.C. 1994. Exercise, upper respiratory infection, and the immune system. *Medicine and Science in Sports and Exercise 26*: 128-39.

41. Pedersen, B.K., & Ullum, H. 1994. NK cell response to physical activity: Possible mechanisms of action. *Medicine and Science in Sports and Exercise 26*: 140-46.

CHAPTER 7: AGING, SOCIAL CONNECTIONS, AND STRESS (PP. 183-203)

1. Marmot, M., & Elliott, P., eds. 1992. *Coronary heart disease epidemiology: From aetiology to public health.* Oxford & New York: Oxford University Press.

2. Berkman, L.F., & Breslow, L. 1983. *Health and ways of living: The Alameda County Study.* New York: Oxford University Press.

3. Carter, H. & Glick, P.C. 1970. Marriage and divorce: A social and economic study. *American Public Health Association, vital and health statistics.* Cambridge, MA: Harvard University Press.

4. Gore, S. 1978. The effect of social support on moderating the health consequences of unemployment. *Journal of Health and Social Behavior 19*: 157-65.

5. Marmot, M., & Elliott, P., eds. 1992. *Coronary heart disease epidemiology: From aetiology to public health.* Oxford & New York: Oxford University Press.

6. Ortmeyer, C.F. 1974. Variations in mortality, morbidity and health care by marital status. In *Mortality and morbidity in the U.S.,* edited by L.L. Erhardt & J.E. Berline. Cambridge, MA: Harvard University Press.

7. Berkman, L.F., & Breslow, L. 1983. *Health and ways of living: The Alameda County Study.* New York: Oxford University Press.

8. Parkes, C.M.; Benjamin, B.; & Fitzgerald, R.F. 1969. Broken heart: A statistical study of increased mortality among widowers. *British Medical Journal I*: 740-43.

9. Pelletier, K.R. 1981. *Longevity, fulfilling our biological potential.* New York: Delacorte Press/Lawrence.

10. Goleman, D. 1992, September 2. Study says anger impairs heart. *New York Times.*

11. Romero, L.M.; Raley-Susman, K.M.; Redish, D.M.; Brooke, S.M.; Sapolsky, R. 1992, November 15. Possible mechanism by which stress accelerates growth of virally derived tumors. *Proceedings of the National Academy of Sciences of the United States 89:* 11084-87.

12. Sapolsky, R.M. 1992. *Stress, the aging brain, and the mechanisms of neuron death.* Cambridge, MA: MIT Press.

13. Sapolsky, R.M. 1994. *Why zebras don't get ulcers: A guide to stress, stress related diseases, and coping.* New York: W.H. Freeman.

14. Landers, D., & Petruzzello, S. 1994. Physical activity, fitness, and anxiety. In *Physical activity, fitness, and health,* edited by C. Bouchard, R.J. Shephard, & T. Stephens. 868-82. Champaign, IL: Human Kinetics.

15. Sapolsky, R.M. 1994. *Why zebras don't get ulcers: A guide to stress, stress related diseases, and coping.* New York: W.H. Freeman.

16. Marmot, M., & Elliott, P., eds. 1992. *Coronary heart disease epidemiology: From aetiology to public health.* Oxford & New York: Oxford University Press.

17. Blair, S.N.; Goodyear, N.N.; Gibbons, L.W.; & Cooper, K.H. 1984. Physical fitness and incidence of hypertension in healthy normotensive men and women. *Journal of the American Medical Association* 252: 487-90.

18. Benson, H. 1975. *The relaxation response.* New York: Morrow.

19. Olsen, E. 1986, August. How running relieves stress. *The Runner,* pp. 38-43, 82.

CHAPTER 8: EXERCISE AND THE MIND (pp. 205-228)

1. College Study data show that among 10,201 alumni who survived through 1988, there were 387 first attacks of physician-diagnosed depression (the figure doesn't include many who were depressed but didn't seek medical help). The rate of cases of depression per 10,000 man-years of observation during the 27 years between 1962, when the first College Study questionnaires went out, and 1988 steadily increased, from 10 cases per 10,000 man-years in the first nine years of observation to 12 to 16 cases in the second, to 18 to 24 cases in the third nine-year increment, as the alumni grew older.

2. Paffenbarger, R.S., Jr.; Lee, I-M.; & Leung, R. 1994. Chronic disease in former college students: LIII. Physical activity and personal characteristics associated with depression and suicide in American college men. In J. Lonnqvist, & T. Sahi, eds., *Acta Psychiatrica Scandinavica* 89 (Suppl. 377): 16-22.

3. Dunn, A.L., & Dishman, R.K. 1991. Exercise and the neurobiology of depression. In J.O. Holloszy, ed., *Exercise and Sports Sciences Reviews* 19: 41-98.

4. Simon, H.B. 1992. *Staying well. Your complete guide to disease prevention.* Boston: Houghton Mifflin.

5. Paffenbarger, R.S., Jr.; Lee, I-M.; & Leung, R. 1994. Chronic disease in former college students: LIII. Physical activity and personal characteristics associated with depression and suicide in American college men. In J.

Lonnqvist, & T. Sahi, eds., *Acta Psychiatrica Scandinavica 89* (Suppl. 377): 16-22.

6. Brown, R., Ramirez, D.E.; & Taub, J.M. 1978, December. The prescription of exercise for depression. *The Physician and Sportsmedicine 6*: 34-45.

7. Greist, J.H.; Klein, M.H.; Eischens, R.R.; & Faris, J.T. 1978, December. Running out of depression. *The Physician and Sportsmedicine 6*: 49-54.

8. Greist, J.H.; Klein, M.H.; Eischens, R.R.; Faris, J.; Gurman, A.S.; & Morgan, W.P. 1979. Running as treatment for depression. *Comprehensive Psychiatry 20*: 41-54.

9. North, T.C.; McCullagh, P.; & Tran, Z.V. 1990. Effect of Exercise on Depression. In K.B. Pandolf and J.O. Holloszy, eds., *Exercise and Sport Sciences Reviews 18*: 379-415.

10. Morgan, W.P. 1994. Physical activity, fitness, and depression. In *Physical activity, fitness, and health,* edited by C. Bouchard, R.J. Shephard, & T. Stephens, 851-67. Champaign, IL: Human Kinetics.

11. Paffenbarger, R.S., Jr.; Lee, I-M.; & Leung, R. 1994. Chronic disease in former college students: LIII. Physical activity and personal characteristics associated with depression and suicide in American college men. In J. Lonnqvist, & T. Sahi, eds., *Acta Psychiatrica Scandinavica 89* (Suppl. 377): 16-22.

12. Raglin, J. 1990. Exercise and mental health: Beneficial and detrimental effects. *Sports Medicine 9* (5): 323-29.

13. Several investigators have begun "mining" the literature of exercise and depression to analyze the conduct of each study in question and to look at trends in results of a variety of studies conducted over time in different places by different investigators. Among the most comprehensive of these "meta-analyses" are W.P. Morgan's own work and that of T.C. North.

14. Fries, J.F., & Crapo, L. 1981. *Vitality and aging.* San Francisco: W.H. Freeman.

15. Shephard, R. 1978. *Physical activity and aging.* Chicago: Croom Helm.

16. Evans, D.A.; Funkenstein, H.H.; Albert, M.S.; Scherr, P.A.; Cook, N.R.; Chown, M.J.; Hebert, L.E.; Hennekens, C.H.; & Taylor, J.O. 1989, November 10. Prevalence of AD in a community population of older persons. *Journal of the American Medical Association 262*: 2551-2556.

17. Scherr, P.A.; Cook, N.R.; Albert, M.S.; Funkenstein, H.H.; Smith, L.A.; Hebert, L.E.; Wetle, T.T.; Branch, L.G.; Chown, M.J.; Hennekens, C.A.; & Taylor, J.O. 1990. Level of formal education may be a risk factor for Alzheimers Disease. New York: The Milbank Memorial Fund.

18. Diamond, M. 1993, March 12. Lecture, *Successful Aging.* University of California-Berkeley.

19. Katzman, R. 1993, January. Education and the prevalence of dementia and Alzheimer's disease. *Neurology 43*: 13-20.

20. Hatfield, B.; Slater, B.A.; SantaMaria, D.L.; & Krotz, A.J. 1992. Aerobic training is associated with increased central nervous system efficiency in older trained males [Abstract of a paper presented at the meeting of the North American society for the Psychology of Sport and Physical Activity, Pittsburgh, PA.]

21. Dustman, R. 1992, August 15. Telephone interview with E. Olsen (co-author).

22. Dustman, R.E.; Ruhling, R.O.; Russell, E.M.; Shearer, D.E.; Bonekat, H.W.; Shigeoka, J.W.; Wood, J.S.; & Bradford, D.C. 1984. Aerobic exercise training and improved neuropsychological function of older individuals. *Neurobiology of Aging 5*: 35-42.

23. Dustman, R.E.; Emmerson, R.; & Shearer, D.E. 1990. Electrophysiology and aging: Slowing, inhibition, and aerobic fitness. In *Cognitive and behavioral performance factors in atypical aging*, edited by M.L. Howe, M.J. Stones, & C.J. Brainerd, 103-49. New York: Springer-Verlag.

24. Dustman, R.; Emmerson, R.Y.; Ruhling, R.O.; Shearer, D.E.; Steinhous, L.A.; Johnson, S.C.; Bonekat, H.W.; & Shigeoka, J.W. 1990, May-June. Age and fitness effects on EEG, ERPs, visual sensitivity, and cognition. *Neurobiology of Aging 11*: 193-200.

25. Simon, H.B. 1992. *Staying well. Your complete guide to disease prevention*. Boston: Houghton Mifflin.

26. Dunn, A.L., & Dishman, R.K. 1991. Exercise and the neurobiology of depression. In *Exercise and Sports Sciences Reviews, edited by J.O. Holloszy, 19*: 41-98.

27. Sasco, A.; Paffenbarger, R.S., Jr.; Gendre, I.; & Wing, A.L. 1992, April. The role of physical exercise in the occurrence of Parkinson's Disease. *Archives of Neurology 49*: 360-65.

28. MacRae, P.G.; Spirduso, W.W.; Walters, T.J.; Farrar, R.P.; & Wilcox, R.E. 1987. Endurance training effects on striatal D2 dopamine receptor binding and striatal dopamine metabolites in presenescent older rats. *Psychopharmacology 92*: 236-40.

29. MacRae, P.G. Spirduso, W.W.; Cartee, G.D.; Farrar. R.P.; & Wilcox, R.E. 1987. Endurance training effects on striatal D2 dopamine receptor binding and striatal dopamine metabolite levels. *Neuroscience Letters 79*: 138-44.

30. Spirduso, W. 1992, August 19. Telephone interview with E. Olsen (coauthor).

31. Dustman, R.E.; Emmerson, R.; & Shearer, D.E. 1990. Electrophysiology and aging: Slowing, inhibition, and aerobic fitness. In *Cognitive and behavioral performance factors in atypical aging*, edited by M.L. Howe, M.J. Stones, & C.J. Brainerd, 103-49. New York: Springer-Verlag.

32. Black, J. 1992, August 2. Telephone interview with E. Olsen (coauthor).

33. Morgan, W.P. 1994. Physical activity, fitness, and depression. In *Physical activity, fitness, and health*, edited by C. Bouchard, R.J. Shephard, & T. Stephens, 851-67. Champaign, IL: Human Kinetics.

CHAPTER 9: FIGURING IT OUT (pp. 231-266)

1. Åstrand, P-O., & Rodahl, K. 1970. *Textbook of work physiology*. New York: McGraw-Hill.

2. Lee I-M., & Paffenbarger, R.S., Jr. 1992. Chronic disease in former college students: LI. Change in body weight and longevity. *Journal of the American Medical Association 268*: 2045-49.

3. Csikszentmihalyi, M. 1991. Leisure and self-actualization. In *Benefits of leisure*, edited by B.L. Driver, P.J. Brown, & G.L. Peterson, 95. State College, PA: Venture.

4. Knapp, D.N. 1988. Behavioral management techniques and exercise promotion. In *Exercise adherence: Its impact on public health*, edited by R.K. Dishman, 203-35. Champaign, IL: Human Kinetics.

5. Leonard, G. 1974. *The ultimate athlete*. New York: Avon Books. 5.

CHAPTER 10: PUTTING IT TOGETHER (pp. 267-303)

1. Hatano, Y. 1993, Summer. Use of the pedometer for promoting daily walking exercise. *International Council on Health, Physical Education and Recreation*, pp. 4-8.

2. Myers, D. 1992. *Pursuit of happiness: Discovering the pathway to fulfillment*. New York: Avon.

3. The "marathon hypothesis" was first proposed over 20 years ago in a letter to the editor of the *Lancet*. This was the notion that running a marathon confers absolute protection against death from CHD. Run a marathon and you'll never have a heart attack. Never. Of course, this was all before marathoner and author Jim Fixx had his fatal heart attack, and well before science caught up with enthusiasm. Later refined, the hypothesis suggests that if you could train for a marathon, and if you adopted the sort of lifestyle necessary to train for a marathon, you were immune from a heart attack. This somewhat more generous refinement meant you didn't actually have to run a marathon as long as you did the requisite training and lived the requisite lifestyle; actually completing a marathon, then, was simply a vivid indication you'd done all the right things. Still, the idea was essentially the same: Run an awful lot and you'll never have a heart attack, and the message left too many with the idea that anything less than training for or completing a marathon was futile. And the result was that many reasonable and well-intentioned men and women went out onto the jogging trails and promptly ran themselves into overuse injuries, or at least into a profound distaste for sweat and exertion.

4. Hatano, Y. 1993, Summer. Use of the pedometer for promoting daily walking exercise. *International Council on Health, Physical Education and Recreation,* pp. 4-8.

5. Wilmore, J. 1994. Interview with E. Olsen (coauthor), American College of Sports Medicine Conference, Indianapolis, IN.

6. Pearl, B., & Moran, G.T. 1986. *Getting stronger.* Bolinas, CA: Shelter.

7. Brennan, B.A. 1988. *Hands of light.* New York: Bantam Books.

8. Capra, F. 1983. *The turning point.* New York: Bantam Books.

9. Eisenberg, D. 1987. *Encounters with Qi.* New York: Penguin Books.

10. Lee, M.; Lee, E.; & Johnson, J. 1989. *Ride the tiger to the mountain: T'ai Chi for health.* Reading, MA: Addison Wesley.

11. Siu, R.G.H. 1974. *Ch'i—a neo-Taoist approach to life.* Cambridge, MA: MIT.

12. Ha, C.F., & Olsen, E. In progress. *The nature of energy: Perspectives on Ch'i.*

13. Lee, M.; Lee, E.; & Johnson, J. 1989. *Ride the tiger to the mountain: T'ai Chi for health.* Reading, MA: Addison Wesley.

14. Anderson, B. 1980. *Stretching.* Bolinas, CA: Shelter Publications.

CHAPTER I I: FOR THE LONG HAUL: SENSIBLE TRAINING, SENSIBLE LIVING (pp. 305-340)

1. Budgett, R. 1994, August 13. The overtraining syndrome. *British Medical Journal 309:* 464-68.

2. Noakes, T. 1991. *Lore of running.* Champaign, IL: Human Kinetics, p. 425.

3. Paffenbarger, R.S.; Hyde, R.T.; Wing, A.L.; & Hsieh, C.-C. 1986. Physical activity, all-cause mortality, and longevity of college alumni. *New England Journal of Medicine 314* (10): 605-12.

4. Rowe, W. 1992, September 19. Extraordinary unremitting endurance exercise and permanent injury to the normal heart. *Lancet 340:* 712-14.

5. Hein, H.O.; Suadicani, P.; Sorensen, H.; & Gyntelberg, F. 1994. Changes in physical activity level and risk of ischaemic heart disease. *Scandinavian Journal of Medicine & Science in Sports 4:* 52-64.

6. Lakka, T.; Venalainen, J.M.; Rauramaa, R.; Salonen, R.; Tuomilehto, J.; & Salonen, J. 1994, June 2. Relation of leisure-time physical activity and cardiorespiratory fitness to the risk of acute myocardial infarction in men. *New England Journal of Medicine 330:* 1549-54.

7. Mittleman, M.; Maclure, M.; Tofler, G.; Sherwood, J.B.; Goldberg, R.J.; & Muller, J.E. 1993. Triggering of acute MI by heavy physical exertion. *New England Journal of Medicine 329* (23): 1677-1731.

8.   Wannamethee, G., & Shaper, A.G. 1992, March 7. Physical activity and stroke in British middle-aged men. *British Medical Journal 304*: 597-601.

9.   Lee, I-M. 1994. Physical activity, fitness, and cancer. In *Physical activity, fitness, and health,* edited by C. Bouchard, R. Shephard, & T. Stephens, 814-31. Champaign, IL: Human Kinetics.

10.   Simon, H. 1990. Discussion: Exercise, immunity, cancer, and infection. In *Exercise, fitness, and health,* edited by C. Bouchard, R.J. Shepard, T. Stephens, J.R. Sutton & B.D. McPherson, 581-88. Champaign, IL: Human Kinetics.

11.   Kohl, H.W.; Powell, K.E.; Gordon, N.F.; Blair, S.N.; & Paffenbarger, R.S. 1992. Physical activity, physical fitness and sudden cardiac death. *Epidemiologic Reviews 14*: 37-58.

12.   Vuori, I. 1986. The cardiovascular risks of physical activity. *Acta Medica Scandinavica 711* (Suppl.): 205-14.

13.   Thompson, P. 1992, May 27. Athletes, athletics and sudden cardiac death. Symposium: Exercise, Physical Activity and Sudden Death: the Cardiac Conundrum, American College of Sports Medicine annual meeting, Dallas, TX.

14.   Rich, B., MD. 1992, June 2. Telephone interview with E. Olsen (coauthor).

15.   Lawrence, R., MD. 1992, June 5. Telephone interview with E. Olsen (coauthor).

16.   Olsen, E. 1990, February. The critical juncture. *Runner's World,* pp. 38-43.

17.   Olsen, E. 1993, May. The wounded knee. *Running Times,* pp. 29-33.

18.   Olsen, E. 1984, December. A real pain in the. . . . *The Runner,* pp. 72-79.

19.   Olsen, E. 1990, June. Watch your back. *Men's Health,* pp. 82-83.

20.   Plato, 1989. *Laws,* VII, 803d. In *Plato: the Collected Dialogues,* edited by E. Hamilton and H. Cairns. Princeton, NJ: Bollingen Series.

additional resources

Aloia, J.F.; Vaswani, A.N.; Yeh, J.; & Cohn, S.H. 1988. Premenopausal bone mass is related to physical activity. *Archives of Internal Medicine 148:* 121-23.

Aneshensel, C.S. 1985. The natural history of depressive symptoms: Implications for psychiatric epidemiology. In *Research in Community and Mental Health*, edited by J.R. Greenley, 47-75. Greenwich, CT: JAI Press.

Bailey, B.K., & Jones, S.S. 1994, August. 10 ways to increase metabolism. *Let's Live*, pp. 18-21.

Ballard-Barbash, R.; Schatzkin, A.; Albanes, D.; Schiffman, M.H.; Kreger, B.E.; Kannel, W.B.; Anderson, K.M.; & Helsel, W.E. 1990. Physical activity and risk of large bowel cancer in the Framingham Study. *Cancer Research 50:* 3610.

Baltes, P.B. 1993, October. The aging mind: Potential and limits. *Gerontologist 33:* 580-94.

Baltes, P.B., & Staudinger, U.M. 1993, June. The search for a psychology of wisdom. *Current Directions in Psychological Science 2:* 75-80.

Begley, S., with Hager, M., & Murr, A. 1990, March 5. The search for the fountain of youth. *Newsweek 115:*44-53.

Beloc, N.B., & Breslow, L. 1972, August. The relation of physical health status and health practices. *Preventive Medicine 1:* 409-21.

Beloc, N.B., & Breslow, L. 1973. Relationship of health practices and mortality. *Preventive Medicine 2:* 67-81.

Benfante, R.J.; Reed, D.M.; MacLean, C.J.; & Yano, K. 1989. Risk factors in middle age that predict early and late onset of coronary heart disease. *Journal of Clinical Epidemiology 42:* 95-104.

Blair, S.N.; Kohl, H.W., III; Barlow, C.E.; Paffenbarger, R.S., Jr.; Gibbons, L.W.; & Macera, C.A. 1995. Changes in physical fitness and all-cause mortality: A prospective study of healthy and unhealthy men. *Journal of the American Medical Association 273:* 1093-98.

Blair, S.N.; Kohl, H.W., III; Gordon, N.F.; & Paffenbarger, R.S., Jr. 1992. How much physical activity is good for health? *Annual Review of Public Health 13:* 99-126.

Blomqvist, C.G., & Saltin, B. 1983. Cardiovascular adaptations to physical training. *Annual Review of Physiology 45:* 169-89.

Bortz, W.M., II. 1993, September. The physics of frailty. *Journal of the American Geriatrics Society 41*: 1004-8.

Bouchard, C.; Shephard, R.J.; & Stephens, T., eds. 1994. *Physical activity, fitness, and health.* Champaign, IL: Human Kinetics.

Brickman, J.B., & Rodgers, T.A. 1988. Exercise in psychiatry. In *Exercise in the practice of medicine,* 2nd rev. ed., edited by G.F. Fletcher, 429-38. Mount Kisco, NY: Futura.

Brownson, R.C.; Zahm, S.H.; Chang, J.C.; & Blair, A. 1989. Occupational risk of colon cancer. An analysis by anatomic subsite. *American Journal of Epidemiology 130*: 675.

Bunker, J.B.; Gomby, P.S.; & Kehrer, B.H. 1989. *Pathways to health: The role of social factors.* Menlo Park, CA: Henry J. Kaiser Foundation.

Butler, R.N.; Ahronheim, J.; Fillit, H.; Rapoport, S.I. 1994, January. Vascular dementia: An updated approach to patient management (part 3) (Panel Discussion). *Geriatrics 49*: 39-44.

Callahan, D. 1987. *Setting limits: Medical goals in an aging society.* New York: Simon & Schuster.

Camacho, T.C.; Roberts, R.E.; Lazarus, N.B.; Kaplan, G.A.; & Cohen, R.D. 1991. Physical activity and depression: Evidence from the Alameda County Study. *American Journal of Epidemiology 134*: 220-31.

Caspersen, C.J.; Bloemberg, B.P.M.; Saris, W.H.M.; Merritt, R.K.; & Kromhout, D. 1991. The prevalence of selected physical activities and their relation with coronary heart disease risk factors in elderly men: The Zutphen Study, 1985. *American Journal of Epidemiology 133*: 1078-92.

Cassel, C.K.; Rudberg, M.A.; & Olshansky, S.J. 1992, Summer. The price of success: Health care in an aging society. *Health Affairs.* 87-99.

Chave, S.P.W.; Morris, J.N.; Moss, S.; & Semmence, A.M. 1978. Vigorous exercise and the death rate: A study of male civil servants. *Journal of Epidemiology & Community Health 32*: 239-43.

Clausen, J.P. 1977. Effect of physical training on cardiovascular adjustments to exercise in man. *Physiological Reviews 57*: 779-815.

Cooper, K.H. 1968. *Aerobics.* New York: Evans.

Cooper, K.H. 1982. *The aerobics program for total well-being.* New York: Evans.

Cooper, K.H. 1985. *Running without fear.* New York: Evans.

Csikszentmihalyi, M. 1990. *Flow.* New York: Harper Perennial.

Cummings, S.R.; Kelsey, J.L.; Nevitt, M.C.; & O'Dowd, K.J. 1985. Epidemiology of osteoporosis and osteoporotic fractures. *Epidemiologic Reviews 7*: 178-208.

Curfman, G.D. 1993. The health benefits of exercise: A critical reappraisal. *New England Journal of Medicine 328*: 574-76.

Delaney, L. 1995, March. A hotter furnace: How to rev up your calorie burn. *Men's Journal,* p. 102.

Dishman, R.K. 1994, *Advances in exercise adherence*. Champaign, IL: Human Kinetics.

Donahue, R.P.; Abbott, R.D.; Reed, D.M.; & Yano, K. 1988. Physical activity and coronary heart disease in middle-aged and elderly men: The Honolulu Heart Program. *American Journal of Public Health 78*: 683-5.

Drinkwater, B.L. 1989. Assessing fitness and activity patterns of women in general population studies. In *Assessing physical fitness and physical activity in population-based surveys*, edited by T. Drury, 261-71. DHHS pub. no. (PHS) 89-1253. Washington, D.C.: U.S. Government Printing Office.

Driver, B.L; Brown, P.J.; & Peterson, G.L., eds. 1991. *Benefits of leisure*. State College, PA: Venture.

Duncan, J.J.; Farr, J.E.; Upton, S.J.; Hagan, R.D.; Oglesby, M.E.; & Blair, S.N. 1985. The effects of aerobic exercise on plasma catecholamines and blood pressure in patients with mild essential hypertension. *Journal of the American Medical Association 254*: 2609-13.

Dustman, R.; Emmerson, R.; & Shearer, D. 1994. Physical activity, age, and cognitive-neuropsychological function. *Journal of Aging and Physical Activity 2*: 143-81.

Dychtwald, K. 1989, February-April. Old age evangelist. In *Special report on health*, edited by K. Bellows, 42-47. Knoxville, TN: Whittle Communications.

Ekelund, L.-G.; Haskell, W.L.; Johnson, J.L.; Whaley, F.S.; Criqui, M.H.; & Sheps, D.S. 1988. Physical fitness as a predictor of cardiovascular mortality in asymptomatic North American men: The Lipid Research Clinics Mortality Follow-up Study. *New England Journal of Medicine 319*: 1379-84.

Eysenk, H.J. 1992, August 22. Psychosocial factors, cancer and ischaemic heart disease. *British Medical Journal 305*:457-59

Farmer, M.E.; Locke, B.Z.; Mosciki, E.K.; Dannenberg, A.L.; Larson, D.B.; & Radloff, L.S. 1988. Physical activity and depressive symptoms: The NHANES I epidemiologic follow-up study. *American Journal of Epidemiology 128*: 1340-51.

Fiatarone, M.A.; O'Neill, E.F.; Ryan, N.D.; Clements, K.M.; Solares, G.R.; Nelson, M.E.; Roberts, S.B.; Keyayias, J.J.; Lipsitz, L.A.; & Evans, W.J. 1994, June 23. Exercise training and nutritional supplementation for physical frailty in very elderly people. *New England Journal of Medicine 330*: 1769-75.

Fischbach, G.D. 1992, September. Mind and brain: The biological foundations of consciousness, memory and other attributes of mind have begun to emerge; an overview of this most profound of all research efforts. *Scientific American 267*: 48-57.

Fletcher, G.F.; Blair, S.N.; Blumenthal J.; Caspersen, C.; Chaitman, B.; Epstein, S.; Falls, H.; Froelicher, E.S.; Froelicher, V.F.; & Pina, I.L. 1992. Statement on exercise: Benefits and recommendations for physical activity programs for all Americans: A statement for health professionals by the Committee on

Exercise and Cardiac Rehabilitation of the Council on Clinical Cardiology, American Heart Association. *Circulation 86*: 340-44.

Folkins, C.H., & Sime, W.E. 1981. Physical fitness training and mental health. *American Psychology 36*: 373-89.

Fredriksson, M.; Bengtsson, N.O.; Hardell, L.; & Axelson, O. 1989. Colon cancer, physical activity, and occupational exposures: A case-control study. *Cancer 63*: 1838.

Fries, J.F. 1990. The compression of morbidity: Near or far? *Milbank Quarterly 67*: 208-32.

Fries, J.F.; Green, L.W.; & Levine, S. 1989. Health promotion and the compression of morbidity. *Lancet 1*: 481-83.

Fuster, V.; Badimon, L.; Badimon, J.J.; & Chesebro, J.H. 1992. The pathogenesis of coronary artery disease and the acute coronary syndromes. *New England Journal of Medicine 326*: 242-50, 310-18.

Godber, G. 1991. Is longevity desirable? *British Medical Journal 302*: 1095-96.

Gordon, D.J., & Rifkind, B.M. 1989. High-density lipoprotein—the clinical implications of recent studies. *New England Journal of Medicine 321*: 1311-16.

Gortmaker, S.L; Must, A.; Perrin, J.N.; Sobol, A.M.; Dietz, W.H. 1993, September 30. Social and economic consequences of overweight in adolescence and young adulthood. *New England Journal of Medicine 329*: 1008-12.

Greenberg, L.J., & Yunis, E.J. 1978, April. Histocompatibility determinants, immune responsiveness and aging in man. *Federal Proceedings*. 1248-62.

Gunby, P. 1994, November 23/30. Graying of America stimulates more research on aging-associated factors. *Journal of the American Medical Association 272*: 1561-66.

Guralnik, J.M., & Kaplan, G.A. 1989. Predictors of healthy aging: Prospective evidence from the Alameda County Study. *American Journal of Public Health 79* (6): 703-8.

Guy, W.A. 1983. Contributions to a knowledge of the influence of employments upon health. *Journal of the Royal Statistical Society 6*: 197-211.

Gyntelberg, F.; Lauridsen, L.; & Schubell, K. 1980. Physical fitness and risk of myocardial infarction in Copenhagen males aged 40-59. *Scandinavian Journal of Work, Environment & Health 6*: 170-78.

Hahn, R.A.; Teutsch, S.M.; Rothenberg, R.B.; & Marks, J.S. 1990. Excess deaths from nine chronic diseases in the United States. *Journal of the American Medical Association 264*: 2654-59.

Hambrecht, R.; Niebauer, J.; Marburger, C.; Grunz, M.; Kalberer, B.; Hauer, K.; Schlierf, G.; Kubler, W.; & Schuler, G. 1993. Various intensities of leisure time physical activity in patients with coronary artery disease: Effects on cardio-respiratory fitness and progression of coronary atherosclerotic lesions. *Journal of the American College of Cardiology 22*: 468-77.

Harvard Medical School. 1992, January. Stress: The "Type A" hypothesis. *Harvard Heart Letter* 2: 1-4.

Harvard Medical School. 1992, August. Alzheimer's disease—Part I. *The Harvard Mental Health Letter* 9: 1-4.

Harvard Medical School. 1994, October. Understanding risk: A tricky business. *Harvard Health Letter* (Special suppl.): 9-12.

Haskell, W.L.; Leon, S.A.; Caspersen, C.J.; Froelicher, V.F.; Hagberg, J.M.; & Harlan, W. 1992. Cardiovascular benefits and assessment of physical activity and physical fitness in adults. *Medicine and Science in Sports and Exercise* 24 (6 Suppl.): S201-S220.

Hatfield, B. 1991. Exercise and mental health: The mechanisms of exercise-induced psychological states. In *Psychology of sports, exercise, and fitness: Social and personal issues*, edited by L. Diamant, 17-49. New York: Hemisphere.

Hatfield, B.; Landers, D.M.; & Ray, W.J. 1987, September. Cardiovascular-CNS interactions during a self-paced, intentional attentive state: Elite marksmanship performance. *Psychophysiology* 24: 542-49.

Hatziandreu, E.L.; Koplan, J.P.; Weinstein, M.C.; Caspersen, C.J.; & Warner, K.E. 1988. A cost-effectiveness analysis of exercise as a health promotion activity. *American Journal of Public Health* 78: 1417-21.

Hedley, O.F. 1939. Analysis of 5,116 deaths reported as due to acute coronary occlusion in Philadelphia, 1933-1936. *Public Health Reports* 54: 972 ff.

Herring, J.L.; Molè, P.A.; Meredith, C.N.; & Stern, J.S. 1992. Effect of suspending exercise training on resting metabolic rate in women. *Medicine and Science in Sports and Exercise* 24: 59-65.

Higdon. H. 1984, November. Jim Fixx: How he lived, why he died. *The Runner*, pp. 32-38.

Hill, A.B. 1971. *Principles of medical statistics*, 9th ed. New York: Oxford University Press.

Hughes, J.F. 1984. Psychological effects of habitual aerobic exercise: A critical review. *Preventive Medicine* 13: 66-78.

Huizinga, J. 1955. *Homo ludens: A study of the play element in culture*. Boston: Beacon Press.

Johns Hopkins Medical Institutions. 1991, April. Seeking the ultimate cure. *Health After 50: The Johns Hopkins Medical Letter* 3: 1-6.

Kaplan, G.A.; Roberts, R.E.; Camacho, T.C.; & Coyne, J.C. 1987. Psychological predictors of depression: Prospective evidence from the Human Population Laboratory Studies. *American Journal of Epidemiology* 125: 206-20.

Karvonen, M.J. 1982. Physical activity in work and leisure time in relation to cardiovascular diseases. *Annals of Clinical Research* 34 (Suppl. 14): 118-23.

Karvonen, M.J. 1989. Determinants of cardiovascular diseases in the elderly. *Annals of Medicine* 21: 3-12.

Katzman, R., & Kawas, C. 1994. The epidemiology of dementia and Alzheimer disease. In *Alzheimer disease,* edited by R.D. Terry, R. Katzman, & K.L. Bick, 105-22. New York: Raven Press.

Kendrick, J.S.; Williamson, D.F.; & Caspersen, C.J. 1991. Letter to the editor re: "A meta-analysis of physical activity in the prevention of coronary heart disease." *American Journal of Epidemiology 134*: 232-34.

Kestin, A.S.; Ellis, P.A.; Barnard, M.R.; Errichetti, A.; Rosner, B.A.; & Michelson, A.D. 1993. Effect of strenuous exercise on platelet activation state and reactivity. *Circulation 88*: 1502-11.

King, A.C. 1991. Mini-series: Exercise and aging. *Annals of Behavioral Medicine 13*: 87-90.

Knowles, J., ed. 1977. *Doing better and feeling worse: Health in the United States.* New York: W.W. Norton.

Lee, I-M. 1995, June. Physical activity and cancer. *Physical activity and fitness research digest.* Washington D.C.: President's Council on Physical Fitness and Sports, Department of Health and Human Services.

Lee, I-M., & Paffenbarger, R.S. 1992. Change in body weight and longevity (from manuscript, Report No. LI in College Study series).

Lee, I-M.; Paffenbarger, R.S., Jr.; & Hsieh, C-C. 1991. Chronic disease in former college students: XLIV. Physical activity and risk of colorectal cancer among college alumni. *Journal of the National Cancer Institute 83:* 1324.

Levy, B., & Langer, E. 1994, June. Aging free from negative stereotypes: Successful memory in China and among the American deaf (Attitudes and Social Cognition). *Journal of Personality and Social Psychology 66*: 989-97.

Lie, H.; Mundal, R.; & Erikssen, J. 1985. Coronary risk factors and incidence of coronary death in relation to physical fitness: Seven-year follow-up study of middle-aged and elderly men. *European Heart Journal 6*: 147-57.

Light, K.E., & Spirduso, W.W. 1990, May. Effects of adult aging on the movement complexity factor of response programming. *Journal of Gerontology 45*: 107-9.

Lin, N., & Ensel, W.M. 1984. Depression-mobility and its social etiology: The role of life events and social support. *Journal of Health and Social Behavior 25*: 176-88.

Macauley, D.A. 1994. History of physical activity, health and medicine. *Journal of the Royal Society of Medicine 87*: 32-35.

Manson, J.E.; Nathan, D.M.; Krolewski, A.S.; Stampfer, M.J.; Willett, W.C.; & Hennekins, C.H. 1992. A prospective study of exercise and incidence of diabetes among U.S. male physicians. *Journal of the American Medical Association 268*: 63-67.

Marans, R.W., & Mohaim, P. 1991. Leisure resources, recreation activity, and the quality of life. In *Benefits of leisure,* edited by B.L. Driver, P.J. Brown, & G.L. Peterson, 351-364. State College, PA: Venture.

Mayo Foundation for Medical Education and Research. 1994, June. Exercise:

Are the risks underplayed and the benefits overdone? *Mayo Clinic Health Letter 12*:1-3.

McGinnis, J.M., & Foege, W.H. 1993. Actual causes of death in the United States. *Journal of the American Medical Association 270* (18): 2207-12.

Miettinen, O.S. 1974. Proportion of disease caused or prevented by a given exposure, trait or intervention. *American Journal of Epidemiology 99*: 325-32.

Montoye, H.J. 1992. The Raymond Pearl Memorial Lecture, 1991: Health, exercise, and athletics: A millenium of observations—a century of research. *American Journal of Human Biology 4*: 69-82.

Montoye, H.J.; Van Huss, W.D.; Olson, H.W.; Pierson, W.R.; & Hudec, A.J. 1957. *The longevity and morbidy of college athletes.* Lansing, MI: Michigan State University.

Moore, T.J. 1993. *Lifespan: Who lives longer and why.* New York: Simon and Schuster.

Morgan, J.E. 1873. *University oars.* London: MacMillan

Morgan, W.P. 1982. Psychological effects of exercise. *Behavioral Medicine Update 4*: 25-30.

Morgan, W.P. 1992, May 28. Psychological outcomes of physical activity: The bright and dark sides. Lecture at the American College of Sports Medicine, Dallas, TX.

Morgan, W.P., & O'Connor, P.J. 1988. Exercise and mental health. In *Exercise adherence: Its impact on public health,* edited by R.K. Dishman, 91-121. Champaign, IL: Human Kinetics.

Morris, J.N.; Chave, S.P.W.; Adam, C.; Sirey, C.; Epstein, L.; & Sheehan, D.J. 1973. Vigorous exercise in leisure-time and the incidence of coronary heart disease. *Lancet i*: 333-39.

Morris, J.N.; Everitt, M.G.; Pollard, R.; Chave, S.P.W.; & Semmence, A.M. 1980. Vigorous exercise in leisure-time: Protection against coronary heart-disease. *Lancet ii*: 1207-10.

Morris, J.N.; Heady, J.A.; Raffle, P.A.B.; Roberts, C.G.; & Parks, J.W. 1953. Coronary heart disease and physical activity of work. *Lancet ii*: 1053-57, 1111-20.

Morris, J.N.; Kagan, A.; Pattison, D.C.; Gardner, M.; & Raffle, P.A.B. 1966. Incidence and prediction of ischaemic heart disease in London busmen. *Lancet ii*: 552-59.

Moss, M.B., & Albert, M.S. 1988. Alzheimer's disease and other dementing disorders. In *Geriatric neuropsychology,* edited by M.S. Albert & M.B. Moss, 145-78. New York: Guilford Press.

Newmann, J.P. 1989. Aging and depression. *Psychology and Aging 4*: 150-65.

Noakes, T.D.; Higginson, L.; & Opie, L.H. 1983. Physical training increases ventricular fibrillation thresholds of isolated rat hearts during normoxia, hypoxia, and regional ischemia. *Circulation 67*: 24-30.

Office of Disease Prevention and Health Promotion. 1988. *Disease prevention/ health promotion.* Palo Alto, CA: Bull.

Olsen, E. 1980, October. Running through the blues. *The Runner,* pp. 50-60.

Olsen, E. 1992, October. Pain: Why it hurts. *Running Times,* pp. 30-34.

Ornish, D. 1993. *Eat more, weigh less: Dr. Dean Ornish's Life Choice Program for losing weight safely while eating abundantly.* New York: HarperCollins.

Oster, G.; Colditz, G.A.; & Kelly, N.L. 1984. The economic costs of smoking and benefits of quitting for individual smokers. *Preventive Medicine 13*: 377-89.

Paffenbarger, R.S., Jr. 1988. Chronic disease in former college students: XXXV. Contributions of epidemiology to exercise and cardiovascular health. *Medicine and Science in Sports and Exercise 20*: 426-38.

Paffenbarger, R.S., Jr. 1994. Chronic disease in former college students: LVIII. Forty years of progress: Physical activity, health, and fitness. *American College of Sports Medicine 40th Anniversary Lectures:* 93-109.

Paffenbarger, R.S., Jr., & Asnes, D.P. 1966. Chronic disease in former college students: III. Precursors of suicide in early and middle life. *American Journal of Public Health 56*: 1026-36.

Paffenbarger, R.S., Jr.; Brand, R.J.; Sholtz, R.I.; & Jung D.L. 1978. Energy expenditure, cigarette smoking, and blood pressure level as related to death from specific diseases. *American Journal of Epidemiology 108*: 12-18.

Paffenbarger, R.S., Jr., & Hale, W.E. 1975. Work activity and coronary heart mortality. *New England Journal of Medicine 292*: 545-50.

Paffenbarger, R.S., Jr.; Hyde, R.T.; Wing, A.L.; Lee, I-M.; & Kampert, J.B. 1994. Chronic disease in former college students: L. Some interrelationships of physical activity, physiological fitness, health, and longevity. In *Physical activity, fitness, and health,* edited by C. Bouchard, R.J. Shephard, & T. Stephens, 119-33. Champaign, IL: Human Kinetics.

Paffenbarger, R.S., Jr.; Hyde, R.T.; Wing, A.L.; & Steinmetz, C.H. 1984. Chronic disease in former college students: XXV. A natural history of athleticism and cardiovascular health. *Journal of the American Medical Associaton 252*: 491-95.

Paffenbarger, R.S., Jr.; Jung, D.L.; Leung, R.W.; & Hyde, R.T. 1991. Chronic disease in former college students: XXXIX. Physical activity and hypertension: An epidemiological view. *Annals of Medicine 23*: 319-27.

Paffenbarger, R.S., Jr.; King, S.H.; & Wing, A.L. 1969. Chronic disease in former college students: IX. Characteristics in youth that predispose to suicide and accidental death in later life. *American Journal of Public Health 59*: 900-8.

Paffenbarger, R.S., & Lee, I-M. In press. Exercise and fitness in the primary prevention of coronary heart disease. In *Prevention of myocardial infarction,* edited by J.E. Manson, P.M. Ridker, J.M. Graziano, & C.H. Hennekens. Columbia, MD: Bermedica Production, Ltd.

Paffenbarger, R.S., Jr.; Lee, I-M; & Leung, R. 1984. Physical activity and personal characteristics associated with depression and suicide in American college men. In J. Lonnqvist & T. Sahi, eds., *Acta Psychiatrica Scandinavica 89* (Suppl. 37): 16-22.

Paffenbarger, R.S., Jr.; Notkin, J.; Krueger, D.E.; Wolf, P.A.; Thorne, M.C.; LeBauer, E.J. 1966. Chronic disease in former college students: II. Methods of study and observations on mortality from coronary heart disease. *American Journal of Public Health 56*: 962-71.

Paffenbarger, R.S., Jr., & Wing, A.L. 1969. Chronic disease in former college students: X. The effects of single and multiple characteristics on risk of fatal coronary heart disease. *American Journal of Epidemiology 90*: 527-35.

Paffenbarger, R.S., Jr.; Wing, A.L.; & Hyde, R.T. 1978. Chronic disease in former college students: XVI. Physical activity as an index of heart attack risk in college alumni. *American Journal of Epidemiology 108*: 161-75.

Paffenbarger, R.S., Jr.; Wing, A.L.; Hyde, R.T.; & Jung, D.L. 1983. Chronic disease in former college students: XX. Physical activity and incidence of hypertension in college alumni. *American Journal of Epidemiology 117*: 245-57.

Paffenbarger, R.S., Jr.; Wolf, P.A.; Notkin, J.; & Thorne, M.C. 1966. Chronic disease in former college students: I. Early precursors of fatal coronary heart disease. *American Journal of Epidemiology 83*: 314-28.

Park, R.J., & McCloy, C.H. 1989. Research lecture: Health, exercise, and the biomedical impulse, 1870-1914. *Research Quarterly for Exercise and Sport 61*: 126-40.

Perlman, D. 1993, November 10. Lifestyle factors called biggest killers. *San Francisco Chronicle*.

Péronnet, F.; Cléoux, J.; Perrault, H.; Coustinearu, D.; de Champian, J.; & Nadeau, R. 1981. Plasma norepinephrine response to exercise before and after training in humans. *Journal of Applied Physiology 51*: 812-15.

Peters, R.K.; Cady, L.D., Jr.; Bischoff, D.P.; Bernstein, L.; & Pike, M.C. 1983. Physical fitness and subsequent myocardial infarction in healthy workers. *Journal of the American Medical Association 249*: 3052-56.

Peters, R.K.; Garabrant, D.Y.; Yu, M.C.; & Mack, T.M. 1989. A case-control study of occupational and dietary factors in colorectal cancer in young men by subsite. *Cancer Research 49*: 5459.

Powell, D.H., & Whitla, D.K. 1994. *Profiles in cognitive aging*. Cambridge, MA: Harvard University Press.

Powell, D.H., & Whitla, D.K. 1994, February. Normal cognitive aging: Toward empirical perspectives. *Current Directions in Psychological Science 3*: 27-31.

Ramazzini, B. 1940. *Diseases of workers*. Translated from the Latin text (1713) and revised, with notes, by W.C. Wright. Chicago: University of Chicago Press.

Rauramaa, R.; Rankinen, T.; Tuomainen, P.; Vaisanen, S.; & Mercuri, M. 1995. Inverse relationship between cardiorespiratory fitness and carotid atherosclerosis. *Atherosclerosis 112* (2): 212-21.

Rich, B., MD. 1992, June 2. Telephone interview with E. Olsen (coauthor).

Richardson, P.D.; Davies, M.J.; & Born, G.V.R. 1989. Influence of plaque configuration and stress distribution on fissuring of coronary atherosclerotic plaques. *Lancet 2*: 941-44.

Roberts, S.B.; Fuss, P.; Heyman, M.B.; Evans, W.J.; Tsay, R.; Rasmussen, H.; Fiatarone, M.; Cortiella, J.; Dallal, G.E.; & Young, V.R. 1994, November 23/30. Control of food intake in older men. *Journal of the American Medical Association 272*: 1601-6.

Rose, G. 1991, December 14. Epidemiology of atherosclerosis. *British Medical Journal 303*: 1537-39.

Ross, C.E., & Hayes, D. 1988. Exercise and psychologic well-being in the community. *American Journal of Epidemiology 127*: 762-71.

Russell, L.B. 1986. *Is prevention better than cure?* Washington, D.C.: Brookings Institute.

Sallis, J.F.; Haskell, W.L.; Wood, P.D.; Fortmann, S.P.; Rogers, T.; Blair, S.N.; & Paffenbarger, R.S., Jr. 1985. Physical activity assessment methodology in the Five-City Project. *American Journal of Epidemiology 121*: 91-106.

Salonen, J.T.; Puska, P.; & Tuomilehto, J. 1982. Physical activity and risk of myocardial infarction, cerebral stroke and death. *American Journal of Epidemiology 115*: 526-37.

Saltin, B. 1992. Sedentary lifestyle: An underestimated health risk. *Journal of Internal Medicine 232:* 467-69.

Sandvik, L.; Erikssen, J.; Thaulow, E.; Erikssen, G.; Mundal, R.; & Rodahl, K. 1993. Physical fitness as a predictor of mortality among healthy, middle-aged Norwegian men. *New England Journal of Medicine 328*: 533-37.

Sarna, S.; Sahi, T.; Koskenvuo, M.; & Kaprio, J. 1993. Increased life expectancy of world-class male athletes. *Medicine and Science in Sports and Exercise 25*: 237-44.

Schaie, K.W. 1992, July-August. The impact of methodological changes in gerontology. *International Journal of Aging & Human Development 35*: 19-29.

Schaie, K.W. 1994, April. The course of adult intellectual development (1993 address, American Psychological Association Award Addresses). *American Psychologist 49*: 304-313.

Schaie, K.W., & Willis, S.L. 1991, November. Adult personality and psychomotor performance: Cross-sectional and longitudinal analysis. *Journal of Gerontology 46*: 275-284.

Schrof, J.M. 1994, November 28. Brain power. *U.S. News & World Report*, pp. 89-97.

Scragg, R.; Stewart, A.; Jackson, R.; & Beaglehole, R. 1987. Alcohol and exercise in myocardial infarction and sudden coronary death in men and women. *American Journal of Epidemiology 126*: 77-85.

Shaper, A.G., & Wannamethee, G. 1991. Physical activity and ischaemic heart disease in middle-aged British men. *British Heart Journal 66*: 384-94.

Shephard, R.J. 1990. Costs and benefits of an exercising versus a nonexercising society. In *Exercise, fitness, and health,* edited by C. Bouchard, R.J. Shephard, T. Stephens, J.R. Sutton, & B.D. McPherson, 49-60. Champaign, IL: Human Kinetics.

Shinton, R., & Sagar, G. 1993. Lifelong exercise and stroke. *British Medical Journal* 307: 231-34.

Siscovick, D.S.; Weiss, N.S.; Fletcher, R.H.; & Lasky, T. 1984. The incidence of primary cardiac arrest during vigorous exercise. *New England Journal of Medicine* 311: 874-77.

Slattery, M.L., & Jacobs, D.R. 1988. Physical fitness and cardiovascular disease mortality: The U.S. Railroad Study. *American Journal of Epidemiology* 127: 571-80.

Slattery, M.L.; Jacobs, D.R., Jr.; & Nichaman, M.Z. 1989. Leisure time physical activity and coronary heart disease death. The U.S. Railroad Study. *Circulation 79*: 304-11.

Slattery, M.L.; Schumacher, M.C.; Smith, K.R.; West, D.W.; & Abd-Elghany, N. 1988. Physical activity, diet, and risk of colon cancer in Utah. *American Journal of Epidemiology 128*: 989.

Snow-Harter, C., & Marcus, R. 1991. Exercise, bone mineral density, and osteoporosis. In J.O. Holloszy, ed., *Exercise and Sport Sciences Reviews 19*: 351-388.

Sobolski, J.; Kornitzer, M.; de Backer, G.; Dramaix, M.; Abramowicz, D.S.; & Denolin, H. 1987. Protection against ischemic heart disease in the Belgian physical fitness study: Physical fitness rather than physical activity? *American Journal of Epidemiology 125*: 601-10.

Solomon, H.A. 1984. *The exercise myth.* San Diego: Harcourt Brace Jovanovich.

Spirduso, W. 1980. Physical fitness, aging, and psychomotor speed: A review. *Journal of Gerontology 35:* 850-65.

Spirduso, W. 1987, June. Exercise and the aging brain. *Research Quarterly for Exercise and Sport 54*: 208-18.

Spirduso, W. & Farrar, R.P. 1981. Effects of aerobic training on reactive capacity: An animal model. *Journal of Gerontology 36:* 654-662.

Spirduso, W., & MacRae, P.G. 1990. Motor performance and aging. In *Handbook of the psychology of aging,* edited by J.E. Birren & K.W. Schaie. San Diego: Academic Press.

Stewart, A.L., & King, A.C. 1991. Evaluating the efficacy of physical activity for influencing quality-of-life outcomes in older adults. *Annals of Behavioral Medicine 13*: 108-16.

Stunkard, A.J., & Sorensen, T. 1993, September 30. Obesity and socioeconomic status. *New England Journal of Medicine 329*: 1036-37.

Sytkowski, P.A.; Kannel, W.B.; & D'Agostini, R.B. 1990. Changes in risk factors and the decline in mortality from cardiovascular disease: The Framingham Study. *New England Jounal of Medicine 322*: 1635-41.

Thomas, G.S.; Lee, P.R.; Franks, P.; & Paffenbarger, R.S., Jr. 1981. *Exercise and health: The evidence and the implications.* Cambridge, MA: Oelgeschlager, Gunn & Hain.

Thompson, P.D.; Funk, E.J.; Carleton, R.A.; & Sturner, W.Q. 1982. Incidence of death during jogging in Rhode Island from 1975 through 1980. *Journal of the American Medical Association 247*: 2535-38.

Weinstein, M.C., & Stason, W.B. 1985. Cost-effectiveness of intervention to prevent or treat coronary heart disease. *Annual Review of Public Health 6:* 41-63.

Weintraub, S.; Powell, D.H.; & Whitla, D.K. 1994. Successful cognitive aging: Individual differences among physicians on a computerized test of mental state. *Journal of Geriatric Psychiatry 27*: 15-34.

Whittemore, A.S.; Wu-Williams, A.H.; Lee, M.; Shu, Z.; Gallagher, R.P.; Deng-ao, J.; Lun, Z.; Xianghui, W.; Kun, C.; Jung, D.; Teh, C-Z.; Chengde, L.; Yao, X.J.; Paffenbarger, R.S., Jr.; & Henderson, B.E. 1990. Diet, physical activity, and colorectal cancer among Chinese in North America and China. *Journal of the National Cancer Institute 82*: 915.

Wilhelmsen, L.; Bjure, L.; Ekström-Jodal, B.; Aurell, M.; Grimby, G.; Svärdsudd, K.; Tibblin, G.; & Wedel, H. 1981. Nine years' follow-up of a maximal exercise test in a random population sample of middle-aged men. *Cardiology 68* (Suppl 2): 1-8.

Williams, R.S.; Schaible, T.F.; Bishop, T.; Morey, M. 1984. Effects of endurance training on cholinergic and adrenergic receptors in the heart rate. *Journal of Molecular and Cellular Cardiology 16*: 395-403.

Willich, S.N.; Lewis, M.; Lowel, H.; Arntz, H-R.; Schubert, F.; & Schroder, R. 1993. Physical exertion as a trigger of acute myocardial infarction. *New England Journal of Medicine 329* : 1684-90.

Willis, S.L. 1990, November. Introduction to the special section on cognitive training in later adulthood. *Developmental Psychology 26*: 875-878.

index

about the authors

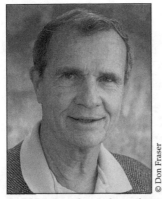

The name **Ralph S. Paffenbarger, Jr.** ("Paff" to his friends) may not be as recognizable as Fonda or Schwarzenegger. But among fitness professionals, Dr. Paffenbarger is considered a true pioneer.

In 1960 Paff embarked on the College Alumni Health Study, commonly known as the "College Study," that investigated the exercise habits of more than 50,000 University of Pennsylvania and Harvard University alumni. The results of this study demonstrated that people who are more physically active live longer and have a lower risk of coronary heart disease.

Paffenbarger holds an MD from the Northwestern University Medical School and a DrPH in epidemiology from the School of Hygiene and Public Health at Johns Hopkins University. His early career was spent in poliomyelitis research as an officer in the United States Public Health Service. Later, when polio was no longer a public health problem, Paff began his landmark study of the relations between physical activity, chronic disease, and longevity.

Paffenbarger maintains a heavy schedule as a professor at both Stanford University School of Medicine and Harvard University School of Public Health and as a research epidemiologist at the University of California at Berkeley. While these activities often keep Paff busy, he still practices what he has long preached, an active and fit way of life. In 1967, at the age of 45, Paff took up jogging: He now has more than 150 marathon and ultra-marathon events to his credit. He has run the Boston Marathon 22 times and the Western States National Endurance Run, a grueling 100-mile race across the Sierra Nevada mountains, 5 times. Although he has slowed down slightly, Paff still walks and jogs regularly.

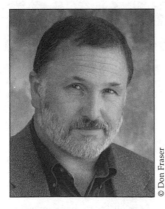

Award-winning journalist **Eric Olsen** is the author of several hundred articles on exercise, fitness, health, and peak performance. A former senior writer for *The Runner* (1977-86), Eric is a contributor to such well-known publications as *Men's Fitness, Hippocrates, American Health, Prime Health and Fitness, Success, Money, Parent Magazine,* and *Reader's Digest.* He also serves as an editor of a community health magazine sponsored by a major medical center in Oakland, California.

Olsen holds an AB in letters and a master of fine arts from the University of Iowa's Writers Workshop. He has been selected as an "outstanding journalist" by the Road Runners Club of America, and he was named a James A. Michener Fellow by the Copernicus Foundation in 1984.

Olsen is firmly committed to exercise, practicing both aerobic and strength training. He also enjoys weight-lifting, martial arts, reading, and writing mystery novels.

Paff and Olsen are neighbors in Berkeley, California.